Clinical Gerontology

Clinical Gerontology

Edited by Oliver Fincher

AMERICAN
MEDICAL PUBLISHERS
www.americanmedicalpublishers.com

American Medical Publishers,
41 Flatbush Avenue,
1st Floor, New York,
NY 11217, USA

Visit us on the World Wide Web at:
www.americanmedicalpublishers.com

ISBN: 978-1-63927-001-9

Cataloging-in-Publication Data

Clinical gerontology / edited by Oliver Fincher.
p. cm.
Includes bibliographical references and index.
ISBN 978-1-63927-001-9
1. Geriatrics. 2. Older people--Diseases. 3. Gerontology. 4. Older people--Diseases--Treatment.
5. Older people--Health and hygiene. 6. Aging. I. Fincher, Oliver.
RC952 .C55 2022
618.97--dc23

Table of Contents

Preface

The scientific study of the phenomena of aging is known as gerontology. It traces the progressive changes that take place in a cell, a tissue, an organ system and a total organism, with the passage of time. However, gerontology has a major focus on the changes that occur between the accomplishment of maturity and the death of the individual and the factors influencing these changes. Social and economic, psychological aspects of aging, physiological basis of aging and general biological aspects of aging in all animal species are the four major categories where the problems of gerontology fall. Gerontology aims to learn about the aging process for the purpose of minimizing the disabilities and handicaps of old age rather than the purpose of extending the life span. The book studies, analyzes and upholds the pillars of gerontology and its utmost significance in modern times. It is compiled in such a manner, that it will provide an in-depth knowledge about the theory and practice of gerontology. This book is appropriate for students seeking detailed information in this area as well as for experts.

This book has been the outcome of endless efforts put in by authors and researchers on various issues and topics within the field. The book is a comprehensive collection of significant researches that are addressed in a variety of chapters. It will surely enhance the knowledge of the field among readers across the globe.

It gives us an immense pleasure to thank our researchers and authors for their efforts to submit their piece of writing before the deadlines. Finally in the end, I would like to thank my family and colleagues who have been a great source of inspiration and support.

Editor

1

Nutritional and Functional Assessment of Hospitalized Elderly: Impact of Sociodemographic Variables

Emam M. M. Esmayel,[1] Mohsen M. Eldarawy,[1] Mohamed M. M. Hassan,[1] Hassan Mahmoud Hassanin,[1] Walid M. Reda Ashour,[2] and Wael Mahmoud[2]

[1] *Department of Internal Medicine, Faculty of Medicine, Zagazig University, Zagazig 44519, Egypt*
[2] *Department of Neurology, Faculty of Medicine, Zagazig University, Zagazig 44519, Egypt*

Correspondence should be addressed to Emam M. M. Esmayel; mmdemmo@yahoo.com

Academic Editor: F. Richard Ferraro

Background. This work was constructed in order to assess the nutritional and functional status in hospitalized elderly and to study the associations between them and sociodemographic variables. *Methods.* 200 elderly patients (>65 years old) admitted to Internal Medicine and Neurology Departments in nonemergency conditions were included. Comprehensive geriatric assessments, including nutritional and functional assessments, were done according to nutritional checklist and Barthel index, respectively. Information was gathered from the patients, from the ward nurse responsible for the patient, and from family members who were reviewed. *Results.* According to the nutritional checklist, 56% of participants were at high risk, 18% were at moderate risk of malnutrition, and 26% had good nutrition. There was a high nutritional risk in patients with low income and good nutrition in patients with moderate income. Also, there was a high nutritional risk in rural residents (61.9%) in comparison with urban residents (25%). Barthel index score was significantly lower in those at high risk of malnutrition compared to those at moderate risk and those with good nutrition. *Conclusions.* Hospitalized elderly are exposed to malnutrition, and malnourished hospitalized patients are candidates for functional impairment. Significant associations are noticed between both nutritional and functional status and specific sociodemographic variables.

1. Introduction

In recent years, there has been a sharp increase in the number of older persons worldwide [1]. It is estimated that almost half of the adults who are hospitalized are 65 years of age or older, although those older than 65 years represent only 12.5 percent of the population [2]. Aging is associated with various physiological changes and needs, which make elderly people vulnerable to malnutrition [3].

Malnutrition is a major geriatric problem associated with poor health status and high mortality, and the impact of a patient's nutritional condition on the clinical outcome has been widely recognized [4]. Application of nutritional support based on nutritional screening results significantly reduced the incidence of complications and the length of hospital stay [5]. The prevalence of malnutrition varies considerably depending on the population studied and the criteria used for the diagnosis [3].

The nutritional screening checklist (NCL) is the most frequently used nutritional screening tool for community-dwelling older adults. It is intended to prevent impairment by identifying and treating nutritional problems before they become a detriment to the lives of older adults [6]. Nutrition and physical activity impact functional changes through changes in body composition [7].

Tanimoto et al. recently reported that sarcopenia, defined by muscle mass, muscle strength, and physical performance, was associated with functional decline over a 2-year period in elderly Japanese [8]. Also, Andre et al. found that the percentage of elderly with dependence was significantly higher in the malnourished (87.6%) than in well-nourished elderly (50.9%) [3].

Dependency interferes with the health and quality of life, not only for the elderly, but also for relatives and healthcare providers [9]. Assessment of functional capacity is a key element in geriatric health, as it can help in identifying what services or programs are needed [10]. The Barthel self-care index (BSI) is proposed as the standard index for clinical and research purposes [11], and it has proved to be a good predictor of in-hospital mortality [12]. Matzen et al. [13] recently concluded that it is a strong independent predictor of survival in older patients admitted to an acute geriatric unit, and they also suggested that it may have a potential role in decision making for the clinical management of frail geriatric inpatients. It is also found useful for evaluating the functional ability of elderly patients being treated in outpatient care [14].

However, less attention is given to the underlying risk of functional decline and the vulnerability to hospital-associated complications [2]. Also, information about the nutritional and functional status and its correlation with sociodemographic variables in Egypt among hospitalized elderly are scarce; the sociodemographic data will focus a bit on which group is at increased risk of nutritional and functional instability, and hence which group deserves more attention. This study was conducted in order to clarify the impact of sociodemographic factors on nutritional and functional status of the elderly in, addition to the interrelationship between both.

2. Methods

This study has been carried out on 200 elderly patients (>65 years old) admitted to Internal Medicine and Neurology Departments, Zagazig University Hospitals, which are educational hospitals serving Sharkia governorate, during the period between October 2009 and October 2010. The admission was due to gastrointestinal troubles in 88 patients, cardiac troubles in 28, chest troubles in 40, neurological in 28, or other causes in 16 patients.

According to age, they were classified into young old (65–74.9 years), old old (75–84.9 years), and oldest old (≥85 years). Patients who required treatment in specialized units such as the intensive care units, were excluded. All participants gave informed consents and the study had approval from local ethical committee.

Information was gathered on admission by the treating physician from the patients, from the ward nurse responsible for the patient, and from family members who reviewed. All the patients were subjected to full history taking and clinical examination.

Nutritional assessment was done by physical examination by searching for clinical signs of nutritional deficiencies. We used the NCL for nutritional screening which included 10 items with a total score of 21 points. A score from 0 to 2 was considered as good nutrition, 3 to 5 as moderate nutritional risk, and 6 or more as high nutritional risk [15]. The nutritional checklist includes illness and tooth or mouth problems affecting feeding, number of meals per day, and types of foods and drinks. Also ability to eating alone, to cook, shop or feed oneself, and weight gain or loss, are included. One study using the NCL was carried out and the researchers found that, when compared to nutritional assessment criteria (anthropometric, dietary, and laboratory data), the NCL identified 83% of the population as being at high risk compared to 74% using the nutritional assessment criteria [16]. It has been suggested that the NCL is more appropriately used in observational epidemiological studies than for population screening [17].

Functional assessment was done using the Barthel self-care index of activities of daily living [18]. The index included bowels, bladder, grooming, toilet use, feeding, transfer, mobility, dressing, stairs, and bathing. Total possible scores range from 0 to 20, with lower scores indicating increased disability. Sociodemographic information and nutritional checklist were collected by direct interviews, while Barthel index was collected using chart reading.

2.1. Statistical Analysis. Data were checked, entered, and analyzed using SPSS version 15 for data processing and statistics. Continuous variables were tested for normal distribution and expressed as mean ± standard deviation and compared by Student's t test. Categorical variables were compared with the chi-square test. For all analyses, P value <0.05 was considered statistically significant.

3. Results

Demographic data of the studied groups are presented in Table 1. A total of 200 elderly patients were included in the study. The large majority of patients were illiterate (84%) and none of them were on regular exercise. As for marital state, 56% were widowed and 40% married with only 4% having no children. 56% had low income with only 2% having means of transportation (Table 2).

According to NCL, 56% of the participants were at high risk and 26% had good nutrition (Table 3). Nutritional checklist score was worst in age group ≥85 years, while age has no significant effect on BSI (Table 4). There was a high nutritional risk in rural residents (61.9%) in comparison with urban residents (25%); the mean of BSI was higher in patients from rural than that of urban areas with no significant difference (Table 5).

High nutritional risk was found in 52.4% of illiterate patients and 75% of educated patients, while there was no association between BSI and education ($P = 0.56$) (Table 6). No significant association was found between BSI and gender ($P = 0.22$) and also between NCL and gender ($P = 0.16$) (Table 7).

There was a significant association between NCL and income ($P = 0.017$), as there was a high nutritional risk in patients with low income and good nutrition in patients with moderate income, in contrast there was no association between BSI and income ($P = 0.47$) (Table 8). A significant association between NCL and BSI (<0.001) indicates that both nutrition and functional ability go together (Table 9).

Table 1: Demographic data of patients.

	N	%
Age		
65 < 75	164	82
75 < 85	28	14
≥85	8	4
Gender		
Male	112	56
Female	88	44
Residence		
Rural	168	84
Urban	32	16

Table 2: Sociodemographic variables in studied patients.

Education		
Illiterate	168	84
Educated	32	16
Vocation		
Retired	64	32
Farmer	52	26
Housewife	72	36
Crafts man	12	6
Habits		
Exercise		
Yes	0	0
No	200	100
Sleep		
Satisfied	84	42
Not satisfied	116	58
Sexual activity		
No	156	78
Satisfied	8	4
Not satisfied	36	16
Substance abuse		
Yes	56	28
No	144	72
Marital status		
Yes	80	40
No	4	2
Widowed	112	56
Divorced	4	2
Children		
Yes	192	96
No	8	4
Presence of close friends		
Yes	136	68
No	64	32
Income		
Low	112	56
Moderate	88	44
High	0	0
Transportation		
Available	196	98
Not available	4	2

4. Discussion

Older patients tend to have multiple organic, psychological, and social problems [19]. Their functional and physiological capacities are often diminished and the adverse effects of drugs are more pronounced. The concept of Comprehensive Geriatric Assessment (CGA) has evolved because of the many problems of elderly subjects [20]. Our study was concerned with patients admitted to Internal Medicine department with age above 65 years. Majority of age group was young old and represented 88% while the oldest old represented 4% of patients included in the study.

As regards assessment of nutrition, considerable number of studies have examined the nutritional status of institutionalized elderly people and reported prevalence figures for malnutrition and nutritional problems [21]. According to the American Dietetic Association (ADA), the nutrient requirements of elderly peopleare not fully understood, although it is known that the physiological and functional changes that occur with agingcan result in changes in nutrient needs [22].

The American Academy of Family Physicians and the National Council of Aging in the United States previously formed the Nutrition Screening Initiative for the development of strategies to detect nutritional risks among older people. One of the strategies included the development of a ten-question checklist, the NCL [23]. This checklist, which was designed to be self-administered, could also be administered by a healthcare professional.

According to NCL, our results showed that about 56% of patients had high nutritional risk. A study conducted in Canada indicated that 37–62% of elderly were at risk of the poor nutrition [24], and the percent was 50.3% in another study in India [25]. A recent study in China [4] found that the overall prevalence of under nutrition and nutritional risk was 17.8% and 41.5%, respectively, using the NCL. Another recent study in Makkah found that among 102 recently hospitalized elderly and according to the mini nutritional assessment (MNA) tool, 22.6% were classified as malnourished, 57.8% were at risk of malnutrition, and 19.6% were well nourished [1]. Also, another study found that 10.2% of elderly individuals were malnourished and 39.9% were at risk of malnutrition according to the MNA screening tool [5]. Differences in prevalence rates of malnutrition among the different studies may be due to difference in selection criteria of elderly, different assessment tools, and differences in sociodemographic variables.

In this study, there was an association between NCL and age group. We found that 100% of oldest old had high nutritional risk and 85.7% of old old have high nutritional risk, but the percent in young old was 48.8%. Our results agree with that obtained by Fang et al. [4] who found that the prevalence of nutritional risk was significantly higher in patients >70 years of age than in patients <70 years (64% versus 32%, $P < 0.001$). Yap et al. found that high nutritional

TABLE 3: Nutritional and functional assessment of studied patients.

Nutritional assessment (NCL)	Good nutrition	52 patients	26%
	Moderate risk of malnutrition	36 patients	18%
	High risk of malnutrition	112 patients	56%
Functional assessment (BSI)	Range	8–20	
	Mean ± SD	16 ± 4.1	

TABLE 4: Association between nutritional checklist (NCL) and Barthel self-care index (BSI) with age.

	NCL						BSI	
	Good nutrition		Moderate risk		High risk		Range	Mean ± SD
	No.	%	No.	%	No.	%		
Age								
Young old (N = 164)	48	29.3	36	22.0	80	48.8	8–20	16.5 ± 3.84
Old old (N = 28)	4	14.3	0	0.0	24	85.7	8–20	13.4 ± 5.2
Oldest old (N = 8)	0	0	0	0	8	100	15–18	16.5 ± 2.1
X^2	10.4						3.65	
P	0.001						0.018	

TABLE 5: Association between nutritional checklist (NCL) and Barthel self-care index (BSI) with residence.

	NCL						BSI	
	Good nutrition		Moderate risk		High risk		Range	Mean ± SD
	N	%	N	%	N	%		
Residence								
Rural N = 168	40	23.8	24	14.3	104	61.9	8–20	15.6 ± 4.6
Urban N = 32	12	37.5	12	37.5	8	25	9–20	7.8 ± 3.67
X^2	8.26						1.81	
P	0.016						0.07	

TABLE 6: Association between nutritional checklist (NCL) and Barthel self-care index (BSI) with education.

	NCL						BSI	
	Good nutrition		Moderate risk		High risk		Range	Mean ± SD
	N	%	N	%	N	%		
Education								
Illiterate N = 168	52	31	28	16.7	88	52.4	8–20	15.97 ± 3.89
Educated N = 32	0	0	8	25	24	75	8–20	16.6 ± 4.9
X^2	6.7						0.85	
P	0.035						0.56	

TABLE 7: Association between nutritional checklist (NCL) and Barthel self-care index (BSI) with gender.

	NCL						BSI	
	Good nutrition		Moderate risk		High risk		Range	Mean ± SD
	N	%	N	%	N	%		
Gender								
Male N = 112	24	21.4	16	14.3	72	64.3	8–20	15.4 ± 4.4
Female N = 88	28	31.8	20	22.7	40	45.5	9–20	16.9 ± 3.4
X^2	3.56						4.35	
P	0.16						0.22	

TABLE 8: Association between nutritional checklist (NCL) and Barthel self-care index (BSI) with financial security (income).

	NCL						BSI	
	Good nutrition		Moderate risk		High risk		Range	Mean ± SD
	N	%	N	%	N	%		
Financial security (income)								
Low $N = 112$	20	17.9	24	21.4	68	60.7	8–20	15.8 ± 3.9
Moderate $N = 88$	36	40.9	8	9.1	44	50	8–20	16.4 ± 4.2
X^2			11.97				0.71	
P			0.017				0.47	

TABLE 9: Association between Barthel self-care index (BSI) with nutritional checklist (NCL).

	NCL			F	P
	Good nutrition	Moderate risk	High risk		
BSI					
$X \pm$ SD	18.4 ± 1.86	18 ± 2.4	14.5 ± 4.3	13.4	<0.001
Range	15–20	13–20	8–20		

risk was more in older patients but with no significant association with age [26].

Also in this study, we found that high nutritional risk represented 52.4% in illiterate patients and about 75% in educated patients; however, we cannot depend on this finding due to the large difference in sample size between illiterate and educated patients (84% versus 16%, resp.). However, the previous study [26] found no significant correlation between NCL and education, and the percent of patients with high nutritional risk was 26.2% and 33.6% in educated versus illiterate patients, respectively. Increased nutritional risk in males was 64.3% versus 45.5% in females (P = 0.16), and this was confirmed by MacLellan and van Til [24]. Contrarily, Rambousková et al. [27] concluded that institutionalized women should be considered a nutritionally vulnerable population group; the reason for this difference may be the higher average age of women versus men (86.1 ± 6.15 versus 81.5 ± 7.97 years) in their study. Meanwhile, Fang et al. [4] found no gender difference in the prevalence of nutritional risk. We found a high nutritional risk in rural residents (61.9%) in comparison with urban residents (25%); this may be due to a higher income and a better nutrition knowledge in urban areas.

High nutritional risk in patients with low income was 60.7%, while it was about 50% in patients with moderate income. A study in Nigeria concluded that males had significantly higher income, higher socioeconomic status scores and were also less vulnerable to malnutrition than females ($P < 0.05$) [28]. Poverty is a nonphysiological cause of under nutrition in older people [29].

As regards functional assessment, the Barthel self care index of activities of daily living, first developed in 1965 [30] and later modified by Granger et al. [31], measures functional disability by quantifying patient performance in 10 activities of daily life. The Barthel Index has been reported to have excellent reliability and validity and adequate responsiveness to change, in measuring neurologic physical disability. Hobart et al. compared psychometric properties of the Barthel index with newer and lengthier scales, the Functional Independence Measure (FIM) and the Functional Independence Measure + Functional Assessment Measure (FIM+FAM), in patients undergoing rehabilitation. This study suggested that the newer and more extensive rating scales of FIM and FIM+FAM offered few advantages over the more practical and economical Barthel index [32]. Similar results were observed in studies of patients with multiple sclerosis and stroke [33, 34].

In this study, we found a significant correlation between disability and age, where functional activity decreased with advancing age. Hairi et al. showed that advancing age was significantly associated with functional limitation [35]. We did not find significant correlation between disability and income, however, a study done ona random sample of persons, 55–85 years of age, drawn from the population registers of 11 municipalities found that low socioeconomic status had been associated with physical disability [36]. Unless low socioeconomic status is associated with handwork, the elderly will be more susceptible to physical inactivity and lack of exercise.

Gender had no effect on functional activity in our study. Bergamini et al. found that older Italian men and women showed similar prevalence of functional limitation, 31% and 28%, respectively [37]. However, Hairi et al. found that female gender was significantly associated with functional limitation; they suggested that disadvantages resulting from limited education may contribute to the greater physical disability and functional limitation burden experienced by older women in their study [35].

Increased incidence of disability was associated with malnutrition in this study. These results are in agreement with Oliveira et al. [38] who assessed the relationship between nutritional status and indicators of functional capacity among recently hospitalized elderly in a general hospital, and showed that these indicators were significantly more deteriorated among the malnourished individuals [38]. Using mini nutritional assessment (MNA) and Barthel index on 123 resident elderly, Cereda et al. showed that the poorer functional status was associated with low nutrition [39]. Also, Chevalier et al., [40] in a study designed to estimate the prevalence of malnutrition in frail elders undergoing rehabilitation and the association between their nutritional status and physical function, showed that there was an interrelationship between nutritional and functional status. It has already been shown that malnutrition compromises the functional status of the individuals [40].

5. Conclusions

Results in this study suggest that the hospitalized elderly are exposed to malnutrition, which emphasizes the importance of early identification of malnutrition among them. High nutritional risk was more with older age, rural areas, educated patients, and low income, while gender had no significant effect. Functional abilities were better with younger age but had no significant correlation with other sociodemographic variables. Malnourished hospitalized patients are candidates for functional impairment. Significant associations were noticed between both nutritional and functional status and specific sociodemographic variables. These interrelationships require further studies to elucidate. Also, it is necessary to pay special attention to functional capacity when planning nutritional care for this vulnerable group.

Limitations of This Study. The patients included in this study were a convenient sample from patients admitted to one hospital, so patients from distant areas were not included. The large percent of illiterate patients (84%) could have an impact on the study. Larger number of patients should be included in future studies.

References

[1] M. A. Elmadbouly and A. M. AbdElhafez, "Assessment of nutritional status of hospitalized elderly patients in Makkah governorate," *Pakistan Journal of Nutrition*, vol. 11, no. 10, pp. 886–892, 2012.

[2] R. M. Kleinpell, K. Fletcher, and B. M. Jennings, "Reducing functional decline in hospitalized elderly," in *Patient Safety and Quality: An Evidence-Based Handbook ForNurses*, R. G. Hughes, Ed., chapter 11, pp. 1–15, AHRQ Publication, 2008.

[3] M. B. Andre, N. Dumavibhat, N. R. Ngatu, M. Eitoku, R. Hirota, and N. Suganuma, "Mini nutritional assessment and functional capacity in community-dwelling elderly in Rural Luozi, Democratic Republic of Congo," *Geriatrics and Gerontology International*, vol. 13, no. 1, pp. 35–42, 2013.

[4] S. Fang, J. Long, R. Tan et al., "A multicenter assessment of malnutrition, nutritional risk, and application of nutritional support among hospitalized patients in Guangzhou hospitals," *Asia Pacific Journal of Clinical Nutrition*, vol. 22, no. 1, pp. 54–59, 2013.

[5] J. - Payne-James, G. Grimble, and D. Silk, "Artificial nutrition support," in *Clinical Practice*, pp. 243–244, GreenwichMedical, London, UK, 2nd edition, 2001.

[6] S. Sinnett, R. Bengle, A. Brown, A. P. Glass, M. A. Johnson, and J. S. Lee, "The validity of nutrition screening initiative DETERMINE checklist responses in older georgians," *Journal of Nutrition for the Elderly*, vol. 29, no. 4, pp. 393–409, 2010.

[7] M. F. Kuczmarski, D. O. Weddle, and E. M. Jones, "Maintaining functionality in later years: a review of nutrition and physical activity interventions in postmenopausal women," *Journal of Nutrition for the Elderly*, vol. 29, no. 3, pp. 259–292, 2010.

[8] Y. Tanimoto, M. Watanabe, W. Sun et al., "Association of sarcopenia with functional decline in community-dwelling elderly subjects in Japan," *Geriatrics & Gerontology International*, 2013.

[9] J. C. Millán-Calenti, M. Gandoy-Crego, M. Antelo-Martelo, M. López-Martinez, M. P. Riveiro-López, and J. M. Mayán-Santos, "Helping the family carers of Alzheimer's patients: from theory to practice. A preliminary study," *Archives of Gerontology and Geriatrics*, vol. 30, no. 2, pp. 131–138, 2000.

[10] A. E. Stuck, J. M. Walthert, T. Nikolaus, C. J. Büla, C. Hohmann, and J. C. Beck, "Risk factors for functional status decline in community-living elderly people: a systematic literature review," *Social Science and Medicine*, vol. 48, no. 4, pp. 445–469, 1999.

[11] D. T. Wade and C. Collin, "The Barthel ADL Index: a standard measure of physical disability?" *International Disability Studies*, vol. 10, no. 2, pp. 64–67, 1988.

[12] A. Supervéa, D. Aranda, M. A. Márquez, A. Aguirre, E. Skaf, and J. Gutiérrez, "Predicting length of hospitalisation of elderly patients, using the Barthel Index," *Age and Ageing*, vol. 37, no. 3, pp. 339–342, 2008.

[13] L. E. -Matzen, D. B. Jepsen, J. Ryg, and T. Masud, "Functional level at admission is a predictor of survival in older patients admitted to an acute geriatric unit," *BMC Geriatr*, vol. 25, pp. 12–32, 2012.

[14] J. Sponton, M. Minosso, F. Amendola, M. R. Alvarenga, and M. A. de Campos Oliveira, "Validation of the Barthel Index in elderly patients attended in outpatient clinics, in Brazil," *ACTA Paulista de Enfermagem*, vol. 23, no. 2, pp. 218–223, 2010.

[15] The Nutrition Screening Initiative, A Project of: American Academy of Family Physicians, The American Dietetic Association, The National Council on the Aging, Washington, DC, USA, 2007.

[16] A. M. Coulston, L. Craig, and A. C. Voss, "Meals-on-wheels applicants are a population at risk for poor nutritional status," *Journal of the American Dietetic Association*, vol. 96, no. 6, pp. 570–573, 1996.

[17] D. Rush, "Nutrition screening in old people: its place in a coherent practice of preventive health care," *Annual Review of Nutrition*, vol. 17, pp. 101–125, 1997.

[18] C. Collin, D. T. Wade, S. Davies, and V. Horne, "The barthel ADL index: a reliability study," *International Disability Studies*, vol. 10, no. 2, pp. 61–63, 1988.

[19] L. Z. Rubenstein, "Geriatric assessment: an overview of its impacts," *Clinics in Geriatric Medicine*, vol. 3, no. 1, pp. 1–15, 1987.

[20] J. K. Luk, K. H. Or, and J. Woo, "Using the comprehensive geriatric assessment technique to assess elderly patients," *Hong Kong Medical Journal*, vol. 6, no. 1, pp. 93–98, 2000.

[21] J. M. Bauer, M. J. Kaiser, P. Anthony, Y. Guigoz, and C. C. Sieber, "The mini nutritional assessment-its history, today's practice, and future perspectives," *Nutrition in Clinical Practice*, vol. 23, no. 4, pp. 388–396, 2008.

[22] ADA Reports, "Position of the American Dietetic Association: liberalization of the diet prescription improves quality of life for older adults in long-term care," *Journal of the American Dietetic Association* , vol. 105, no. 12, pp. 1955–1965, 2005.

[23] B. M. Posner, A. M. Jette, K. W. Smith, and D. R. Miller, "Nutrition and health risks in the elderly: the nutrition screening initiative," *American Journal of Public Health*, vol. 83, no. 7, pp. 972–978, 1993.

[24] D. L. MacLellan and L. D. van Til, "Screening for nutritional risk among community-dwelling elderly on Prince Edward Island,"

Canadian Journal of Public Health, vol. 89, no. 5, pp. 342–346, 1998.

[25] S. Baweja, H. Agarwal, A. Mathur et al., "Assessment of nutritional status and related risk factors in community dwelling elderly in Western Rajastha," *Journal of the Indian Academy of Geriatrics*, vol. 4, no. 1, pp. 5–13, 2008.

[26] K. B. Yap, M. Niti, and T. P. Ng, "Nutrition screening among community-dwelling older adults in Singapore," *Singapore Medical Journal*, vol. 48, no. 10, pp. 911–916, 2007.

[27] J. Rambousková, M. Slavíková, A. Krsková, B. Procházka, and A. Dlouhý, "Nutritional Status Assessment of Institutionalized Elderly in Prague, Czech Republic," *Annals of Nutrition & Metabolism*, vol. 62, no. 3, pp. 199–204, 2013.

[28] O. Ibiyemi, O. Ketiku, and A. Olubode, "Socio-demographic and nutritional assessment of the elderly Yorubas in Nigeria," *Asia Pacific Journal of Clinical Nutrition*, vol. 15, no. 1, pp. 95–101, 2006.

[29] C. MacIntosh, J. E. Morley, and I. M. Chapman, "The anorexia of aging," *Nutrition*, vol. 16, no. 10, pp. 983–995, 2000.

[30] F. I. Mahoney and D. W. Barthel, "Functional evaluation: the barthel index," *Maryland state medical journal*, vol. 14, pp. 61–65, 1965.

[31] C. V. Granger, L. S. Dewis, N. C. Peters, C. C. Sherwood, and J. E. Barrett, "Stroke rehabilitation: analysis of repeated barthel index measures," *Archives of Physical Medicine and Rehabilitation*, vol. 60, no. 1, pp. 14–17, 1979.

[32] J. C. Hobart, D. L. Lamping, J. A. Freeman et al., "Evidence-based measurement: which disability scale for neurologic rehabilitation?" *Neurology*, vol. 57, no. 4, pp. 639–644, 2001.

[33] I.-P. Hsueh, J.-H. Lin, J.-S. Jeng, and C.-L. Hsieh, "Comparison of the psychometric characteristics of the functional independence measure, 5 item Barthel index, and 10 item Barthel index in patients with stroke," *Journal of Neurology Neurosurgery and Psychiatry*, vol. 73, no. 2, pp. 188–190, 2002.

[34] J. J. van der Putten, J. C. Hobart, J. A. Freeman, and A. J. Thompson, "Measuring change in disability after inpatient rehabilitation: comparison of the responsiveness of the Barthel index and the functional independence measure," *Journal of Neurology Neurosurgery and Psychiatry*, vol. 66, no. 4, pp. 480–484, 1999.

[35] N. N. Hairi, A. Bulgiba, R. G. Cumming, V. Naganathan, and I. Mudla, "Prevalence and correlates of physical disability and functional limitation among community dwelling older people in rural Malaysia, a middle income country," *BMC Public Health*, vol. 10, article 492, 2010.

[36] A. Koster, H. Bosma, M. I. Broese van Groenou et al., "Explanations of socioeconomic differences in changes in physical function in older adults: results from the longitudinal aging study Amsterdam," *BMC Public Health*, vol. 6, article 244, 2006.

[37] L. Bergamini, M. Burgoni, G. Federzoni et al., "Multidimensional evaluation of home-dwelling elderly: the impact of medical and social factors on health status indices," *Archives of Gerontology and Geriatrics*, vol. 44, supplement, pp. 75–81, 2007.

[38] M. R. Oliveira, K. C. Fogaça, and V. A. Leandro-Merhi, "Nutritional status and functional capacity of hospitalized elderly," *Nutrition Journal*, vol. 8, no. 1, article 54, 2009.

[39] E. Cereda, L. Valzolgher, and C. Pedrolli, "Mini nutritional assessment is a good predictor of functional status in institutionalised elderly at risk of malnutrition," *Clinical Nutrition*, vol. 27, no. 5, pp. 700–705, 2008.

[40] S. Chevalier, F. Saoud, K. Gray-Donald, and J. A. Morais, "The physical functional capacity of frail elderly persons undergoing ambulatory rehabilitation is related to their nutritional status," *Journal of Nutrition, Health and Aging*, vol. 12, no. 10, pp. 721–726, 2008.

2

Mood Disorders among Older Adults Participating in Individual and Group Active Environments: "Me" versus "Us," or Both?

Rachael C. Stone,[1] Brad A. Meisner,[2] and Joseph Baker[1]

[1] *School of Kinesiology & Health Science, York University, Toronto, ON, Canada M3J 1P3*
[2] *Department of Psychology, Ryerson University, Toronto, ON, Canada M5B 2K3*

Correspondence should be addressed to Rachael C. Stone, raystone@yorku.ca

Academic Editor: Wojtek Chodzko-Zajko

Involvement in physical activity is associated with improved mental health including better social skills, coping mechanisms, and lower rates of depression. However, evidence on whether group or individual active environments better facilitate these benefits remains inconsistent. This cross-sectional cohort study examined the mental health reports of older adults (aged 50+) in relation to participation in group or individual active environments. Logistic multivariate regression analyses were conducted on the Canadian Community Health Survey (cycle 4.1, 2007-2008, $n = 44,057$). Results illustrated that those active in both group and individual environments were 59% less likely to have a mood disorder than those who were not participating in either ($P < 0.001$). Also, those active in both environments were 31% less likely to have a mood disorder than those active in an individual environment ($P < 0.001$). Participating in only group or only individual environments had a similar effect compared to individuals not active in any environments for reducing rates of reported mood disorders (22% and 28%, resp.). However, the findings related to only group environments were not significant. These findings reveal that participating in both group and individual physical activities may have important implications for maintaining older adults' mental health status.

1. Introduction

Older adults in Canada are the fastest growing cohort of the population [1], a trend echoed in other industrialized nations [2]. Currently, over 35% of the Canadian population is comprised of individuals aged 50 years and above, a number expected to rise as the baby boom generation progresses further into older age [2, 3]. Research has concluded that older individuals who are living longer often do so with a reduced quality of life and a greater disease/disability burden [4]. With these outcomes in mind, a growing field of research has begun to focus on how to facilitate "successful aging" amongst the aging population.

A vital component of many successful aging models pertains to maintaining one's psychological and mental health [5, 6].

Mood disorders are a growing health concern for an aging population. For example, the percentage of Canadians reporting a diagnosed mood disorder rose from 5.3% in 2003 to 6.3% in 2009; 43% of those reporting a mood disorder in 2009 were 50 years of age and greater [7, 8]. A major mood disorder is an umbrella term for a range of depressive and manic disorders, and their variants. Depressive disorders are marked by experiencing negative affect, loss of interest in usual enjoyable activities, irritability, and catastrophizing mentalities for at least two weeks. Dysthymia is a more severe and chronic form of depression [9]. On the other hand, manic disorders, which include mania and bipolar disorders, tend to persist for at least a week and are characterized by distinct fluctuations in one's disposition (e.g., being unusually talkative, loud, egomaniacal, paranoid, and reckless) [9]. Mood disorders are most commonly treated with pharmacological agents and/or psychological treatments [9]. Recently, more cost-effective treatments have begun to be explored, including physical activity [10, 11].

Physical activity has been found to lessen the negative and maladaptive symptoms of mood disorders on biochemical, physiological, and psychological levels [11]. Interestingly, evidence from clinical studies has shown that the psychological benefits associated with participating in exercise and physical activities are comparable to those found with standard forms of psychotherapy [12, 13]. Moreover, there is a considerable amount of literature demonstrating the important psychological benefits that consistent exercise participation can offer the aging population including improvements in cognitive function, positive affect, self-efficacy, social skills, cohesion, networking, and engagement, life and sexual satisfaction, as well as reduced incidences of psychological chronic conditions including mood disorders such as depression and schizophrenia [14–23].

The "active environment" describes whether one participates in exercise within a group or an individual setting, and it facilitates mental health benefits [13, 15, 24–28]. However, much of the previous research on exercise environments has focused on how individual *versus* group physical activities affect adoption of, and adherence to, exercise or physical activity among the older adult population. The evidence on whether older individuals prefer exercising in a group or individual activities has been inconsistent and somewhat contradictory. For instance, Beauchamp et al. (2007) found that 68% of adults aged 50 or more preferred participating alone in a one-year aerobic program [13]. In contrast, Fox et al. (2007) noted that European older adults preferred exercising in a group environment during a one-year aerobic program [26]. Although these two studies are contradictory in terms of older adult preferences for exercise, both studies highlight similar mental health benefits from physical activity participation in group and individual environments.

In addition to active environment preferences, previous research has shown inconsistent findings in relation to maintaining exercise participation within a specific mode of an active environment (i.e., group versus individual). Researchers, (e.g., [15, 24, 25, 28]) have highlighted that participating in group exercise produces superior attendance rates among older adults aged 50+ compared to exercising alone. This effect appears to be adjunct to perceptions of group cohesion and belonging as participants felt strongly that they were part of a team, producing an average attendance rate of 85% for group exercise programs. However, in contrast, King et al. (1993) found that adherence rates were slightly higher when participants aged 50+ were placed in an individual, home-based exercise program compared to a group-based program. The success was attributed to participants perceiving greater internal locus of control over their health [27].

Research regarding the accruement of mental health benefits among older adults has also been mixed in regards to the active environment. King et al. (1993) found no significant differences in positive mental health outcomes between group and individual exercise environments during a one-year randomized control trial of aerobic exercise, and it was claimed that group exercise was unnecessary as older adults could receive similar benefits from more convenient forms of individual exercise [27]. In contrast, Brawley et al.'s (2000) nine-month randomized control trial of group versus individual exercise environment interventions found that self-efficacy, social skills, and general mental health were significantly greater among those in the group active environment than the individual one [24].

It is important to note that these previous data are based on structured exercise single-blind interventions rather than voluntary or natural participation in less regimented physical activity or sport. Recent discussions of the role physical activity and sport in promoting healthy aging, (e.g., [29, 30]) have advocated that sport and physical activity produce improvements in health and functioning above and beyond those obtained via standardized exercise routines.

Considering the potential mental health concerns for the aging population and the contradictory findings in previous research in this area of research, the current study examined a mental health outcome among Canadian older adults who were physically active in group and/or individual active environments. The primary objective of this analysis was to examine whether these modes of active environments are associated with mental health. An important secondary goal was to determine the prevalence of these two active environments among older adults in Canada, an objective that contributes to the research on exercise and physical activity preferences among older adults.

2. Methods

2.1. Participants. Cross-sectional data from the Canadian Community Health Survey (CCHS, cycle 4.1) were used. Information collected in the CCHS considers diseases, health, lifestyle, and social conditions, which was collected from December to January of 2007 and 2008. The CCHS contains specific data on sport participation and physical activity behaviours. Cycle 4.1 of the CCHS has a sample size of 131,061 voluntary participants, both male and female, aged 12 and greater. Volunteers were randomly recruited from all provinces and territories. Participants completed the survey via computer-assisted interviews, over the telephone, or their personal computers. The CCHS is praised for having a high nation-wide response rate (86%) and for being representative of the Canadian population. Participants in the current study were a subsample of the overall dataset, as some questionnaire content was optional (i.e., exercise habits, perceived life stress, and drinking/smoking behaviours) [3]. As a result, analyses were first limited to respondents who had a complete set of data for the variables under investigation. The sample was further limited to individuals 50 years of age or greater in correspondence with much of the existing research in this research area. The final sample included 44,057 participants. Ethics approval for the current study was granted by the York University Research Ethics Committee.

2.2. Measurements

2.2.1. Outcome Variable. Mental health was defined by the presence of a mood disorder. The question in the CCHS assessed whether an individual had been diagnosed with depression, bipolar disorder, mania, or dysthymia by a healthcare professional in the past 12 months (yes/no). This question was mandatory for all CCHS participants.

2.3. Main Predictor Variable

2.3.1. Active Environment. This variable was divided into four categories based on self-reported leisure physical activity and sport participation: those participating in only group active environments, those participating in only individual active environments, those participating simultaneously in both environments, and those participating in neither. This variable, which is not available in the CCHS, was calculated using Microsoft Excel 2003 to identify the respondents in each category. Group active environments were defined as physical activities or sports that *require* interactions among individuals when participating. The activities meeting this criterion in the CCHS were ice hockey, baseball/softball, volleyball, basketball, and soccer. Individual active environments were defined as activities or sports that *do not require* interactions among individuals when participating. The activities meeting this criterion in the CCHS were walking, gardening, swimming, bicycling, jogging, golf, and tennis/racquetball. Classification of this variable was captured by summing the total number of participants who responded "yes" to participating in one or more group or individual activities. Furthermore, those participating in both environments simultaneously responded "yes" to one or more activities from group *and* individual categories while others responded "no" to both sets of activities were not participating in either of the specified active environments. Resulting from this classification were four possible categorical responses for the active environments variable: (1) those participating in only group active environments, (2) those participating in only individual active environments, (3) those participating simultaneously in both active environments, and (4) those participating in neither active environment. These specific activities were chosen as the present study aimed to assess purposeful physical activity respondents completed in their leisure time. As such, the present study does not assess incidental physical activity (i.e., transportation, occupational, or house work).

2.4. Covariates. Based on previous research [31–35], a number of covariates were included in the analyses to minimized their confounding effects on the key associations under investigation. First, sociodemographic variables, such as age, sex, and marital status were included. Age was classified in the CCHS in five-year groups, beginning from 50–54 years to 75–79 years with a final group of those aged 80 and greater. Sex was reported as "male" or "female," and marital status was defined as being "married," "common-law," "divorced/widowed," or "single." Second, given that negative health behaviours such as alcohol consumption and smoking are linked with decreases in physical activity [36], they were also included as health behavioural covariates. Regarding the alcohol consumption variable, six categories represented the frequency of binge drinking (i.e., consuming five or more drinks in one sitting): "never," "less than once per month," "once per month," "2-3 times per month," "once per week," and "more than once per week." Three categories represented smoking status: "daily," "occasional," and "not at all." Moreover, considering sport participation intensity can vary considerably and may moderate the likelihood of having or developing a mood disorder, the participant's intensity of physical activity was controlled for in the analyses using the Physical Activity Index variable available within the CCHS based on energy expenditure. Energy expenditure was calculated using average metabolic equivalent values (a measure of intensity) and self-reported frequencies and durations of participants' physical activity endeavours. This variable categorizes respondents as being "active," "moderately active," or "inactive" in their leisure time activities based on the total daily energy expenditure values over the last three months (kcal/kg of body weight/day). "Active" was defined as burning 3 or more kcal/kg/day, "moderately active" as burning between 1.5 and 2.9 kcal/kg/day, and "inactive" as burning between 0 and 1.4 kcal/kg/day [3, 26]. Finally, given that the dependent variable relates to the mental health domain, a variable on psychological stress was also included as a covariate to control for this variable's potential influence on the relationships examined. Five categories represented individuals' perceptions of life stress: "not at all," "not very," "a bit," "quite a bit," and "extremely."

2.5. Analyses. A bivariate logistic regression analysis was used to examine the relationships between the active environments and the presence of a mood disorder (Model A). Subsequently, a multivariate logistic regression analysis was estimated to examine the aforementioned relationship, controlling for the sociodemographic, health behavioural, and psychological stress covariates (Model B). Given that this was a subsample of the overall CCHS sampling strategy due to the optional content within the CCHS included in this analysis, population weights were not applied. Effect sizes were reported as odds ratios (OR), and the significance levels were represented by 95% confidence interval (CI) for all analyses. Analyses were conducted using SPSS version 19.0 software.

3. Results

Table 1 displays descriptive information of the sample. The majority of the older adults were aged 50–64 years (57.6%), female (54.4%), married (55.4%), nonbinge drinkers (71.8%), nonsmokers (81.4%), inactive (52.2%), and perceived their lives to be "a bit" stressed (35.2%). Seven percent of the sample reported the presence of a diagnosed mood disorder. The vast majority of older adults in this sample were participating in individual active environments only (83.2%). Participation in group environments only was reported by an extremely small proportion of participants in this sample (0.1%) while a relatively larger proportion of these older adults participated in both group and individual active environments (3.1%). In comparison, many more reported not participating in either group or individual active environments (13.6%). It should be noted that although 13.6% did not participate in either of the two active environments, 52.2% of the participants were classified as "inactive" according to the Physical Activity Index (i.e., expending less than or equal to 1.4 kcal/kg/day, Table 1). This finding is a result of the fact that a participant can be involved in the specified active environments, but not at

Table 1: Sample descriptive statistics for all variables in the analyses ($N = 44,057$).

Variable and category	n	(%)
Mood disorders		
Yes	3073	7.0
No	40,984	93.0
Active environment		
Group only	41	0.1
Individual only	36,659	83.2
Group + individual	1356	3.1
Neither	6001	13.6
Age (years)		
50–54	8776	19.9
55–59	8767	19.9
60–64	7850	17.8
65–69	5949	13.5
70–74	4809	10.9
75–79	3866	8.8
80 years and greater	4040	9.2
Sex		
Males	20,095	45.6
Females	23,962	54.4
Marital status		
Married	24,406	55.4
Common law	2315	5.3
Widowed/divorced	13,720	31.1
Single	3616	8.2
Physical activity index		
Active (≥3.0 kcal/kg/day)	9597	21.8
Moderately active (1.5–2.9 kcal/kg/day)	11,482	26.1
Inactive (0–1.4 kcal/kg/day)	22,978	52.2
Frequency of binge drinking		
Never	31,652	71.8
Less than once/month	6881	15.6
Once/month	1727	3.9
2-3 times/month	1342	3.0
Once/week	1342	3.0
More than once/week	1113	2.5
Type of smoker		
Daily	7034	16.0
Occasional	1161	2.6
Never	35,862	81.4
Perceived life stress		
Not at all	8612	19.5
Not very	13,011	29.5
A bit	15,508	35.2
Quite a bit	5806	13.2
Extremely	1120	2.5

a high enough intensity level to be considered "active" or "moderately active." It is interesting to note, however, that 73.0% of participants active in group environments were

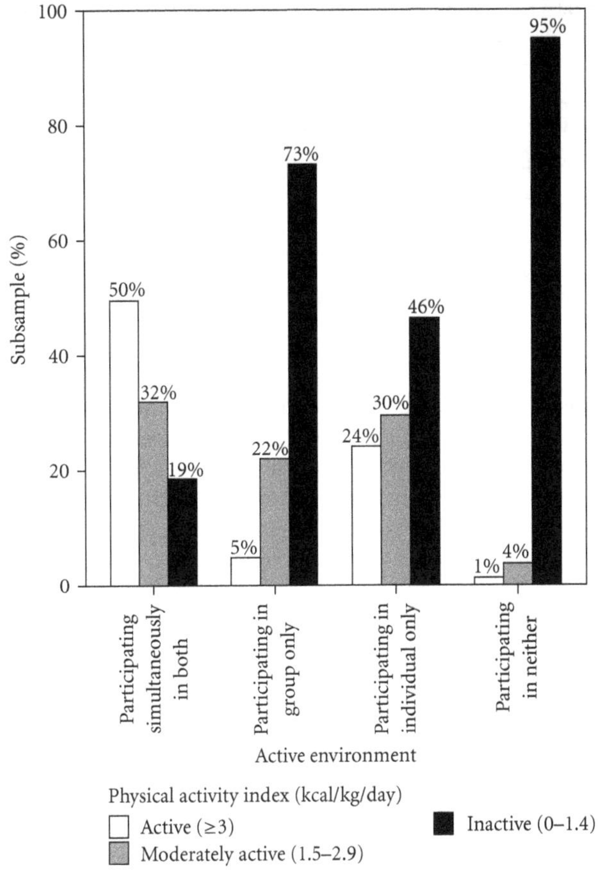

Figure 1: Percentage of participants participating in active environments stratified by daily energy expenditure levels.

classified as "inactive" (Figure 1). On the other hand, 1.0% and 4.0% of the participants who are not active in either environment classified as "active" and "moderately active," respectively (Figure 1), suggesting that these individuals expended energy outside of the leisure activities included in the current study.

The bivariate (Model A) and multivariate (Model B) associations between active environment and the likelihood of having a mood disorder are presented in Table 2. At the bivariate level, older adults participating in both group and individual active environments were 59.0% less likely to have a mood disorder than those who are not participating in any group or individual active environments (OR = 0.41, CI = 0.31–0.55). In addition, those participating in both types of active environments were 31.0% and 37.0% less likely to have a mood disorder than those participating in individual-only or group-only active environments, respectively (CIs = 0.65–0.79 and 0.24–2.5). These findings echo data presented in Figure 1 as 50.0% of participants engaged in both types of active environments were physically active at the most intense level, compared to all other types of active environments. Those participating in individual active environments only were 28.0% less likely to have a mood disorder than those who did not participate in either active environments (OR = 0.72, CI = 0.65–0.79). There were no

Table 2: Results of logistic regression analysis for the relationship between active environments and likelihood of having a mood disorder ($N = 44,057$).

Variable	Model A: OR (95% CI)	Model B: OR (95% CI)
Group only	0.78 (0.24, 2.5)‡	0.83 (0.25, 2.8)‡
Individual only	0.72 (0.65, 0.79)	0.85 (0.77, 0.95)
Group + individual	0.41 (0.31, 0.55)	0.55 (0.41, 0.74)
Neither	1.00 (referent)	1.00 (referent)

All $P \leq 0.01$, except ‡$P \geq 0.05$ (not significant), Model A: bivariate, unadjusted associations. Model B: multivariate, adjusted associations independent of age, sex, marital status, binge drinking, type of smoker, physical activity index, and perceived life stress.

statistically significant differences between those participating in group active environments and nonactive environment participants regarding the presence of a mood disorder (CI = 0.24–2.5). After adjusting for the covariates (i.e., age, sex, marital status, binge drinking, smoking, physical activity index, and life stress), comparable results were found. More specifically, only small decreases were observed in the effect sizes regarding the likelihood of having a mood disorder in the adjusted model, and all of the significance values remained.

4. Discussion

The present investigation found that most of the older adult Canadian population preferred to participate in individual active environments compared to group active environments. This finding is supported by previous research that describes older adults' preferences for individual activities, possibly to maintain their functional independence [13]. The result that older adults active in individual environments experience a decreased likelihood of reporting a mood disorder may be due to increased levels of self-efficacy that many older adults experience when participating in these activities via an internally focused locus of control of one's health [13, 15, 24–28]. This effect would allow older individuals to attribute their physical and psychological health improvements to their own actions rather than to external forces. Other evidence suggests that participation in individual active environments may promote the development of intrapersonal coping mechanisms to counter the psychological stresses, allowing individuals to adjust the stressors, maladaptive behaviours, and emotions associated with mood disorders [9, 37].

Regarding the results on whether participating in group and/or individual active environments had an influence on older adult's mental health outcomes, it was found that exercising solely in individual active environments decreased the likelihood of having a mood disorder, while participating in group environments had no significant effect. The present study does not question whether group active environments are beneficial to health in general; however, it does suggest that the benefits older adults derive from this mode of active environments *alone* may not pertain to mental health or the prevalence of the mood disorders included in the current investigation. Despite the fact that participating in group-only active environments was not statistically associated with the odds of having a mood disorder, older adults who participated in both group and individual active environments were the least likely to have a mood disorder. This finding suggests the beneficial nature of participating in individual activities in conjunction with group activities.

The notion that individual and group activities function together (i.e., via an additive effect) to promote mental health in later life is supported by previous research. Studies have shown similar benefits associated with each environment upon mental health outcomes. For example, improved self-efficacy is a benefit of participating in individual active environments among older adults [24], and this association is also observed among those active in group environments [15, 16]. It is also possible that individuals who participated in both group and individual active environments had a greater involvement in physical activity and sport, therefore, having a greater energy expenditure per day than those active in either environment alone (Figure 1). This possibility may explain why this particular group is the least likely to have a mood disorder (Table 2). Much like previous research [38–41], the present findings suggest that the more active environments one participates in at a moderate-vigorous intensity level, the better symptoms of mood disorders are attenuated. However, it is important to note that the relationship between active environment and the likelihood of having a mood disorder remained significant even after controlling for the physical activity index, a general measure of exercise intensity (Table 2; Model B).

4.1. Limitations. The CCHS contains self-reported data and may be prone to social desirability bias. As well, the cross-sectional nature of these data prevents an analysis of the cause and effect directionality of the relationships under investigation. In addition, due to the fact that several variables were included in the CCHS as optional content, the available subsample comprised of only 30 percent of the overall CCHS sample size, which may limit the generalizability of these findings. Also, regarding the classification of the active environments variable, it is possible that participants participated in individual activities as part of a group environment. For instance, swimming was coded as an individual activity because it does not *require* interactions with others to participate; however, participants could belong to a swimming group. Unfortunately, the structure of the CCHS does not provide these distinctive qualities of these two active environments.

4.2. Future Research. There is a need for continued research in the field of active environments and mental health outcomes for older adults, not only to address the limitations of the current study, but to discern the relative, and perhaps additive, contributions that different modes of active environments have at promoting successful aging in the mental health domain. This field of research would benefit from objective measures and designs, such as randomized control trials, that include individual and group activities to establish a clear cause-and-effect relationship between active environments and mental health in later life. As many of the previous studies have represented active environments as separate entities in their research designs, future studies should include experimental groups that assess group and individual active environments both separately and in conjunction with one another. Furthermore, as much of the current research on active environments focuses on structured exercise regimes, physical activity and sport-related research is lacking, yet such studies are required to validate the findings of the present study.

5. Conclusion

The present study revealed findings consistent with previous literature on mental health outcomes and active environments. Using a large dataset of older adults, this study supports the notion that participation in individual active environments can have benefits on one's mental health. However, this investigation has shown that participation in individual active environments along with group active environments may be even more effective at fostering positive mental health outcomes in later life. These findings suggest that engagement in multimodal active environments may be an important protective strategy against mood disorders among older adults. Overall, these findings have interesting and important implications on promoting successful aging among older Canadian adults [42]. These results should facilitate further research on the topic of active environments to clarify its relationship to mental health and other domains of health as well.

Conflict of Interests

The authors declared that there is no conflict of interests.

References

[1] Statistics Canada, "Population projections for Canada, provinces and territories, 2005–2031," (Catalogue No. 91-520-XIE), http://www.statcan.gc.ca/pub/91-003-x/2007001/4129904-eng.htm , 2005.

[2] United Nations, *World Population Ageing: 1950–2050*, Department of Economic and Social Affairs Population Division, New York, NY, USA, 2002.

[3] Statistics Canada, *Canadian Community Health Survey (CCHS)*, Statistics Canada, Ottawa Canada, 2008.

[4] Y. Hellström and I. R. Hallberg, "Perspectives of elderly people receiving home help on health, care and quality of life," *Health and Social Care in the Community*, vol. 9, no. 2, pp. 61–71, 2001.

[5] J. W. Rowe and R. L. Kahn, "Human aging: usual and successful," *Science*, vol. 237, no. 4811, pp. 143–149, 1987.

[6] W. J. Strawbridge, R. D. Cohen, S. J. Shema, and G. A. Kaplan, "Successful aging: predictors and associated activities," *American Journal of Epidemiology*, vol. 144, no. 2, pp. 135–141, 1996.

[7] R. M. Crum, J. C. Anthony, S. S. Bassett, and M. F. Folstein, "Population-based norms for the Mini-Mental State Examination by age and educational level," *Journal of the American Medical Association*, vol. 269, no. 18, pp. 2386–2391, 1993.

[8] Statistics Canada, "Health indicator profile, annual estimates, by age group and sex, Canada, provinces, territories, health regions (2011 boundaries) and peer groups," (Table 105-0501), http://www5.statcan.gc.ca/cansim/a05?lang=engandid=01050501, 2011.

[9] American Psychiatric Association, *Diagnostic and Statistical Manual of Mental Disorders*, American Psychiatric, Washington, DC, USA, 4th edition, 2000.

[10] J. A. Blumenthal, M. A. Babyak, K. A. Moore et al., "Effects of exercise training on older patients with major depression," *Archives of Internal Medicine*, vol. 159, no. 19, pp. 2349–2356, 1999.

[11] R. Robertson, A. Robertson, R. Jepson, and M. Maxwell, "Walking for depression or depressive symptoms: a systematic review and meta-analysis," *Mental Health and Physical Activity*, vol. 5, no. 1, pp. 66–75, 2012.

[12] M. Babyak, J. A. Blumenthal, S. Herman et al., "Exercise treatment for major depression: maintenance of therapeutic benefit at 10 months," *Psychosomatic Medicine*, vol. 62, no. 5, pp. 633–638, 2000.

[13] M. R. Beauchamp, A. V. Carron, S. McCutcheon, and O. Harper, "Older adults' preferences for exercising alone versus in groups: considering contextual congruence," *Annals of Behavioral Medicine*, vol. 33, no. 2, pp. 200–206, 2007.

[14] K. Andriessen and K. Krysinska, "Can sports events affect suicidal behavior? A review of the literature and implications for prevention," *Crisis*, vol. 30, no. 3, pp. 144–152, 2009.

[15] S. M. Burke, A. V. Carron, M. A. Eys, N. Ntoumanis, and P. A. Estabrooks, "Group versus individual approach? A meta-analysis of the effectiveness of interventions to promote physical activity," *Sport and Exercise Psychology Review*, vol. 2, no. 1, pp. 19–35, 2006.

[16] P. Callaghan, "Exercise: a neglected intervention in mental health care?" *Journal of Psychiatric and Mental Health Nursing*, vol. 11, no. 4, pp. 476–483, 2004.

[17] A. J. Daley, "Exercise therapy and mental health in clinical populations: is exercise therapy a worthwhile intervention?" *Advances in Psychiatric Treatment*, vol. 8, no. 4, pp. 262–270, 2002.

[18] A. C. King, W. L. Haskell, C. Barr Taylor, H. C. Kraemer, and R. F. DeBusk, "Group vs home-based exercise training in healthy older men and women. A community-based clinical trial," *Journal of the American Medical Association*, vol. 266, no. 11, pp. 1535–1542, 1991.

[19] S. K. Powers and E. T. Howley, *Exercise Physiology: Theory and Application to Fitness and Performance*, McGraw Hill, New York, NY, 6th edition, 2007.

[20] Y. Netz, "Physical activity and three dimensions of psychological functioning in advanced age: cognitive, affect and self-perception," in *Handbook of Sport Psychology*, G. Tenenbaum and R. C. Ecklund, Eds., pp. 492–508, John C. Wiley and Sons, Hoboken, NJ, USA, 3rd edition, 2007.

[21] C. B. Taylor, J. F. Sallis, and R. Needle, "The relation of physical activity and exercise to mental health," *Public Health Reports*, vol. 100, no. 2, pp. 195–202, 1985.

[22] A. V. Carron, K. S. Spink, and H. Prapavessis, "Team building and cohesiveness in the sport and exercise setting: use of indirect interventions," *Journal of Applied Sport Psychology*, vol. 9, no. 1, pp. 61–72, 1997.

[23] B. A. Meisner, S. Dogra, A. J. Logan, J. Baker, and P. L. Weir, "Do or decline? Comparing the effects of physical inactivity on biopsychosocial components of successful aging," *Journal of Health Psychology*, vol. 15, no. 5, pp. 688–696, 2010.

[24] L. R. Brawley, W. J. Rejeski, and L. Lutes, "A group-mediated cognitive-behavioral intervention for increasing adherence to physical activity in older adults," *Journal of Applied Biobehavioral Research*, vol. 5, no. 1, pp. 47–65, 2000.

[25] P. A. Estabrooks and A. V. Carron, "Group cohesion in older adult exercisers: prediction and intervention effects," *Journal of Behavioral Medicine*, vol. 22, no. 6, pp. 575–588, 1999.

[26] K. R. Fox, A. Stathi, J. McKenna, and M. G. Davis, "Physical activity and mental well-being in older people participating in the Better Ageing Project," *European Journal of Applied Physiology*, vol. 100, no. 5, pp. 591–602, 2007.

[27] A. C. King, C. B. Taylor, and W. L. Haskell, "Effects of differing intensities and formats of 12 months of exercise training on psychological outcomes in older adults," *Health Psychology*, vol. 12, no. 4, pp. 292–300, 1993.

[28] W. J. Rejeski and B. C. Focht, "Aging and physical disability: on integrating group and individual counseling with the promotion of physical activity," *Exercise and Sport Sciences Reviews*, vol. 30, no. 4, pp. 166–170, 2002.

[29] J. Baker, J. Fraser-Thomas, R. A. Dionigi, and S. Horton, "Sport participation and positive development in older persons," *European Review of Aging and Physical Activity*, vol. 7, no. 1, pp. 3–12, 2010.

[30] S. A. Hawkins, R. A. Wiswell, and T. J. Marcell, "Exercise and the master athlete—a model of successful aging?" *Journals of Gerontology A*, vol. 58, no. 11, pp. 1009–1011, 2003.

[31] J. Cairney and N. Krause, "The social distribution of psychological distress and depression in older adults," *Journal of Aging and Health*, vol. 17, no. 6, pp. 807–835, 2005.

[32] M. Afifi, "Gender differences in mental health," *Singapore Medical Journal*, vol. 48, no. 5, pp. 385–391, 2007.

[33] K. Lasser, J. W. Boyd, S. Woolhandler, D. U. Himmelstein, D. McCormick, and D. H. Bor, "Smoking and mental illness: a population-based prevalence study," *Journal of the American Medical Association*, vol. 284, no. 20, pp. 2606–2610, 2000.

[34] C. A. Okoro, R. D. Brewer, T. S. Naimi, D. G. Moriarty, W. H. Giles, and A. H. Mokdad, "Binge drinking and health-related quality of life: do popular perceptions match reality?" *American Journal of Preventive Medicine*, vol. 26, no. 3, pp. 230–233, 2004.

[35] N. Steverink, R. Veenstra, A. J. Oldehinkel, R. O. B. Gans, and J. G. M. Rosmalen, "Is social stress in the first half of life detrimental to later physical and mental health in both men and women?" *European Journal of Ageing*, vol. 8, no. 1, pp. 21–30, 2011.

[36] K. McCaul, J. Baker, and J. K. Yardley, "Predicting substance use from physical activity intensity in adolescents," *Pediatric Exercise Science*, vol. 16, no. 3, pp. 277–289, 2004.

[37] T. A. Judge and J. E. Bono, "Relationship of core self-evaluations traits—self-esteem, generalized self-efficacy, locus of control, and emotional stability—with job satisfaction and job performance: a meta-analysis," *Journal of Applied Psychology*, vol. 86, no. 1, pp. 80–92, 2001.

[38] K. A. Barbour, T. M. Edenfield, and J. A. Blumenthal, "Exercise as a treatment for depression and other psychiatric disorders: a review," *Journal of Cardiopulmonary Rehabilitation and Prevention*, vol. 27, no. 6, pp. 359–367, 2007.

[39] J. B. Bartholomew, D. Morrison, and J. T. Ciccolo, "Effects of acute exercise on mood and well-being in patients with major depressive disorder," *Medicine and Science in Sports and Exercise*, vol. 37, no. 12, pp. 2032–2037, 2005.

[40] A. L. Dunn, M. H. Trivedi, and H. A. O'Neal, "Physical activity dose-response effects on outcomes of depression and anxiety," *Medicine and Science in Sports and Exercise*, vol. 33, supplement 6, pp. S587–S597, 2001.

[41] A. Ströhle, "Physical activity, exercise, depression and anxiety disorders," *Journal of Neural Transmission*, vol. 116, no. 6, pp. 777–784, 2009.

[42] J. Baker, B. A. Meisner, A. J. Logan, A. M. Kungl, and P. Weir, "Physical activity and successful aging in canadian older adults," *Journal of Aging and Physical Activity*, vol. 17, no. 2, pp. 223–235, 2009.

3

Social Activity and Cognitive Functioning Over Time: A Coordinated Analysis of Four Longitudinal Studies

Cassandra L. Brown,[1] Laura E. Gibbons,[2] Robert F. Kennison,[3] Annie Robitaille,[1] Magnus Lindwall,[4,5] Meghan B. Mitchell,[6] Steven D. Shirk,[6] Alireza Atri,[6] Cynthia R. Cimino,[7] Andreana Benitez,[8] Stuart W. S. MacDonald,[1] Elizabeth M. Zelinski,[9] Sherry L. Willis,[10] K. Warner Schaie,[10] Boo Johansson,[5] Roger A. Dixon,[11] Dan M. Mungas,[12] Scott M. Hofer,[1] and Andrea M. Piccinin[1]

[1] *Department of Psychology, University of Victoria, P.O. Box 3050 STN CSC, Victoria, BC, Canada V8W 3P5*
[2] *Harborview Medical Center and General Internal Medicine, University of Washington, Box 359780, 325 Ninth Avenue, Seattle, WA 98104, USA*
[3] *Department of Psychology, California State University, Los Angeles, 5151 State University Drive, Los Angeles, CA 90032, USA*
[4] *Department of Food and Nutrition, and Sport Science and Department of Psychology, University of Gothenburg, P.O. Box 100, SE 405 30 Gothenburg, Sweden*
[5] *Department of Psychology, University of Gothenburg, P.O. Box 500, SE 405 30 Gothenburg, Sweden*
[6] *Bedford Veterans Affairs Medical Center, Massachusetts General Hospital, Harvard Medical School, 200 Springs Rd, Bedford, MA 01730, USA*
[7] *Department of Psychology and Neurology, University of South Florida, 4202 E. Fowler Avenue, Tampa, FL 33620, USA*
[8] *Center for Biomedical Imaging, Medical University of South Carolina, 68 President St, MSC 120, Charleston, SC 29425, USA*
[9] *Andrus Gerontology Center and Leonard Davis School of Gerontology, University of Southern California, Los Angeles, CA 90089-0191, USA*
[10] *Department of Psychiatry and Behavioral Sciences, University of Washington, 180 Nickerson, Suite 206, Seattle, WA 98109, USA*
[11] *Department of Psychology, University of Alberta, P-217 Biological Sciences Building, Edmonton, AB, Canada T6G 2E9*
[12] *Davis Lawrence J. Ellison Ambulatory Care Center, University of California, 4860 Y Street, Ste 0100, Sacramento, CA 95817, USA*

Correspondence should be addressed to Cassandra L. Brown, clb@uvic.ca and Andrea M. Piccinin, piccinin@uvic.ca

Academic Editor: Denis Gerstorf

Social activity is typically viewed as part of an engaged lifestyle that may help mitigate the deleterious effects of advanced age on cognitive function. As such, social activity has been examined in relation to cognitive abilities later in life. However, longitudinal evidence for this hypothesis thus far remains inconclusive. The current study sought to clarify the relationship between social activity and cognitive function over time using a coordinated data analysis approach across four longitudinal studies. A series of multilevel growth models with social activity included as a covariate is presented. Four domains of cognitive function were assessed: reasoning, memory, fluency, and semantic knowledge. Results suggest that baseline social activity is related to some, but not all, cognitive functions. Baseline social activity levels failed to predict rate of decline in most cognitive abilities. Changes in social activity were not consistently associated with cognitive functioning. Our findings do not provide consistent evidence that changes in social activity correspond to immediate benefits in cognitive functioning, except perhaps for verbal fluency.

1. Introduction

Cognitive decline in older adulthood remains an area of great concern as the population ages. Some changes in cognitive function, such as decreased processing speed, are considered normative aspects of the aging process [1]. However, the impact of even mild cognitive impairment on functional capacity highlights the importance of maintaining cognitive function for as long as possible [2]. Substantial evidence suggests that lifestyle factors and cognitive function in older adulthood are related [3]. Sometimes summarized by the adage "use it or lose it," current evidence suggests that leading an active lifestyle "using it" may buffer the effects of age-related cognitive decline "losing it" [3–5]. The mechanisms by which an active and engaged lifestyle may be related to better or preserved cognitive function in older adulthood remain to be fully elucidated. However, the cognitive reserve hypothesis predicts that some individuals are better able to withstand the physiological insults to the brain without measurable cognitive deficits because they had greater capacity to begin with [6]. Individuals may be able to actively increase their "reserve" through engaging in cognitively stimulating activities [3].

Social activities are considered part of what constitutes an active and engaged lifestyle, alongside cognitive and physical activities [3, 4, 7–9]. However, the evidence for a relationship between social activity participation and cognitive function is mixed. Some studies have found a relationship between social activities and cognitive function [10], while others have failed to do so [11]. In an intervention study, older adults living in residential care with normal cognitive function, after participation in daily short duration social and physical activity sessions, performed better cognitively than they had during their baseline assessment. However, the study design confounded physical and social activity [12]. Conversely, Aartsen et al. [11] found no relationship between social activities and cognitive function six years later using a cross-lagged regression approach that attempted to elucidate the strongest causal pathway. Similarly, Green et al. [13] did not find support for the hypothesis that social contact is protective against later cognitive decline.

The inconclusiveness of results has been acknowledged previously and suggested to relate to differences in statistical techniques [4, 8]. However, among studies that have used similar analytical methods, such as logistic regression, results are still mixed (e.g., [14–17]). Research examining whether social engagement can predict cognitive function and change in cognitive function over time, using growth modeling techniques, has also lacked a consistent finding. James and colleagues [10] found that social activity at baseline was associated with a higher baseline level of global cognitive function and lower rate of decline. Ertel et al. [18] found that baseline social integration was associated with a slower rate of memory decline, but not baseline memory performance. In a study of Danish twins, McGue and Christensen [19] found that social activity at baseline was related to level of cognitive function but not to change in cognitive function over time. They also found that, within monozygotic same-sex twin pairs, there was no evidence that the more socially active twin was less likely to experience cognitive decline than the less active cotwin. Overall, these studies demonstrate that many questions remain about the relationship between social activity and cognitive function [4, 7].

It is not clear whether it is a lifetime of social engagement (the effects of social activity accrued over time) that is protective, or if changes in social activity are related to cognitive function. Small and colleagues [20] examined the relationship between changes in social activity and changes in cognitive function and found stronger evidence for changes in cognitive function predicting changes in social activity than the reverse. Other studies have included only baseline social activity as predictor. Yet, social relations have been found to change qualitatively as people age [21]. Changes in social activity at any point in time may correlate with changes in cognitive functioning after controlling for its overall trend.

The current paper builds on previous work by exploring whether including social activity as a variable that changes over time can clarify the relationship between social activity and cognitive function in older adulthood. Using multilevel growth modeling with social activity as a time-varying covariate allows an examination of the relations between time-specific changes in cognition and social activity. This allows for a detailed test of whether the impact of social activity on cognitive function is accrued over time or whether changing social activity levels might relatively quickly impact cognitive function. Examining the temporal relationship between social engagement and cognitive function is needed to inform theories of possible mechanisms.

The current analysis examines the relationship between social activity, change in social activity, and four domains of cognition including: reasoning, memory, fluency, and semantic knowledge in four different populations. The same models are tested with data from four different longitudinal studies: the Long Beach Longitudinal Study (LBLS), the Seattle Longitudinal Study (SLS), the Victoria Longitudinal Study (VLS), and the Origins of Variance in the Oldest-Old: Octogenarian Twins Study (OCTO-Twin). This addresses the possibility that differing analytical methods may produce differing results and provides the opportunity for immediate replication and direct comparison of results. The diversity of the samples, two American, one Canadian, and one Swedish, increases the generalizability of the results and decreases the possibility that findings might be due to the particular features of one country or community.

2. Method

This research, initiated as a partnership between the Advanced Psychometric Methods Workshop series (Mungas et al., NIA conference grant) and the Integrative Analysis of Longitudinal Studies on Aging (IALSA) network [22], brought workshop participants together with researchers from four IALSA member studies. These studies were specifically selected based on their collection of cognitive, physical, and social activity data along with a range of cognitive functioning measures over multiple occasions held in common across the four studies. While the activity and cognitive functioning variables are not always identical, the subsets of variables in each study were chosen based on the rationale that they tapped similar domains at the construct level (e.g., Fluid Reasoning (Gf), Crystallized Knowledge (Gc), Short-term Memory (Gsm), and Long-term Storage and Retrieval (Glr; e.g., category fluency)) [23]. In some cases the measures are the same, but more often they differ, providing opportunities for both strict and conceptual replication. An exception to this is the OCTO-Twin dataset, for which a fluency measure was not available.

2.1. Origins of Variance in the Oldest-Old (OCTO-Twin) Participants (Sweden). The OCTO-Twin study is based on the oldest cohort of the Swedish Twin Registry and includes 702 participants aged 80 years and older at the time of the first assessment. Beginning in 1991–1993, the longitudinal design included a maximum of five measurement occasions at 2-year intervals. All individuals with a dementia diagnosis at baseline were excluded from the analyses ($n = 98$). The total sample includes 604 individuals, of whom 524 had the social activity measure and at least one of the cognitive measures. Approximately 20% of the sample was lost to followup at each wave (10% per year), but most of this attrition was due to death. The ratios for gender, education, socioeconomic status, marital status, and housing of the OCTO-Twin sample correspond to population statistics for this age range of the Swedish population [24]. Demographic information for the sample appears in Table 1.

2.1.1. OCTO-Twin Measures and Procedure

OCTO-Twin Cognitive Measures. Reasoning was assessed using Koh's Block Design Test [25]. In this task, participants are presented with red and white blocks and several patterns on cards and asked to construct the design on the card with the blocks. *Memory* was assessed using the Prose Recall test in which participants are asked for immediate free recall of a brief (100 words) story that has a humorous point [26]. Responses are coded for the amount of information recalled in a manner similar to the Wechsler Memory Scale [27]. *Semantic knowledge* was assessed using the Swedish version of the Information Task [28], which includes questions of general knowledge.

OCTO-Twin Social Activity. Participants were asked at each wave: "*How many people do you see?*" The possible response was: "none" (0); "1-2" (1); "3–5" (2); "6–10" (3), or "11 or more" (4).

2.2. Long Beach Longitudinal Study Participants (CA, USA). The LBLS was initiated in 1978 when participants were recruited from the Family Health Plan Health Maintenance Organization (HMO), including mainly residents of Long Beach and Orange County. This first panel included 583 individuals aged 28–36 or 55–87. The ethnic composition of the older group (98% Caucasian) was similar to the 65+ population for the area based on the 1970 census. Panel 2, initiated in 1992, included 633 individuals contacted from the same HMO (64 were excluded due to frank dementia or serious sensory or neurological problems).

In order to include the same measures as those in the Seattle Longitudinal Study, LBLS Panel 1 ($n = 106$) and Panel 2 ($n = 631$) data from 1994 to 2003 were used in the current analysis, excluding individuals younger than age 55 in 1994 (baseline $n = 565$). During this period, data were collected at 3-year intervals. Attrition was approximately 50% over each interval, or 17% per year. Dementia incidence is not known. Descriptive information for the sample is presented in Table 2. Additional information on the LBLS design, measures, and participants can be found elsewhere [29, 30].

2.2.1. LBLS Measures and Procedure

LBLS Cognitive Measures. Reasoning was assessed using a composite score of the Schaie-Thurstone Adult Mental Abilities Test (STAMAT; Schaie, [31]) Letter and Number Series tests. In Letter Series, participants view a series of letters (e.g., a b c c b a d e f f) and are asked to discover the rule that governs the series by identifying the letter that should come next in the series. Participants were to complete as many of the 30 items as possible within six minutes. Word Series was a parallel test to Letter Series but the letters were replaced with months (e.g., January) and days of the week (e.g., Monday). *Memory* involved immediate written recall of a list of 20 concrete high-frequency nouns studied for 3.5 minutes. *Fluency* was assessed by a word fluency task where participants were instructed to write down as many words as possible in five minutes that begin with the letter "s." Participants were instructed that they could not use proper nouns or create words by changing endings of other listed words (e.g., if the letter was "w" and you already said "want," you should not also say "wants," "wanting," or "wanted"). *Semantic knowledge* consisted of the STAMAT Recognition Vocabulary test. Participants were given a word and asked to circle a synonym of that word from four possible alternatives. The test included 50 items that were to be completed in five minutes.

LBLS Social Activity Measure. A measure of social activity was derived from a modified version of the Life Complexity Scale that was originally developed for the Seattle Longitudinal Study [32]. Participants were asked to record the number of "hours per week on average" they spent doing various activities (e.g., "going to parties"). The LBLS version of the scale included 34 specific activities, 7 of which were considered social. In the current study, these activity measures were dichotomized in order to distinguish those who reported no activity (coded as 0) from those who reported one or more hours of activity per week (coded as 1). This was done because the range of scores varied greatly within and between measures, and because some scores were highly deviant (skewed) from expected values (e.g., reporting more than 100 hours of reading per week).

The social activity variable was created by selecting questions from the Life Complexity Scale that fit the social activity construct. That is, a composite score was formed by summing up the number of social activity items that were endorsed as having one or more hours of activity per week. The measure consisted of seven questions including: phone conversations, voluntary activities, going to parties, going to dances, playing cards, visiting others, and attending church. The range of possible scores was 0 to 7. A social activity change variable was computed by subtracting the social activity measure in 1994 from social activity in 1994, 1997, 2000, and 2003. This resulted in a difference score that references the baseline testing in 1994.

TABLE 1: OCTO-twin participant characteristics.

Measure	Baseline (n = 524) M (SD)	Year 2 (n = 424) M (SD)	Year 4 (n = 326) M (SD)	Year 6 (n = 245) M (SD)	Year 8 (n = 175) M (SD)
			Year of testing		
Retention from previous testing (%)		82.9	76.7	76.2	72.8
Age	83.2 (2.9)	85.2 (2.8)	86.9 (2.5)	88.8 (2.5)	90.7 (2.4)
Education	7.2 (2.3)	7.3 (2.4)	7.3 (2.3)	7.2 (2.1)	7.2 (2.3)
Sex, female [n (%)]	365 (66)	299 (65)	233 (66)	193 (72)	146 (74)
Reasoning	11.6 (7.1)	11.6 (7.1)	11.5 (7.0)	10.2 (7.3)	10.2 (7.3)
Memory	9.6 (4.0)	9.5 (4.2)	9.5 (4.2)	9.1 (4.4)	9.1 (4.4)
Semantic knowledge	28.2 (11.1)	28.8 (11.1)	28.8 (11.1)	26.1 (11.4)	26.1 (11.4)
Social activity	3.0 (1.0)	3.0 (1.0)	3.1 (0.9)	2.8 (1.0)	2.8 (0.9)
Social activity change	—	−0.1 (1.0)	−0.0 (1.1)	−0.2 (1.1)	−0.4 (1.2)

M: mean, SD: standard deviation. The range for each measure with a defined upper limit is as follows: reasoning = 0–42, memory = 0–16, semantic knowledge = 0–44, and social activity = 0–4. Higher scores represent higher activity.

TABLE 2: LBLS participant characteristics.

Measure	Baseline (n = 565) M (SD)	Year 3 (n = 300) M (SD)	Year 6 (n = 143) M (SD)	Year 9 (n = 102) M (SD)
		Year of testing		
Retention from previous testing (%)		53	48	71
Age	73.8 (9.1)	75.5 (8.7)	75.29 (8.01)	76.4 (7.2)
Education	13.7 (3.0)	13.9 (2.8)	14.2 (2.70)	14.1 (2.7)
Sex, female [n (%)]	278 (49)	148 (49)	74 (52)	50 (49)
Reasoning	22.1 (11.7)	23.7 (11.5)	25.2 (11.63)	25.0 (11.1)
Fluency	32.3 (11.7)	33.5 (11.1)	33.3 (13.29)	34.3 (11.7)
Memory	11.4 (4.0)	11.5 (4.2)	11.6 (4.52)	11.1 (4.7)
Semantic knowledge	38.4 (10.2)	39.3 (9.8)	40.8 (8.95)	39.4 (9.9)
Social activity	3.3 (1.5)	3.5 (1.6)	3.5 (1.4)	3.5 (1.5)
Social activity change	—	0.0 (1.4)	0.1 (1.5)	−0.0 (1.4)

M: mean, SD: standard deviation. The range for each measure with a defined upper limit is as follows: education = 0–20, reasoning = 0–30, memory = 0–20, semantic knowledge = 0–36, and social activity = 0–7.

2.3. Seattle Longitudinal Study Participants (WA, USA). The SLS is a very long-running longitudinal study initiated by Schaie, who first recruited members of a local Health Maintenance Organization in 1956 [33]. Current analyses used up to four waves of SLS data from 1984 to 2005, which include an expanded set of measures that also overlap with the LBLS. Only participants of 55 years and older at baseline were included in the analysis. Baseline was defined as each participant's first study visit, and time was measured in all analyses as years in study (coded as 0, 7, 14, and 21). Attrition during these 7-year intervals was approximately 50%, or 7% per year. Dementia prevalence and incidence are not known. See Table 3 for SLS participant characteristics over the four waves of data analyzed here.

2.3.1. SLS Measures and Procedure

SLS Cognitive Measures. In order to model roughly equivalent cognitive outcomes across the four studies included in this coordinated effort, our analysis included measures of reasoning, fluency, memory, and semantic knowledge from a larger battery of tests. *Reasoning* was assessed with the Word Series test from the Schaie-Thurstone Adult Mental Abilities Test (STAMAT [31]), in which participants were asked to determine a rule that governs a series of words (months or days of the week) by identifying what word should come next in a given series. Participants were provided with a printed word series and instructed to choose the next word in the series in multiple-choice format. The test consists of 30 items and total score is based on number of correct responses completed in 6 minutes. As in LBLS, *Fluency* was assessed with the word fluency test from the Primary Mental Abilities test [34]. *Memory* was assessed with a task in which participants were asked to study a list of 20 printed words for 3.5 minutes and provide immediate written recall of the items. *Semantic knowledge* was assessed with the Educational Testing Service (ETS) test of Advanced Vocabulary, in which participants were asked to identify synonyms for printed words from 5 choices [35]. Total score was based on number of correctly identified synonyms out of 36 test items completed within 4 minutes.

SLS Social Activity Measure. We followed the methodology described in the LBLS method portion of this paper in

TABLE 3: SLS participant characteristics.

Measure	Year of testing			
	Baseline (n = 1657) M (SD)	Year 7 (n = 940) M (SD)	Year 14 (n = 446) M (SD)	Year 21 (n = 181) M (SD)
Retention from previous testing (%)		57	47	41
Age	67.1 (8.2)	73.0 (7.23)	78.0 (6.4)	81.9 (4.9)
Education	14.6 (2.9)	14.7 (2.8)	14.8 (2.7)	14.8 (2.8)
Sex, female [n (%)]	861 (52)	507 (54)	256 (57)	108 (60)
Reasoning	15.6 (5.8)	15.2 (5.6)	14.3 (5.5)	14.0 (5.25)
Fluency	38.5 (12.8)	37.5 (13.1)	36.7 (12.7)	38.8 (14.5)
Memory	12.5 (4.0)	12.0 (4.1)	11.5 (4.1)	11.6 (4.0)
Semantic knowledge	25.0 (6.7)	25.3 (6.6)	25.8 (6.2)	25.9 (5.9)
Social activity	3.5 (1.6)	3.5 (1.6)	3.5 (1.6)	3.3 (1.6)
Social activity change	—	−0.1 (1.5)	−0.2 (1.6)	−0.4 (1.7)

M: mean, SD: standard deviation. The range for each measure with a defined upper limit is as follows: education = 0–20, reasoning = 0–30, memory = 0–20, semantic knowledge = 0–36, and social activity = 0–7.

order to generate a roughly equivalent index of social activity (see LBLS section for a detailed description). Following this methodology, we created a composite activity measure by summing dichotomized responses from a modified version of the Life Complexity Scale [32] creating a seven-item social activity composite (volunteering, playing cards, phone conversations, visiting others, attending church, dancing, and partying). *Social activity change* was computed by subtracting baseline activity from each follow-up activity measure.

2.4. Victoria Longitudinal Study Participants (Victoria BC, Canada). The Victoria Longitudinal Study began in 1986-1987 with a sample of 484 community residing volunteers and three-year retest intervals. Using a longitudinal sequential design, second and third independent samples began in 1992-1993 (n = 530) and 2001-2002 (n = 550) [36]. Each sample is tested at three-year intervals. To date, Sample 1 has been tested on seven occasions (over 18 years), Sample 2 on five (over 12 years), and Sample 3 on two occasions (over 6 years). Participants in all three samples were recruited between the ages of 55 and 85 years.

Data from seven waves of Sample 1 and five waves of Sample 2 were included in the current investigation. Characteristics of the subsample analyzed here are provided in Table 4. Approximately 25% of the sample was lost to followup at each wave, or 8% per year. Dementia prevalence and incidence are not known. Further detail on the VLS design, measures, and participants can be found elsewhere [36].

2.4.1. VLS Materials and Procedure

VLS Cognitive Ability Measures. Fluency was measured by performance on a Similarities task [35]. In this timed task, participants were presented with target words and asked to write as many words as possible with the same or nearly the same meaning within six minutes. *Memory* was indexed using a 30 item, noun list learning task comprised of five semantic categories. Participants studied the word list for two minutes followed by a five minute free recall task [37]. *Reasoning* was indexed by Letter Series [35] in which participants were presented with a series of letters and asked to identify the next letter in the sequence that was consistent with the sequence rule. Participants were given six minutes to complete the task. *Semantic knowledge* was assessed using a 54-item recognition vocabulary test. This task was adapted from the ETS Kit of Factor Referenced Tests [35].

VLS Social Activity/Lifestyle Measure. The social activity/lifestyle measure used in the presented investigation included a subset of items from the VLS Activity Lifestyle Questionnaire. Individual item distributions were reviewed and a small number of poorly distributed items were eliminated. Seven items were selected due to their social nature (Eat at restaurants, visit friend/relative, give dinner party, attend church, meetings of service organizations, meetings of clubs, and do volunteer work). For each item, participants indicated the frequency of engagement in that activity over the past two years on a scale from 0 to 9 (i.e., *never, less than once a year, about once a year, 2 or 3 times a year, about once a month, 2 or 3 times a month, about once a week, 2 or 3 times a week, daily*).

2.5. General Analytic Approach. The current analysis was conducted as part of a larger effort to examine the effects of lifestyle activities on cognitive function using the same analytic approach across studies from the Integrative Analysis of Longitudinal Studies on Aging (IALSA) network [22]. Thus, final models were selected in part to maintain consistency across lifestyle activities.

In order to improve ease of interpretation of our results, age, education, and social activity measures were mean centered for each study. The means for baseline age, education, and social activity were subtracted from their baseline values for each individual. This centered the covariates so that the intercept and linear slope terms would be interpreted as the expected value for an individual at the mean age and with the

TABLE 4: VLS participant characteristics.

Measure	Baseline (n = 977) M (SD)	Year 3 (n = 723) M (SD)	Year 6 (n = 571) M (SD)	Year 9 (n = 411) M (SD)	Year 12 (n = 275) M (SD)	Year 15 (n = 91) M (SD)	Year 18 (n = 52) M (SD)
Retention from previous testing (%)[a]	—	74	79	72	67	79	57
Age	68.6 (6.7)	71.3 (6.6)	73.7 (6.4)	76.5 (5.9)	79.3 (5.2)	82.2 (4.6)	85.1 (3.6)
Years of education at baseline	14.9 (3.3)	15.4 (3.2)	15.6 (3.1)	15.9 (3.1)	15.8 (3.1)	15.2 (3.1)	14.8 (2.8)
Sex, female [n (%)]	614 (62.8)	450 (62.2)	346 (60.6)	251 (61.1)	170 (61.8)	60 (65.9)	35 (67.3)
Reasoning[b]	11.2 (4.7)	11.7 (4.2)	10.3 (4.7)	10.3 (4.6)	9.9 (4.6)	7.5 (4.7)	6.5 (4.2)
Fluency	17.7 (4.3)	17.9 (4.4)	17.7 (4.5)	17.2 (4.8)	16.3 (4.9)	14.7 (5.8)	13.8 (5.4)
Memory[c]	13.7 (5.9)	14.7 (6.0)	14.7 (6.1)	14.9 (6.4)	11.7 (5.4)	13.0 (6.3)	—
Semantic knowledge	43.7 (7.4)	44.7 (6.2)	44.3 (6.0)	44.2 (5.8)	43.5 (5.7)	42.7 (7.1)	42.6 (6.6)
Social activity	23.0 (6.9)	23.2 (7.2)	22.8 (7.3)	22.5 (7.2)	21.2 (7.1)	22.8 (7.7)	21.1 (7.2)
Social activity change	—	−0.1 (5.4)	−0.3 (6.0)	−0.9 (6.4)	−2.5 (6.9)	−3.5 (7.5)	−5.3 (8.1)

M: mean, SD: standard deviation. The range for each measure with a defined upper limit is as follows: reasoning = 0–20, Memory = 0−30, and Semantic knowledge 0−54.
[a]The 1986 cohort was followed for up to 18 years, the 1993 cohort for up to 12.
[b]The reasoning measure was not given until year 6 for the 1986 cohort.
[c]The memory measure was not given in year 18.

mean level of education for the study. The reference category for sex was male.

In order to examine the effects of social activity on cognition, a series of multilevel models was fit with social activity as a baseline and a time varying covariate [38], with time specified as time since baseline, using multilevel mixed-effects regression in StataCorp [39], the restricted maximum likelihood estimator (REML), and an unstructured covariance matrix. In the OCTO-Twin study, participants were nested within their twin pair. In the VLS, we controlled for enrolment cohort. Model assumptions were verified by examining the residuals. Separate models were fit for each of the four cognitive measures (reasoning, fluency, memory, and semantic knowledge) resulting in four reported models for each study. While the "familywise" alpha rate within each individual study may be somewhat liberal, given our use of $P < .05$ as significance criterion, our focus on repetition of findings across studies imposes a strict limit to any reliance on chance findings. Formal meta-analytic methods, which would require identical measures and a larger number of studies, were not used. Instead we relied on comparison of the conclusions derived from each study.

An initial 19-term model included the following terms: (1) baseline age, (2) sex, (3) education, (4) baseline social activity, (5) baseline social activity × age, (6) baseline social activity × sex, (7) baseline social activity × education, (8) individually defined time since baseline, (9) time × baseline age, (10) time × sex, (11) time × education, (12) time × baseline social activity, (13) time × baseline social activity × baseline age, (14) time × baseline social activity × sex, (15) time × baseline social activity × education, (16) change in social activity from baseline (activity change), (17) social activity change × baseline age, (18) social activity change × sex, and (19) social activity change × education. However, several terms were not significant for most of the studies and outcomes and so were trimmed to facilitate model interpretation. This process eliminated 7 of the 19 terms, first the 3-way interactions were eliminated, then the interactions with change in social activity. Last, the baseline social activity by sex interaction was dropped. This resulted in a 12-term final model, presented in Table 5 for separate cognitive constructs of reasoning, memory, semantic knowledge, and fluency.

3. Results

Significant between person age differences were seen at the first occasion of measurement for all memory, reasoning, and fluency tests, with older adults performing less well than their younger counterparts (all $P < .01$). Semantic knowledge results were less consistent, with SLS showing no age differences, $b = 0.02$, $P = .35$, LBLS and OCTO-Twin suggesting the older individuals score worse, $b = -0.28$, $P < .01$, and $b = -0.55$, $P < .01$, respectively, and VLS finding that older individuals performed slightly better, $b = 0.08$, $P = .02$.

At baseline, individuals with more years of education had significantly higher cognitive performance on all tasks, across all studies (all $P < .01$). Women at the mean baseline age had higher memory scores than did same aged men across all studies (all $P < .01$). LBLS and SLS women scored higher than men on all measures (reasoning: $P = .02$ and $P < .01$; fluency: both $P < .01$), except for LBLS semantic knowledge ($P = .13$, SLS $P = .02$). OCTO-Twin women had significantly lower Information scores, considered semantic knowledge, at baseline than OCTO-Twin men ($b = -4.20$, $P < .01$).

Significant within person declines were seen over time in study in all cognitive abilities and all studies (all $Ps < .01$). A significant time ∗ age interaction indicated that within each sample, those who were older at baseline declined

Table 5: Mixed model results of four longitudinal studies.

	OCTO-Twin			LBLS			SLS			VLS		
	b	SE	*P*	*b*	SE	*P*	*b*	SE	*P*	*b*	SE	*P*
Reasoning												
Intercept	10.89	0.55	<.01	21.43	0.53	<.01	14.65	0.17	<.01	9.52	0.59	<.01
Age	−0.33	0.12	.01	−0.62	0.04	<.01	−0.35	0.01	<.01	−0.26	0.02	<.01
Female	0.68	0.67	.31	1.86	0.77	.02	1.57	0.24	<.01	−0.15	0.31	.62
Education	0.56	0.13	<.01	1.30	0.13	<.01	0.52	0.04	<.01	0.32	0.05	<.01
Social activity	1.01	0.28	<.01	0.08	0.25	.74	0.11	0.08	.14	0.05	0.02	.03
Age × social activity	−0.02	0.11	.83	0.08	0.03	<.01	0.01	0.01	.15	0.00	0.00	.40
Education × social activity	0.04	0.11	.71	−0.04	0.08	.67	−0.03	0.03	.26	−0.01	0.01	.69
Slope	−0.44	0.08	<.01	−0.50	0.08	<.01	−0.25	0.02	<.01	−0.25	0.03	<.01
Age	−0.02	0.02	.28	−0.03	0.01	<.01	−0.01	0.00	<.01	−0.01	0.00	<.01
Female	0.08	0.09	.42	0.08	0.11	.48	0.01	0.02	.51	0.01	0.03	.76
Education	0.01	0.02	.56	−0.05	0.02	<.01	−0.01	0.00	.11	−0.01	0.00	.08
Social activity	0.06	0.05	.24	0.04	0.04	.30	0.02	0.01	.02	0.00	0.00	.44
Social activity change	0.65	0.15	<.01	0.04	0.17	.83	0.13	0.06	.04	0.03	0.00	.02
Fluency												
Intercept				31.01	0.61	<.01	36.11	0.44	<.01	11.5	0.56	<.01
Age				−0.30	0.05	<.01	−0.34	0.04	<.01	−0.10	0.03	<.01
Female				3.39	0.88	<.01	3.36	0.60	<.01	0.51	0.36	.16
Education				1.05	0.15	<.01	1.31	0.11	<.01	0.63	0.05	<.01
Social activity				0.99	0.29	<.01	0.24	0.19	.20	0.04	0.03	.12
Age × social activity				0.03	0.03	.40	0.00	0.02	.89	−0.01	0.01	.29
Education × social activity				−0.11	0.10	.24	0.04	0.07	.59	−0.01	0.01	.07
Slope				−0.24	0.11	.02	−0.43	0.04	<.01	−0.12	0.03	<.01
Age				−0.03	0.01	<.01	−0.02	0.00	<.01	−0.01	0.01	<.01
Female				−0.20	0.15	.18	0.11	0.05	.02	0.06	0.04	.16
Education				−0.01	0.03	.65	−0.01	0.01	.15	−0.01	0.01	.74
Social activity				0.07	0.05	.15	0.02	0.02	.26	0.01	0.01	.83
Social activity change				0.73	0.25	<.01	0.18	0.15	.21	0.06	0.02	<.01
Memory												
Intercept	8.70	0.32	<.01	10.80	0.20	<.01	11.56	0.13	<.01	17.28	0.41	<.01
Age	−0.20	0.06	<.01	−0.19	0.02	<.01	−0.18	0.01	<.01	−0.19	0.02	<.01
Female	0.99	0.39	.01	1.50	0.28	<.01	1.59	0.17	<.01	1.45	0.27	<.01
Education	0.34	0.07	<.01	0.29	0.05	<.01	0.32	0.03	<.01	0.31	0.04	<.01
Social activity	0.34	0.07	<.01	0.00	0.09	.98	0.14	0.06	.01	0.06	0.02	<.01
Age × social activity	−0.09	0.06	.10	0.01	0.0	.61	0.00	0.01	.51	−0.01	0.01	.95
Education × social activity	0.01	0.06	.91	−0.02	0.03	.57	−0.02	0.02	.18	−0.01	0.01	.19
Slope	−0.26	0.07	<.01	−0.18	0.05	<.01	−0.17	0.01	<.01	−0.27	0.03	<.01
Age	0.00	0.02	.97	0.00	0.01	.46	−0.01	0.00	<.01	−0.01	0.01	<.01
Female	0.05	0.08	.55	−0.03	0.07	.64	0.02	0.02	.15	−0.02	0.03	.56
Education	−0.01	0.02	.73	0.01	0.01	.40	0.00	0.00	.58	−0.01	0.01	.15
Social activity	0.07	0.04	.07	0.03	0.02	.15	0.01	0.01	.37	0.01	0.01	.25
Social activity change	0.47	0.11	<.01	0.11	0.10	.30	0.12	0.06	.03	0.06	0.01	<.01
Semantic knowledge												
Intercept	30.49	0.86	<.01	38.19	0.54	<.01	24.08	0.22	<.01	43.77	0.71	<.01
Age	−0.55	0.17	<.01	−0.28	0.04	<.01	0.02	0.02	.35	0.08	0.03	.02
Female	−4.20	1.05	<.01	1.19	0.78	.13	0.70	0.30	.02	−0.01	0.46	.99
Education	1.43	0.19	<.01	1.03	0.14	<.01	1.12	0.05	<.01	0.77	0.07	<.01
Social activity	0.87	0.40	.03	0.10	0.25	.70	−0.22	0.10	.02	0.02	0.03	.63
Age × social activity	−0.10	0.15	.47	0.08	0.03	<.01	−0.01	0.01	.61	0.01	0.01	.77
Education × social activity	0.03	0.17	.84	−0.06	0.09	.50	−0.05	0.03	.15	0.01	0.01	.61

Table 5: Continued.

	OCTO-Twin			LBLS			SLS			VLS		
	b	SE	P	b	SE	P	b	SE	P	b	SE	P
Slope	−0.85	0.11	<.01	−0.46	0.08	<.01	−0.12	0.01	<.01	−0.16	0.03	<.01
Age	−0.05	0.02	.03	−0.04	0.01	<.01	−0.01	0.00	<.01	−0.01	0.01	<.01
Female	0.19	0.13	.15	0.12	0.12	.30	0.06	0.02	<.01	0.03	0.04	.42
Education	0.03	0.03	.29	−0.02	0.02	.32	0.00	0.00	.78	−0.01	0.01	.18
Social activity	0.11	0.07	.12	0.01	0.04	.95	0.01	0.01	.01	−0.01	0.01	.40
Social activity change	0.86	0.19	<.01	0.17	0.17	.33	0.08	0.06	.13	−0.01	0.01	.93

Values represent model coefficients and their standard error. Across all studies, time was measured in years since baseline visit and activity change was entered as a time-varying covariate. All other variables represent baseline measurements alone, in interaction with one another, or in interaction with time.

significantly faster than the younger participants on all VLS, SLS, and LBLS measures except LBLS immediate memory. Except for the Information test, evidence for differential decline in older individuals was not seen in OCTO-Twin, which has a much narrower age range.

Women showed less decline than men in the SLS data only, and only for the fluency and semantic knowledge measures. Evidence for differential decline related to education was seen only for the LBLS reasoning measure.

Higher social activity levels at baseline, for individuals of average age and education, were associated with higher scores on reasoning within the VLS and OCTO-Twin studies, $b = 0.05$, $P = .03$, and $b = 1.01$, $P < .01$, respectively. The most consistent finding was that individuals with higher social activity levels at baseline also had higher memory scores. This was true for the SLS, VLS, and OCTO-Twin studies, $b = 0.14$, $P = .01$, $b = 0.06$, $P < .01$, $b = 0.34$, $P < .01$, respectively. Baseline social activity was also positively related to fluency in the LBLS (though the same measure was not significant in SLS sample). Social activity at baseline and semantic knowledge was positively related in the OCTO-Twin sample (operationalized as information; $b = 0.87$, $P = .03$), but negatively related in the SLS sample (operationalized as vocabulary; $b = -0.22$, $P = .02$). The OCTO-Twin sample was the only one where all cognitive measures considered had a positive association with baseline social activity levels.

The Baseline Age ∗ Social Activity interaction terms were significant and positive for LBLS reasoning ($b = 0.08$, $P < .01$) and semantic knowledge ($b = 0.08$, $P < .01$), indicating a stronger effect of social activity for older participants than for younger participants. However, the interaction of age and social activity was not significant for any other studies or cognitive measures ($Ps > .05$). The interaction between education and social activity at baseline was not significantly associated with any cognitive measure within any of the samples.

In terms of within person age changes, social activity at baseline was significantly related to the slope of semantic knowledge for SLS participants such that higher social activity at baseline was associated with less semantic knowledge decline ($P = .01$). There were no other significant relationships between social activity at baseline and rate of change for any cognitive measure within any of the samples (all $P > .05$).

In examining associations with change in social activity as a time-varying covariate in each of the models, several significant relationships were found. A reported increase in social activity was positively associated with performance on the fluency measures in all studies except SLS (LBLS $P < .01$, VLS $P < .01$, SLS $P = .21$), such that individuals who increased their level of social activity from their own baseline level exhibited higher occasion-specific fluency performance relative to their expected linear trajectory over time. In VLS and SLS, a significant relationship was also found between change in social activity and the reasoning (VLS $P = .02$, SLS $P = .04$) and memory (VLS $P < .01$, SLS $P = .03$) measure, indicating that participants who increased their social activity level also scored higher relative to their expected trajectory on the reasoning or memory measure. Changes in social activity were related to all cognitive measures in the OCTO-Twin study (all $P < .05$), such that OCTO-Twin participants who increased their social activity level from baseline had higher occasion-specific cognitive scores relative to their own linear trajectory in all domains tested.

4. Discussion

Comparing results of the same statistical model across four longitudinal studies of aging, we observed relatively few consistent associations between social activity and cognitive functioning. Looking at within person change in social activity and the four cognitive measures, the most consistent finding was an association with fluency in two of the three studies measuring it, after adjusting for linear effects of time and other covariates. Change in social activity was associated with memory performance in only half of the four studies (SLS and VLS). In only one study, OCTO-Twin, change in social activity was significantly related to performance in all three of the cognitive domains considered (fluency measure not available). The OCTO-Twin sample was the oldest and had the narrowest range of ages. Social activity in the OCTO-Twin study was defined by the number of people with whom participants had contact, whereas the other studies included a range of activities with a social component. Given that within person decreases in performance were seen across all cognitive measures in all studies, the positive relationships generally represent attenuated decline, rather than improvement in cognitive performance.

The use of within person change in social activity as a time-varying predictor of cognitive function is somewhat unique. However, in another study examining the temporal relations of social activity change and cognitive function, Small and colleagues [20] found significant coupling of social activity change and three cognitive domains: semantic decision speed (similar to our fluency measure), episodic memory, and semantic memory. They, however, found greater support for models where cognitive measures predicted changes in social activity levels, than the reverse.

There was little evidence that initial levels of social activity were related to within person rate of decline in cognitive function. Although higher initial levels of social activity were associated with less decline on the SLS semantic knowledge measure, this was not evident in any other samples. SLS has the widest interval between measurements and so correspondingly greater attrition between waves (though a similar yearly rate), but this does not suggest an obvious reason for the difference. The findings from the other studies are consistent with McGue and Christensen [19], who found that social activity at the first assessment was related to initial level of cognitive function but not change in cognitive function. However, other groups have found that social activity levels are associated with both baseline cognitive function and a reduced rate of decline over time [10]. Contrary to our findings, but similarly examining specific cognitive domains, Ertel et al. [18] found that social integration was related to a slower rate of memory decline. We did not include a composite measure of general cognitive function, but our results, and the results of others who have examined specific facets of cognition, suggest that it is important to examine cognitive domains separately.

Several between person differences were found. Specifically, individuals with higher initial levels of social activity performed better on the memory measures in three of the four samples. Interestingly, the sample that did not show the effect was the LBLS, which used the same measure as the SLS study. This suggests the discrepancy is not a function of different memory measures being used, or how social activity was characterized in the study. It is perhaps related to differences in samples, although both were similar in average years of education and were American, although from different regions. It is possible that how well a measure captures social activity varies by community. This, and the accessibility of the activities, may influence the association with cognitive function. However, such differences would not likely be specific to memory performance. The mean age of LBLS participants was about six years older and the first wave of LBLS assessment included in the present study was conducted ten years later than the first assessment of the SLS. The age differences are not an obvious explanation, because the mean age of LBLS participants is only slightly older than SLS and VLS participants and is nearly ten years younger than OCTO-Twin participants. The LBLS is the only study for which the majority of participants are not female, though this difference is slim (49% female in the LBLS versus 52% in SLS at baseline). It is possible another factor, such as attrition, is playing a role. The LBLS does have the highest yearly rate of attrition (17% versus 10%, 7%, and 8%), although the loss at each measurement wave is similar to that of SLS. It is unclear how this would affect the association between baseline social activity and memory performance; however, particularly considering that the mean social activity and memory measure scores for the LBLS and SLS were similar. It would be interesting in future work to consider general health and its age gradient in each of the studies. The lack of obvious reasons for discrepant findings, however, supports the importance of considering the reproducibility of results in coordinated, rather than pooled, analyses.

Social integration has been posited to influence general health through multiple pathways that may overlap with those influencing cognition [40]. Unfortunately, our findings do not strongly suggest that increased engagement in social activities confers immediate benefit in terms of cognitive function. Nor do they suggest that social participation reduces risk of cognitive decline in any domain apart from fluency. The cognitive reserve hypothesis suggests that, over time, "reserve" can be built up through stimulating activities and that individuals with high reserve can withstand more physiological deterioration before cognitive decline is observable [6]. That social participation does not reduce the risk of cognitive decline in a broad range of measures suggests that it is not conferring "reserve."

One possible mechanism through which social engagement and cognitive function are related may be the cognitively stimulating nature of social activities [20]. The cognitive training literature has found that training in specific tasks (e.g., memory tasks) does not necessarily transfer to other cognitive domains [3]. This may be similarly true of social activity participation, whereby a relationship is only seen in cognitive domains that are being challenged by the social activity. Social interactions do typically involve verbal communication, and thus fluency, likely specifically verbal fluency, may be the cognitive domain most similar to our participants' social activities.

Discrepancies in which activities are considered social may contribute to the lack of consistent association between social activity and cognitive function. For example, some activities (e.g., card games) may generally be more cognitively demanding than others (e.g., visits from family members), or primarily tax different cognitive skills, but this is likely to differ across individuals and situations. Although plausible, further research would need to confirm the validity of such hypothesis. In the context of physical health, others [40] have suggested that different social factors (e.g., social influence, social engagement, and social support) may act primarily through different behavioral, psychological, and physiological pathways. Similarly, cognitive function may be differentially influenced depending on the particular combination of social factors and pathways. In this way, how social activity is conceptualized and measured may be related to the mechanistic pathway and thus differentially related to various domains of cognitive function. These effects may have contributed to the discrepancies between OCTO-Twin and the other three studies in the current analysis, as OCTO-Twin focused on frequency of contact with people as the social activity measure, whereas the other three encompassed a variety of activities. However, the lack of consistency between the two studies employing the same measures suggests that conceptualization of social activity does not fully explain the findings. A clue to the source of inconsistency across LBLS and SLS may be the very small average change in the LBLS social activities measure, though its variance is comparable to those of SLS and OCTO-Twin. The association between cognition and social activity in LBLS in particular also seems to vary by age more than in the other studies.

A considerable strength of our analysis is the replication of the models across four longitudinal studies from geographically separate regions. This limits the possibility of spurious findings taking on undue importance and provides an opportunity to examine consistencies and inconsistencies between sample groups.

In terms of potential methodological limitations, Hertzog et al. ([41] for slope covariances; [42] for variance components) suggest that the power to detect correlated change is extremely low. However, analysis of longitudinal studies on aging, including those used in the current paper, has consistently reported statistically significant variances and covariances in rates of change in cognitive outcomes ([43–54], for summary see [55]). In addition, the tests used by Hertzog et al. are based on significance tests for variance components whereas change was evaluated in our paper by examining fixed effects which will generally have greater power [56]. Lending support to the argument that analyses in the current paper were adequately powered are the findings of significant associations between the identical set of cognitive outcomes in these same studies and physical and cognitive activities [57, 58].

Another limitation to our analysis is that while the study samples were restricted to initially healthy older adults, efforts were not made to exclude individuals who developed dementia over the course of the study periods (dementia diagnosis was available only in the OCTO-Twin study). We cannot assume that any protective effects of social activity on cognitive function would be equivalent across healthy and dementing older adults. Including individuals whose cognitive decline may have been driven by the dementia process may impact the associations between social activity and cognitive function over time in nondementing individuals, and this may also contribute to inconsistencies in the literature.

Finally, it is difficult to rule out the possibility that individuals decrease their social activities because their declining cognitive abilities make it more difficult for them to maintain social ties. The difficulty of determining the directionality of the relationship has been well acknowledged in the literature and it is similarly difficult to determine causal pathways in the current analysis [4, 5, 10]. Some attempts have been made to determine the most likely direction of the relationship, but the evidence is limited [20]. The longitudinal nature of the studies considered here, and allowing social activity to vary across time, have narrowed the temporal distance between the social activity and cognitive performance, at least partially disentangling whether the relationship is primarily based on historical activity levels or whether the two tracks over time.

Across four studies in three countries, baseline social activity levels failed to predict rate of decline in most cognitive abilities, and changes in social activity were not consistently associated with within person fluctuations in cognitive functioning. Our findings leave little support for the hypothesis that changes in social activity correspond to immediate benefits in cognitive functioning, except perhaps for fluency.

Acknowledgments

The research was supported by the Integrative Analysis of Longitudinal Studies of Aging (IALSA) research network (NIA AG026453, S. M. Hofer and A. M. Piccinin, PIs) and by the *Conference on Advanced Psychometric Methods in Cognitive Aging Research* (NIA R13AG030995, D. M. Mungas, PI). Dr. L. E. Gibbons was supported by a grant from the NIH (AG05136, Murray Raskind, PI). Drs. A. Atri, S. D. Shirk, and M. B. Mitchell were supported by NIA Grant AG027171 (Alireza Atri, PI). The LBLS was funded by NIA Grants AG10569 and AG00037 (Elizabeth M. Zelinski, PI). The OCTO-Twin study was funded by NIA AG08861 (Boo Johansson, PI). SLS was funded by the National Institute of Child Health and Human Development (HD00367, 1963–1965; HD04476, 1970–1973) and the National Institute of Aging (AG00480, 1973–1979; AG03544, 1982–1986; AG04470, 1984–1989; AG08055, 1980–2006; AG027759, 2006–2008; currently AG024102, 2005–2015; Sherry L. Willis, PI). The VLS is currently funded by NIA Grant AG008235 (R. A. Dixon, PI). Finally, and most importantly, the authors express their deep gratitude for the commitment of the study participants across all four studies. The content of this study is solely the responsibility of the authors and does not necessarily represent the views of the National Institutes of Health, the Department of Veterans Affairs, or the United States Government. The authors report no conflict of interests with the present study.

References

[1] F. I. M. Craik and T. A. Salthouse, *The Handbook of Aging and Cognition*, Psychology Press, New York, NY, USA, 2007.

[2] C. L. Burton, E. Strauss, D. Bunce, M. A. Hunter, and D. F. Hultsch, "Functional abilities in older adults with mild cognitive impairment," *Gerontology*, vol. 55, no. 5, pp. 570–581, 2009.

[3] C. Hertzog, A. F. Kramer, R. S. Wilson, and U. Lindenberger, "Enrichment effects on adult cognitive development: can the functional capacity of older adults be preserved and enhanced?" *Psychological Science in the Public Interest, Supplement*, vol. 9, no. 1, pp. 1–65, 2008.

[4] A. A. M. Bielak, "How can we not "lose it" if we still don't understand how to "use it"? unanswered questions about the influence of activity participation on cognitive performance in older age—a mini-review," *Gerontology*, vol. 56, no. 5, pp. 507–519, 2010.

[5] D. F. Hultsch, C. Hertzog, B. J. Small, and R. A. Dixon, "Use it or lose it: engaged lifestyle as a buffer of cognitive decline in aging?" *Psychology and Aging*, vol. 14, no. 2, pp. 245–263, 1999.

[6] Y. Stern, "Cognitive reserve," *Neuropsychologia*, vol. 47, no. 10, pp. 2015–2028, 2009.

[7] L. Fratiglioni, S. Paillard-Borg, and B. Winblad, "An active and socially integrated lifestyle in late life might protect against dementia," *Lancet Neurology*, vol. 3, no. 6, pp. 343–353, 2004.

[8] P. Ghisletta, J. F. Bickel, and M. Lövdén, "Does activity engagement protect against cognitive decline in old age? Methodological and analytical considerations," *Journals of Gerontology—Series B*, vol. 61, no. 5, pp. P253–P261, 2006.

[9] D. A. Bennett, J. A. Schneider, Y. Tang, S. E. Arnold, and R. S. Wilson, "The effect of social networks on the relation between Alzheimer's disease pathology and level of cognitive function in old people: a longitudinal cohort study," *Lancet Neurology*, vol. 5, no. 5, pp. 406–412, 2006.

[10] B. D. James, R. S. Wilson, L. L. Barnes, and D. A. Bennett, "Late-life social activity and cognitive decline in old age," *Journal of the International Neuropsychological Society*, vol. 17, no. 6, pp. 998–1005, 2011.

[11] M. J. Aartsen, C. H. M. Smits, T. Van Tilburg, K. C. P. M. Knipscheer, and D. J. H. Deeg, "Activity in older adults: cause or consequence of cognitive functioning? A longitudinal study on everyday activities and cognitive performance in older adults," *Journals of Gerontology—Series B*, vol. 57, no. 2, pp. P153–P162, 2002.

[12] S. Benloucif, L. Orbeta, R. Ortiz et al., "Morning or evening activity improves neuropsychological performance and subjective sleep quality in older adults," *Sleep*, vol. 27, no. 8, pp. 1542–1551, 2004.

[13] A. F. Green, G. Rebok, and C. G. Lyketsos, "Influence of social network characteristics on cognition and functional status with aging," *International Journal of Geriatric Psychiatry*, vol. 23, no. 9, pp. 972–978, 2008.

[14] H. Agüero-Torres, E. Von Strauss, M. Viitanen, B. Winblad, and L. Fratiglioni, "Institutionalization in the elderly: the role of chronic diseases and dementia. Cross-sectional and longitudinal data from a population-based study," *Journal of Clinical Epidemiology*, vol. 54, no. 8, pp. 795–801, 2001.

[15] M. K. Andrew and K. Rockwood, "Social vulnerability predicts cognitive decline in a prospective cohort of older Canadians," *Alzheimer's and Dementia*, vol. 6, no. 4, pp. 319–325, 2010.

[16] S. S. Bassuk, T. A. Glass, and L. F. Berkman, "Social disengagement and incident cognitive decline in community- dwelling elderly persons," *Annals of Internal Medicine*, vol. 131, no. 3, pp. 165–173, 1999.

[17] I. Kåreholt, C. Lennartsson, M. Gatz, and M. G. Parker, "Baseline leisure time activity and cognition more than two decades later," *International Journal of Geriatric Psychiatry*, vol. 26, no. 1, pp. 65–74, 2011.

[18] K. A. Ertel, M. M. Glymour, and L. F. Berkman, "Effects of social integration on preserving memory function in a nationally representative US elderly population," *American Journal of Public Health*, vol. 98, no. 7, pp. 1215–1220, 2008.

[19] M. McGue and K. Christensen, "Social activity and healthy aging: a study of aging Danish twins," *Twin Research and Human Genetics*, vol. 10, no. 2, pp. 255–265, 2007.

[20] B. J. Small, J. J. McArdle, R. A. Dixon, and K. J. Grimm, "Do changes in lifestyle engagement moderate cognitive decline in normal aging? Evidence from the Victoria Longitudinal Study," *Neuropsychology*, vol. 26, no. 2, pp. 144–155, 2012.

[21] B. A. Shaw, N. Krause, J. Liang, and J. Bennett, "Tracking changes in social relations throughout late life," *Journals of Gerontology—Series B*, vol. 62, no. 2, pp. S90–S99, 2007.

[22] S. M. Hofer and A. M. Piccinin, "Integrative data analysis through coordination of measurement and analysis protocol across independent longitudinal studies," *Psychological Methods*, vol. 14, no. 2, pp. 150–164, 2009.

[23] J. L. Horn and S. M. Hofer, "Major abilities and development in the adult period," in *Intellectual Development*, R. J. Sternberg and C. A. Berg, Eds., pp. 44–99, Cambridge University Press, New York, NY, USA, 1992.

[24] S. F. Simmons, B. Johansson, S. H. Zarit, B. Ljungquist, R. Plomin, and G. E. Mcclearn, "Selection bias in samples of older twins?: a comparison between octogenarian twins and singletons in Sweden," *Journal of Aging and Health*, vol. 9, no. 4, pp. 553–567, 1997.

[25] I. Dureman and H. Sälde, *Psykometriska och experimentalpsykologiska metoder för klinisk tillämpning*, Almqvist & Wiksell, Uppsala, Sweden, 1959.

[26] B. Johansson, S. H. Zarit, and S. Berg, "Changes in cognitive functioning of the oldest old," *Journals of Gerontology*, vol. 47, no. 2, pp. P75–P80, 1992.

[27] D. Wechsler, *Manual for the Wechsler Adult Intelligence Scale-Revised*, Psychological Corporation, New York, NY, USA, 1991.

[28] C. O. Jonsson and L. Molander, *Manual Till CVB-Skalen [Manual of the CVB Scales]*, Psykologi Forlaget, Stockholm, Sweden, 1964.

[29] E. M. Zelinski and K. P. Burnight, "Sixteen-year longitudinal and time lag changes in memory and cognition in older adults," *Psychology and Aging*, vol. 12, no. 3, pp. 503–513, 1997.

[30] E. M. Zelinski and K. L. Lewis, "Adult age differences in multiple cognitive functions: differentiation, dedifferentiation or process-specific change?" *Psychology and Aging*, vol. 18, no. 4, pp. 727–745, 2003.

[31] K. W. Schaie, *Schaie-Thurstone Adult Mental Abilities Test*, Consulting Psychologists Press, Palo Alto, Calif, USA, 1985.

[32] K. W. Schaie, *Intellectual Development in Adulthood*, Cambridge University Press, Cambridge, UK, 1996.

[33] K. W. Schaie, *Developmental Influences on Adult Intelligence: The Seattle Longitudinal Study*, Oxford University Press, New York, NY, USA, 2005.

[34] L. Thurstone and T. Thurstone, *Examiner Manual for the SRA Primary Mental Abilities Test (Form 10–14)*, Science Research Associates, Chicago, Ill, USA, 1949.

[35] R. B. Ekstrom, J. W. French, H. H. Harman, and D. Derman, *Kit of Factor-Referenced Cognitive Tests*, Educational Testing Service, Princeton, NJ, USA, 1976.

[36] R. A. Dixon and C. M. de Frias, "The Victoria Longitudinal Study: from characterizing cognitive aging to illustrating changes in memory compensation," *Aging, Neuropsychology, and Cognition*, vol. 11, no. 2-3, pp. 346–376, 2004.

[37] D. F. Hultsch, C. Hertzog, and R. A. Dixon, "Ability correlates of memory performance in adulthood and aging," *Psychology and Aging*, vol. 5, no. 3, pp. 356–368, 1990.

[38] D. Hedeker and R. D. Gibbons, "Application of random-effects pattern-mixture models for missing data in longitudinal studies," *Psychological Methods*, vol. 2, no. 1, pp. 64–78, 1997.

[39] StataCorp, "Stata statistical software: release 12," StataCorp LP, College Station, Tex, USA, 2011.

[40] L. F. Berkman, T. Glass, I. Brissette, and T. E. Seeman, "From social integration to health: durkheim in the new millennium," *Social Science and Medicine*, vol. 51, no. 6, pp. 843–857, 2000.

[41] C. Hertzog, U. Lindenberger, P. Ghisletta, and T. Von Oertzen, "On the power of multivariate latent growth curve models to detect correlated change," *Psychological Methods*, vol. 11, no. 3, pp. 244–252, 2006.

[42] C. Hertzog, T. Von Oertzen, P. Ghisletta, and U. Lindenberger, "Evaluating the power of latent growth curve models to

detect individual differences in change," *Structural Equation Modeling*, vol. 15, no. 4, pp. 541–563, 2008.

[43] K. J. Anstey, S. M. Hofer, and M. A. Luszcz, "A latent growth curve analysis of ate life cognitive and sensory function over eight years: evidence for specific and common factors underlying change," *Psychology and Aging*, vol. 18, no. 4, pp. 714–726, 2003.

[44] H. Christensen, A. Mackinnon, A. F. Jorm et al., "The Canberra Longitudinal Study: design, aims, methodology, outcomes and recent empirical investigations," *Aging, Neuropsychology, and Cognition*, vol. 11, no. 2-3, pp. 169–195, 2004.

[45] P. Ghisletta and U. Lindenberger, "Age-based structural dynamics between perceptual speed and knowledge in the Berlin aging study: direct evidence for ability dedifferentiation in old age," *Psychology and Aging*, vol. 18, no. 4, pp. 696–713, 2003.

[46] C. Hertzog, R. A. Dixon, D. F. Hultsch, and S. W. S. MacDonald, "Latent change models of adult cognition: are changes in processing speed and working memory associated with changes in episodic memory?" *Psychology and Aging*, vol. 18, no. 4, pp. 755–769, 2003.

[47] S. M. Hofer, H. Christensen, A. J. Mackinnon et al., "Change in cognitive functioning associated with ApoE genotype in a community sample of older adults," *Psychology and Aging*, vol. 17, no. 2, pp. 194–208, 2002.

[48] D. F. Hultsch, C. Hertzog, B. J. Small, L. McDonald-Miszczak, and R. A. Dixon, "Short-term longitudinal change in cognitive performance in later life," *Psychology and Aging*, vol. 7, no. 4, pp. 571–584, 1992.

[49] B. Johansson, S. M. Hofer, J. C. Allaire et al., "Change in memory and cognitive functioning in the oldest-old: The effects of proximity to death in genetically related individuals over a six-year period," *Psychology and Aging*, vol. 19, no. 1, pp. 145–156, 2004.

[50] A. Mackinnon, H. Christensen, S. M. Hofer, A. E. Korten, and A. F. Jorm, "Use it and still lose it? The association between activity and cognitive performance established using latent growth techniques in a community sample," *Aging, Neuropsychology, and Cognition*, vol. 10, no. 3, pp. 215–229, 2003.

[51] M. J. Sliwinski, S. M. Hofer, and C. Hall, "Correlated and coupled cognitive change in older adults with and without clinical dementia," *Psychology and Aging*, vol. 18, no. 4, pp. 672–683, 2003.

[52] M. J. Sliwinski, S. M. Hofer, C. Hall, H. Buschke, and R. B. Lipton, "Modeling memory decline in older adults: The importance of preclinical dementia, attrition and chronological age," *Psychology and Aging*, vol. 18, no. 4, pp. 658–671, 2003.

[53] R. S. Wilson, L. A. Beckett, L. L. Barnes et al., "Individual differences in rates of change in cognitive abilities of older persons," *Psychology and Aging*, vol. 17, no. 2, pp. 179–193, 2002.

[54] P. Rast and S. M. Hofer, "Substantial power to detect variance and covariance among rates of change: simulation results based on current longitudinal studies," *Psychological Methods*. In press.

[55] D. Zimprich and M. Martin, "Can longitudinal changes in processing speed explain longitudinal age changes in fluid intelligence?" *Psychology and Aging*, vol. 17, no. 4, pp. 690–695, 2002.

[56] T. A. B. Snijders and R. J. Bosker, *Multilevel Analysis: An Introduction to Basic and Advanced Multilevel Modeling*, Sage Publications, London, UK, 1999.

[57] M. Lindwall, C. R. Cimino, L. E. Gibbons et al., "Dynamic associations of change in physical activity and change in cognitive function: coordinated analyses of four longitudinal studies," *Journal of Aging Research*. In press.

[58] M. Mitchell, C. R. Cimino, A. Benitez et al., "Cognitively stimulating activities: effects on cognition across four studies with up to 21 years of longitudinal data," *Journal of Aging Research*. In press.

4

Association of Social Engagement with Brain Volumes Assessed by Structural MRI

Bryan D. James,[1] Thomas A. Glass,[2] Brian Caffo,[3] Jennifer F. Bobb,[3] Christos Davatzikos,[4] David Yousem,[5] and Brian S. Schwartz[2,6,7]

[1] *Rush Alzheimer's Disease Center, Department of Internal Medicine, Rush University Medical Center, Chicago, IL 60612, USA*
[2] *Department of Epidemiology, Johns Hopkins Bloomberg School of Public Health, Baltimore, MD 21205, USA*
[3] *Department of Biostatistics, Johns Hopkins Bloomberg School of Public Health, Baltimore, MD 21205, USA*
[4] *Department of Radiology, University of Pennsylvania School of Medicine, Philadelphia, PA 19104, USA*
[5] *Department of Radiology, Johns Hopkins School of Medicine, Baltimore, MD 21205, USA*
[6] *Department of Environmental Health Sciences, Johns Hopkins Bloomberg School of Public Health, Baltimore, MD 21205, USA*
[7] *Department of Medicine, Johns Hopkins School of Medicine, Baltimore, MD 21205, USA*

Correspondence should be addressed to Bryan D. James, bryan_james@rush.edu

Academic Editor: Alan J. Gow

We tested the hypothesis that social engagement is associated with larger brain volumes in a cohort study of 348 older male former lead manufacturing workers ($n = 305$) and population-based controls ($n = 43$), age 48 to 82. Social engagement was measured using a summary scale derived from confirmatory factor analysis. The volumes of 20 regions of interest (ROIs), including total brain, total gray matter (GM), total white matter (WM), each of the four lobar GM and WM, and 9 smaller structures were derived from T1-weighted structural magnetic resonance images. Linear regression models adjusted for age, education, race/ethnicity, intracranial volume, hypertension, diabetes, and control (versus lead worker) status. Higher social engagement was associated with larger total brain and GM volumes, specifically temporal and occipital GM, but was not associated with WM volumes except for corpus callosum. A voxel-wise analysis supported an association in temporal lobe GM. Using longitudinal data to discern temporal relations, change in ROI volumes over five years showed null associations with current social engagement. Findings are consistent with the hypothesis that social engagement preserves brain tissue, and not consistent with the alternate hypothesis that persons with smaller or shrinking volumes become less socially engaged, though this scenario cannot be ruled out.

1. Introduction

Social engagement, the performance of meaningful social roles for either leisure or productive activity, has been shown to be associated with better cognitive function and lowered rates of cognitive decline and dementia in older adults [1–4]. Yet many questions remain regarding how social engagement can potentially get "under the skull" to preserve cognitive abilities. Inconsistencies in measurement across studies is frequent with a number of overlapping constructs such as social activity [1, 5], social networks [6, 7], and social support [8] linked to cognitive outcomes; each has been theorized to affect the brain through separate mechanisms. Yet the neurological mechanisms that could lead to preservation of cognitive function remain unclear and perhaps the largest obstacle is a lack of research to directly explore the biological effects of social engagement on the brain. A popular hypothesis is that social engagement helps to build a brain reserve capacity that allows the brain to tolerate neuropathologic damage due to aging or disease without deterioration of cognitive abilities [9, 10]. In a case of "use it or lose it," remaining socially engaged as one ages may build this brain reserve through neuroplastic changes in the brain such as attenuated neuronal loss, or increased synaptic count [11–13] or the growth of new neurons [14]—all of which could be reflected in an increase or attenuated shrinking of brain volume. In the context of aging, larger brain volumes are associated with better cognitive function [15, 16], and preservation of cognitive function in the face of neuropathology [17]. Demonstrating a link between social engagement and larger brain volumes would provide support for the brain reserve hypothesis and our understanding of the neurological mechanisms at play.

We examined the relationship between social engagement and brain volumes using two complementary methods, a region-of-interest (ROI) analysis to investigate recognized anatomical brain regions, and voxel-based morphometry (VBM) to explore unbiased associations across the entire brain. Utilizing available longitudinal MRI data, we were also able to evaluate whether change in ROI volumes over five years prior to assessment of social engagement was associated with current level of social engagement in order to better discern temporal relations. We hypothesized that more socially engaged persons have larger brain volumes, especially for GM, which was found to evidence larger age-related declines in volume compared to WM in this population [18].

2. Methods

2.1. Study Population and Design. We used data from a study of lead exposure and cognitive function in former employees of a chemical manufacturing plant in the eastern United States and population-based controls with no history of occupational lead exposure [19]. The controls were selected from the same geographical residential as the former lead workers resided in using random selection from a telephone database and frequency-matched to lead workers for age, education, and race [20]. We used data from the third phase of this study when assessment of social engagement and a second MRI were obtained from study participants; an initial baseline structural MRI was acquired in phase 2, on average 5 years earlier. Detailed methods for study design and recruitment in phases 1 (1994–1997; 703 former lead workers and 130 controls, mean age 56 years) [20, 21] and 2 (2001–2003; 589 of 979 former lead workers and 67 of 131 controls completed MRI; mean age 56 at enrollment) [22] are described elsewhere. During phase 3 (2005–2008), 396 participants returned for an additional study visit. All phases of the study were reviewed and approved by the Johns Hopkins Bloomberg School of Public Health Committee on Human Research and written informed consent was obtained from all participants.

During phase 3, participants who completed the first MRI in phase 2 (589 former lead workers and 67 controls) were invited for a second MRI; 317 (54%) former lead workers and 45 (67%) controls completed a second MRI. Thus, two MRIs were obtained from 362 participants, representing 91% of the 396 participants who returned for phase 3 of the study. Nine of these had poor quality scans, leaving 353 participants with useable MRIs. Participants with phase 3 MRIs were on average younger than participants with no MRI or only a phase 2 MRI [18]. Five participants had missing data on social engagement; our final analysis included 348 participants.

2.2. Structural Magnetic Resonance Imaging Acquisition. A 3 T General Electric scanner was utilized for the phase 3 MRI. T1-weighted images were acquired using spoiled gradient recalled acquisition (SPGR) in steady state sequence (repetition time (TR) = 21 ms, echo time (TE) = 8 ms, field of view (FOV) = 24 cm, flip angle = 30° one excitation, voxel size = 0.9375 mm by 0.9375 mm by 1.5 mm, field of view 24 cm, matrix size 256 × 256). Methods for phase 2 MRI have been previously published [22].

2.3. Image Analysis. Quantitative analysis of MR volumes was completed using previously published methods [23]. First, extracranial tissue and brainstem structures were stripped. A validated specialized image analysis method was employed to segment the images into GM and WM. The CLASSIC algorithm [24] employs a 4-dimensional segmentation framework in which the first and second scans are considered jointly to minimize discrepancies between the two segmentations. The segmented images provide quantitative volumetric measures of total GM, WM, and brain (GM plus WM) matter.

To obtain volumes of predefined ROIs, regional analysis was performed via computerized template matching techniques previously reported and validated [22, 25]. In brief, a computerized image analysis algorithm based on pattern matching was used to warp a reference digital brain atlas to each participant's MRI. The resulting 20 nonmutually exclusive ROIs included the volumes of total brain, total GM, total WM, major lobar subdivisions, and a number of smaller structures.

For the voxel-wise approach, regional analysis of volumes examined in normalized space (RAVENS) was used to yield brain maps for analysis of local volumetric differences not constrained by *a priori* anatomic definitions [23]. This method can provide confirmatory evidence of associations in predefined regions or provide additional insights into areas of the brain linked to social engagement that are not apparent from using the ROI approach. Using previously published methods [25], segmented images were transformed into a standard coordinate space using an elastic deformation algorithm. This procedure yields tissue density maps for GM and WM whose values are direct measurements of local tissue volumes. Associations of predictor variables with GM and WM volumes could then be examined on a voxel-by-voxel basis, not constrained by arbitrary anatomical boundaries, thereby revealing spatial patterns of such associations.

2.4. Social Engagement. Social engagement was measured for the first time in phase 3 of this study (i.e., at the time of the second MRI). The measure of social engagement came from the enacted function profile (EFP), a 20-item scale designed to measure multiple domains of enacted functional performance in older adults based on pre-existing theory regarding the measurement of actual functional performance (rather than theoretical functional capacity) in daily life [26]. The EFP asks respondents how often they have engaged in a number of common daily activities over the past week or month. To test our measurement theory and to correct for random measurement error, we used confirmatory factor analysis to examine the conditional independence of four domains of enacted function (social engagement, community involvement, self-care, and productive activities) and to derive factor scores to represent our theorized latent constructs. For the analysis, a factor-based score based on the 8 social engagement items was generated using MPLUS version 5. The social engagement items and scale details are included in the appendix.

2.5. Statistical Analysis

2.5.1. ROI-Based Approach. We first evaluated whether higher social engagement was associated with larger volumes of predefined anatomical ROIs (dependent variable) in a cross-sectional analysis of phase 3 data. Associations between social engagement and brain volumes were examined using linear ordinary least squares regression modeling, with a separate model for each ROI. Because tibia lead is associated with smaller brain volumes [22], but was only available for lead workers, we first evaluated whether tibia lead level altered the association of interest or if it was appropriate to include both lead workers and controls in our main analyses without adjusting for lead. Tibia lead was not associated with social engagement and there was no evidence that the association of social engagement and brain volumes differed by control status or by tibia lead level, so we combined former lead workers and controls in all subsequent analyses.

All models were adjusted for intracranial volume, handedness, and control status (versus former lead workers). Demographic and health factors that could confound the relationship between social engagement and brain volume included age (centered), race/ethnicity (all minorities versus whites), education (five categories, with high school plus trade school as the reference group), cardiovascular disease risk factors known to be associated with brain pathology (hypertension and diabetes), and tibia lead level (measured in lead workers only). Effect modification by age, education, race/ethnicity, cardiovascular risk factors, and control status was evaluated using models with cross-product terms. To facilitate comparisons across ROIs, standardized regression coefficients are presented. Model diagnostics were performed to examine model fit and influential points. Because the 20 ROIs are not independent, we did not adjust for multiple comparisons in this analysis choosing instead to report standard errors and unadjusted tests of associations. Analyses were performed with SAS 9.1 statistical software.

2.5.2. ROI-Based Analysis to Address Temporality. To discern temporal relations, we performed secondary analyses using the available longitudinal data from the first and second MRI. We modeled social engagement (measured at the time of the second MRI) as the *outcome variable* regressed upon the change in ROI volumes from first to second MRI (to address whether change in brain volumes over five years is associated with social engagement at the end of the interval). Standardized regression coefficients are presented. Strength of association and model fit for these models were compared to our main models.

2.5.3. Voxel-Wise Approach. We next used voxel-based analysis to identify areas of GM and WM associated with social engagement. At each voxel we conducted linear regression of the voxel volume versus social engagement controlling for the aforementioned covariates. From the regression output we obtained a t-statistic for each voxel. We identified 3-dimensional clusters of 100 or more contiguous voxels exceeding the statistical threshold $t > 3.11$ (corresponding to an uncorrected P value <0.001). To address multiplicity, we conducted a permutation test to assess the statistical significance of each cluster with respect to the permutation distribution of the largest cluster of suprathreshold t-statistics. More specifically, for 250 repetitions, we permuted the brain images (e.g., voxel volumes) across subjects, keeping the covariate data fixed. Then for each permuted dataset, we performed the same analysis as was done on the original dataset, identifying the largest cluster of contiguous voxels exceeding $t > 3.11$. We finally obtained a P value for each cluster by calculating the proportion of repetitions for which the size of the cluster in question was greater than or equal to the largest cluster of the permuted data. This voxel-wise analysis was conducted separately for the gray and white matter maps.

3. Results

3.1. Descriptive Summary of Study Participants. Study participants were 48 to 82 years of age (mean (S.D.) = 65.2 (7.9)); the majority were white/non-Hispanic, had a high school education plus trade school, were hypertensive, and not diabetic (Table 1). The oldest individuals and the most educated were more socially engaged. Younger participants, white non-Hispanic persons, and those without hypertension or diabetes had larger brain volumes. There was a complex pattern of association between brain volumes and levels of education, as persons with a graduate degree had brain volumes similar to those with less than high school education; both groups had smaller total brain volumes compared with the high school plus trade school reference group. Participants in both the lowest and highest education groups were an average of 3.5 years older than participants in the middle categories. Former lead workers were less socially engaged than population-based controls but had larger brain volumes on average.

3.2. Associations of Social Engagement with Brain Volumes

3.2.1. ROI-Based Method. Inferences did not significantly differ for base models and fully adjusted models, so only fully adjusted models are presented. Higher social engagement was significantly associated with larger total brain volume and total GM volume, as well as larger temporal and occipital GM lobar volumes (Table 2), but not with total or lobar WM ROIs. Among the other ROIs evaluated, social engagement was only significantly associated with corpus callosum volume. There was no evidence of effect modification by age, education, race/ethnicity, or cardiovascular risk factors on relations of social engagement with ROI volumes.

3.2.2. Analysis to Discern Temporal Relationships. We evaluated whether changes in ROI volumes from the first to second MRI were associated with social engagement at the time of the second MRI. Information on changes in brain volumes

Table 1: Descriptive statistics.

	N	(%)	Social Engagement (Range −0.79, 1.09)	(SD)	Total brain volume (Range 880.6, 1449.3)	(SD)
All	348	(100%)	0.01	(0.33)	1137.4	(100.4)
Age						
48–59	82	(23.6%)	−0.07	(0.35)	1187.5	(94.6)
60–64	92	(26.4%)	0.04	(0.32)	1161.3	(90.6)
65–69	84	(24.1%)	0.02	(0.29)	1123.9	(81.8)
70–82	90	(25.9%)	0.07	(0.33)	1079.7	(100.4)
			$P = 0.028$		$P < 0.001$	
Race/ethnicity						
White/Non-Hispanic	315	(90.5%)	0.02	(0.32)	1141.6	(99.9)
All other	33	(9.6%)	−0.05	(0.40)	1097.1	(97.9)
			$P = 0.25$		$P = 0.015$	
Educational attainment						
<High school	25	(7.2%)	−0.05	(0.41)	1083.1	(74.7)
High school	90	(25.9%)	−0.05	(0.32)	1139.8	(97.4)
High school + trade school	167	(48.0%)	0.03	(0.30)	1135.8	(101.6)
College degree	56	(16.1%)	0.04	(0.34)	1171.6	(92.2)
Graduate degree	10	(2.9%)	0.28	(0.41)	1086.1	(137.9)
			$P = 0.018$		$P = 0.002$	
Hypertension						
Yes	180	(51.7%)	0.01	(0.32)	1116.6	(97.5)
No	168	(48.3%)	0.01	(0.33)	1159.6	(99.0)
			$P = 0.97$		$P < 0.001$	
Diabetes						
Yes	54	(15.5%)	−0.01	(0.29)	1098.8	(90.5)
No	294	(84.5%)	0.02	(0.34)	1144.4	(100.7)
			$P = 0.59$		$P = 0.002$	
Control status						
Population-based control	43	(12.4%)	0.12	(0.29)	1103.5	(100.5)
Former lead worker	305	(87.6%)	0.00	(0.33)	1142.1	(99.6)
			$P = 0.018$		$P = 0.018$	

All P-values from analysis of variance (ANOVA) tests.

in this cohort has been previously reported [18]. Changes in brain volumes over five years were not associated with social engagement at the end of the interval, except for temporal WM ($P = 0.034$) (Table 3).

3.2.3. Voxel-Based Method. Clusters of voxels were identified in both GM and WM where social engagement was associated with larger voxel volume after adjustment for the aforementioned covariates (Table 4, Figure 1). There were twelve GM clusters of 100 or more voxels exceeding a statistical threshold of $t = 3.11$ ($P < 0.001$). The largest GM cluster was 4581 voxels (peak $t = 4.23$, $P < 0.0001$) and the second largest was 2501 voxels (peak $t = 4.23$, $P < 0.0001$). The permutation test-based P values for the largest two clusters were 0.05 and 0.14, respectively. Although social engagement was not associated with total or lobar WM ROIs, the VBM analysis identified six suprathreshold WM clusters of more than 100 contiguous voxels. The largest two WM clusters consisted of 3221 voxels (peak $t = 3.95$, $P < 0.001$) and 2592 voxels (peak $t = 4.06$, $P < 0.0001$), respectively. These clusters were localized to the interior regions near the cerebral fissure. Applying the cluster-based permutation test, the P value for the largest cluster was 0.10.

As the VBM analysis was not constrained by anatomical regions, there were a number of similarities as well as differences. Significant GM clusters were observed in the temporal lobe (Figure 1), the region found to have the strongest association with social engagement in the ROI analysis, but a number of clusters were observed in regions not identified by the ROI analysis, including clusters in the parietal lobe and cerebellum. Furthermore, there were no

Table 2: Adjusted associations between social engagement (independent variable) and ROI volumes (dependent variables).

ROI	Mean volume (cc)	Social engagement standardized coefficient	P value
Total brain volume	**1137.96**	**0.037**	**0.011**
Total gray matter (GM)	**534.14**	**0.072**	**0.007**
Total white matter (WM)	603.82	0.001	0.975
Gray matter lobes			
Frontal GM	134.85	0.037	0.273
Temporal GM	**96.58**	**0.083**	**0.009**
Parietal GM	65.40	0.068	0.081
Occipital GM	**45.56**	**0.076**	**0.048**
White matter lobes			
Frontal WM	201.47	0.008	0.761
Temporal WM	119.03	0.021	0.501
Parietal WM	106.08	0.026	0.456
Occipital WM	58.22	0.007	0.869
Smaller structures			
Cerebellum	119.63	−0.013	0.763
Medial structures	80.63	0.047	0.135
Cingulate gyrus	21.02	0.045	0.269
Insula	13.94	0.008	0.865
Corpus callosum	**11.89**	**0.127**	**0.004**
Internal capsule	9.85	0.026	0.520
Hippocampus	7.42	−0.004	0.923
Amygdala	2.43	0.037	0.453
Entorhinal cortex	2.37	−0.016	0.756

From models adjusted for age, education, intracranial volume, race/ethnicity, hypertension, diabetes, handedness, and control status.
Bold: $P \leq 0.05$.

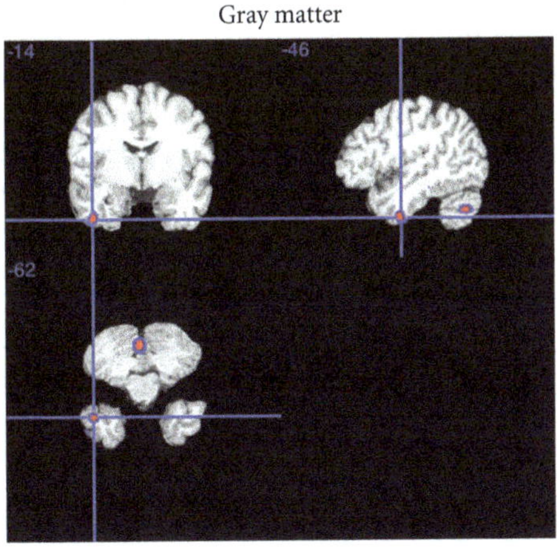

(a) Gray matter

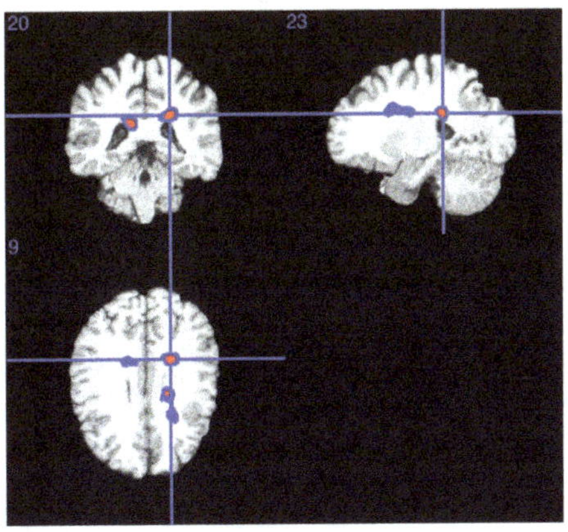

(b) White matter

Figure 1: The highlighted zones indicate regions in which higher social activity was associated with larger brain volumes from voxel-based morphometry analysis. Only clusters of 100+ voxels shown. See Table 4 for cluster-specific statistics.

significant associations with lobar WM volumes in the ROI analysis, but large significant clusters were observed in WM in the VBM analysis. These were in the corpus callosum, which aligns with the ROI analysis.

4. Discussion

These findings provide some of the first published evidence that higher social engagement is associated with larger brain volumes as assessed by structural MRI using ROI- and voxel-based methods. In contrast, change in brain volumes over the five-year-period was not associated with social engagement. Therefore, these findings are consistent with the hypothesis that social engagement preserves brain tissue, and provide some evidence against the alternate hypothesis that persons with smaller or shrinking volumes become less socially engaged, although we cannot rule out the possibility that changes in social engagement over a longer period than five

TABLE 3: Adjusted associations between change in ROI volumes (independent variable) and social engagement (dependent variable).

ROI	ΔROI standardized coefficient[1]	P value
Total brain volume	0.023	0.713
Total gray matter (GM)	0.062	0.299
Total white matter (WM)	−0.039	0.494
Gray matter lobes		
Frontal GM	0.032	0.599
Temporal GM	0.112	0.055
Parietal GM	0.092	0.133
Occipital GM	−0.011	0.849
White matter lobes		
Frontal WM	0.010	0.851
Temporal WM	**−0.115**	**0.034**
Parietal WM	−0.035	0.526
Occipital WM	0.046	0.416
Other structures (GM and WM)		
Cerebellum	0.022	0.695
Medial structures	0.005	0.937
Cingulate gyrus	−0.023	0.696
Insula	−0.014	0.803
Corpus callosum	−0.019	0.730
Internal capsule	0.067	0.244
Hippocampus	0.005	0.934
Amygdala	0.050	0.368
Entorhinal cortex	0.027	0.633

From models adjusted for age, education, intracranial volume, race/ethnicity, hypertension, diabetes, handedness, and control status.
[1]Social engagement at time of 2nd MRI was the dependent variable.
Bold: $P \leq 0.05$.

years may be associated with later volumes. The primary associations were with temporal and occipital lobar GM volumes, and likely as a result of this, with total GM and total brain volumes. There were no associations with lobar WM volumes. The findings support the brain reserve hypothesis by providing evidence that social engagement is associated with larger brain volumes in specific regions, which may in turn help to preserve cognitive function at older ages.

There are a number of proposed biological mechanisms by which social engagement could affect cognitive function through changes in brain volume, especially in GM, the site of the neuronal cell bodies and a variety of connections between neural and glial tissues. Total brain volume loss [27], GM loss [28], neuronal shrinkage [29], and synaptic loss [30] are common consequences of aging. Neuronal and synaptic loss, as well as accelerated gross atrophy, are well-documented pathophysiologic correlates of early Alzheimer's disease [31]. Brain areas with larger volumes may be able to tolerate more loss caused by aging or disease before exhibiting declines in cognitive function because of a higher number of remaining healthy neurons and synapses [32]. Social engagement may lead to larger brain volumes through a decrease in neuronal death or shrinkage, neurogenesis in certain areas of the brain [12], increased dendritic spine growth or axonal rearrangement [33]. Other lines of research provide support for a link between social engagement and larger brain volumes, including associations between social engagement and other aspects of brain pathology or function and demonstrated neuroplastic increases in volume due to human behavior such as activity and learning. Furthermore, experiments with animals placed in enriched environments with increased opportunity for learning, activity, and interaction with other animals have demonstrated neurogenesis, synaptogensis, and reduced neuronal loss [11, 13, 34–36].

The localization of the social engagement-volume relationship should be interpreted with caution, but some initial conjectures can be made. The association with social engagement was strongest in GM in the right temporal lobe. Facial and verbal recognition, long-term memory, and personality features reside in the temporal lobe [37]. Loss of GM in this area occurs during aging [28]. GM was not significantly associated with social engagement in the frontal lobe, which displays the most loss during brain aging [38]. Furthermore, no significant associations were found for the hippocampus, a structure important to memory and cognition and vulnerable to aging [39], though some studies have shown preservation of hippocampal volumes with aging [40]. Research on enriched environments in animal models have found evidence of neurogenesis in the hippocampus, [14] and a study in humans showed larger hippocampi in socially engaged persons [41]. However, the hippocampus is a small structure and it is likely measured with less accuracy due to greater proportional error. The only WM structure found to be significantly associated with social engagement in the ROI-based analysis was the corpus callosum. There is some evidence that hemispheric asymmetry is a marker of reserve [42], and it is hypothesized that larger corpus callosum volume (which facilitates communication across hemispheres) may compensate for psychomotor slowing in later life [43]. Moreover, it is possible that preservation of lobar GM volumes could also preserve inter-hemispheric connections between those areas resulting in a larger corpus callosum.

Strengths of this study include the relatively large number of subjects with MRIs, the robustness of brain imaging analysis, the use of a rigorous measure of social engagement, the availability of longitudinal data, and the ability to control for important confounders. Conducting analyses using both ROIs and VBM gave us two separate but complimentary ways to examine the association between social engagement and tissue volume in specific areas of the brain [15]. The ROI analysis was informed by recognized anatomical structures while the VBM analysis did not rely on *a priori* structural boundaries but rather examined the entire brain in an unbiased region-by-region basis.

One important limitation was the lack of a baseline social engagement measure, preventing us from examining the association between social engagement and change in brain structure or the association of change in social engagement with later brain structure. Another limitation is the unique nature of this cohort, which includes persons with past

TABLE 4: Cluster statistics from voxel-wise analysis.

X	Y	Z	Maximum t-statistic	Unadjusted P value	Cluster size	Cluster P value
Gray matter						
−42	50	−54	4.23	0.00002	4581	0.05
−3	51	−66	4.23	0.00001	2501	0.14
−65	−17	21	3.97	0.00004	1278	0.34
64	4	15	3.78	0.00009	1029	0.43
−46	−14	−63	4.16	0.00002	908	0.48
−56	−32	−64	4.08	0.00003	892	0.49
−65	17	−14	3.86	0.00007	511	0.68
−57	66	−25	3.9	0.00006	315	0.74
57	1	−46	3.73	0.00011	272	0.76
17	71	−31	3.54	0.00023	227	0.79
30	−37	32	3.47	0.00029	162	0.82
−50	14	−39	3.26	0.00062	119	0.82
White matter						
24	−21	12	3.95	0.00005	3221	0.10
−14	18	3	4.06	0.00003	2592	0.14
23	20	9	4.12	0.00002	1904	0.23
13	−47	−15	3.45	0.00031	797	0.44
35	45	−21	3.46	0.00030	198	0.77
27	41	−6	3.33	0.00048	102	0.83

Displays cluster centroid (x-, y-, and z- MNI coordinates), maximum t-statistic within the cluster, P value (unadjusted) of the maximum t-statistic, cluster size in number of contiguous voxels, and permutation test-based cluster P value. The cluster P-value compares the size of each suprathreshold cluster to the permutation distribution of the largest cluster, thereby accounting for multiple comparisons. Only results from clusters of 100+ voxels shown.

TABLE 5: Social engagement assessment.

Item: in the last week/month have you...	Response scale	Mean (std dev)
(i) been in touch with friends or relatives by phone or by letters?	W	2.6 (1.2)
(ii) gotten your hair [MEN cut WOMEN done] or dressed up to go out at least once?	M	2.5 (1.3)
(iii) done any unpaid volunteer work or community service?	M	0.9 (1.5)
(iv) been out to have lunch or dinner with someone?	M	2.8 (1.4)
(v) been to a meeting at a club, senior center, or organization in which you are active other than religious institution?	M	0.8 (1.2)
(vi) been out socially with friends or relatives, for example, to see a show, a party or holiday celebration, or some other social event?	M	1.2 (1.1)
(vii) gone shopping for food, clothes, or something else you needed?	M	2.8 (1.2)
(viii) done any indoor or outdoor recreational activity like bowling, working out, fishing, hiking, boating, swimming, golfing?	M	1.8 (2.0)

occupational lead exposure. Although we found no evidence that associations differed after control for lead dose or in comparing former lead workers to controls, the findings may not be generalizable to the general older adult population. The cohort is also racially and occupationally homogenous, and all male. Thus, we have no information on social engagement and the older female brain or differences across race/ethnic groups. However, homogeneity in occupation and socioeconomic status in this cohort may increase internal validity by lessening concerns of confounding by other factors linked to brain reserve and correlated with social engagement. Some potential confounders we were not able to adjust for include genes, IQ, stress response, personality, history of head injury, and MCI or prodromal dementia, all of which could be associated with both social engagement and brain structure. Finally, a limitation that could in part relate to the observed lack of an association between social engagement and WM is that we did remove white matter lesions from volumetric measures prior to analysis.

For more than a decade, recommendations have been made for older adults to stay socially engaged to keep their brains healthy based on evidence from epidemiologic studies of cognition and dementia. These studies have not addressed the "black box" regarding how social engagement may be related to the neuroanatomical substrate. Ours is an example, in a community-dwelling older adult population, of this

TABLE 6: The 8 social engagement items form one factor, of four, in the 20-item enacted function profile. Measurement properties of the enacted function profile follow.

Chi-square test of model fit	
Value	68.437
Degrees of freedom	46
P value	0.018
CFI/TLI	
Comparative fit index (CFI)	0.950
Tucker-lewis fit index (TLI)	0.946
RMSEA (Root mean square error of approximation)	
Estimate	0.035
WRMR (Weighted root mean square residual)	
Value	0.676

necessary piece to the puzzle of why socially engaged persons are more cognitively intact at advanced ages.

Acknowledgments

The authors would like to thank the participants and staff of the former lead workers study. This research was supported by Grant R01 AG10785 from the National Institute on Aging. Its content is solely the responsibility of the authors. B. D. James was supported by training grant T32 AG000247 from the National Institute on Aging and the Illinois Department of Public Health. There are no disclosures to report.

References

[1] B. D. James, R. S. Wilson, L. L. Barnes, and D. A. Bennett, "Late-life social activity and cognitive decline in old age," *Journal of the International Neuropsychological Society*, vol. 17, no. 6, pp. 998–1005, 2011.

[2] K. A. Ertel, M. M. Glymour, and L. F. Berkman, "Effects of social integration on preserving memory function in a nationally representative US elderly population," *American Journal of Public Health*, vol. 98, no. 7, pp. 1215–1220, 2008.

[3] S. S. Bassuk, T. A. Glass, and L. F. Berkman, "Social disengagement and incident cognitive decline in community—dwelling elderly persons," *Annals of Internal Medicine*, vol. 131, no. 3, pp. 165–173, 1999.

[4] L. Fratiglioni, S. Paillard-Borg, and B. Winblad, "An active and socially integrated lifestyle in late life might protect against dementia," *Lancet Neurology*, vol. 3, no. 6, pp. 343–353, 2004.

[5] A. Karp, S. Paillard-Borg, H. X. Wang, M. Silverstein, B. Winblad, and L. Fratiglioni, "Mental, physical and social components in leisure activities equally contribute to decrease dementia risk," *Dementia and Geriatric Cognitive Disorders*, vol. 21, no. 2, pp. 65–73, 2006.

[6] L. L. Barnes, C. F. Mendes De Leon, R. S. Wilson, J. L. Bienias, and D. A. Evans, "Social resources and cognitive decline in a population of older African Americans and whites," *Neurology*, vol. 63, no. 12, pp. 2322–2326, 2004.

[7] R. E. Holtzman, G. W. Rebok, J. S. Saczynski, A. C. Kouzis, K. W. Doyle, and W. W. Eaton, "Social network characteristics and cognition in middle-aged and older adults," *Journals of Gerontology B*, vol. 59, no. 6, pp. P278–P284, 2004.

[8] T. E. Seeman, T. M. Lusignolo, M. Albert, and L. Berkman, "Social relationships, social support, and patterns of cognitive aging in healthy, high-functioning older adults: MacArthur studies of successful aging," *Health Psychology*, vol. 20, no. 4, pp. 243–255, 2001.

[9] L. Fratiglioni and H. X. Wang, "Brain reserve hypothesis in dementia," *Journal of Alzheimer's Disease*, vol. 12, no. 1, pp. 11–22, 2007.

[10] M. J. Valenzuela and P. Sachdev, "Brain reserve and cognitive decline: a non-parametric systematic review," *Psychological Medicine*, vol. 36, no. 8, pp. 1065–1073, 2006.

[11] G. Kempermann, D. Gast, and F. H. Gage, "Neuroplasticity in old age: Sustained fivefold induction of hippocampal neurogenesis by long-term environmental enrichment," *Annals of Neurology*, vol. 52, no. 2, pp. 135–143, 2002.

[12] N. W. Milgram, C. T. Siwak-Tapp, J. Araujo, and E. Head, "Neuroprotective effects of cognitive enrichment," *Ageing Research Reviews*, vol. 5, no. 3, pp. 354–369, 2006.

[13] M. C. Diamond, "Response of the brain to enrichment," *Anais da Academia Brasileira de Ciências*, vol. 73, pp. 211–220, 2001.

[14] G. Kempermann, H. G. Kuhn, and F. H. Gage, "More hippocampal neurons in adult mice living in an enriched environment," *Nature*, vol. 386, no. 6624, pp. 493–495, 1997.

[15] B. S. Schwartz, S. Chen, B. Caffo et al., "Relations of brain volumes with cognitive function in males 45 years and older with past lead exposure," *NeuroImage*, vol. 37, no. 2, pp. 633–641, 2007.

[16] N. T. Aggarwal, R. S. Wilson, J. L. Bienias et al., "The association of magnetic resonance imaging measures with cognitive function in a biracial population sample," *Archives of Neurology*, vol. 67, no. 4, pp. 475–482, 2010.

[17] R. Katzman, R. Terry, R. DeTeresa et al., "Clinical, pathological, and neurochemical changes in dementia: a subgroup with preserved mental status and numerous neocortical plaques," *Annals of Neurology*, vol. 23, no. 2, pp. 138–144, 1988.

[18] B. S. Schwartz, B. Caffo, W. F. Stewart et al., "Evaluation of cumulative lead dose and longitudinal changes in structural magnetic resonance imaging in former organolead workers," *Journal of Occupational and Environmental Medicine*, vol. 52, no. 4, pp. 407–414, 2010.

[19] B. S. Schwartz, K. I. Bolla, W. Stewart, D. P. Ford, J. Agnew, and H. Frumkin, "Decrements in neurobehavioral performance associated with mixed exposure to organic and inorganic lead," *American Journal of Epidemiology*, vol. 137, no. 9, pp. 1006–1021, 1993.

[20] B. S. Schwartz, W. F. Stewart, K. I. Bolla et al., "Past adult lead exposure is associated with longitudinal decline in cognitive function," *Neurology*, vol. 55, no. 8, pp. 1144–1150, 2000.

[21] W. F. Stewart, B. S. Schwartz, D. Simon, K. I. Bolla, A. C. Todd, and J. Links, "Neurobehavioral function and tibial and chelatable lead levels in 543 former organolead workers," *Neurology*, vol. 52, no. 8, pp. 1610–1617, 1999.

[22] W. F. Stewart, B. S. Schwartz, C. Davatzikos et al., "Past adult lead exposure is linked to neurodegeneration measured by brain MRI," *Neurology*, vol. 66, no. 10, pp. 1476–1484, 2006.

[23] A. F. Goldszal, C. Davatzikos, D. L. Pham, M. X. H. Yan, R. N. Bryan, and S. M. Resnick, "An image-processing system for qualitative and quantitative volumetric analysis of brain

images," *Journal of Computer Assisted Tomography*, vol. 22, no. 5, pp. 827–837, 1998.

[24] Z. Xue, D. Shen, and C. Davatzikos, "CLASSIC: consistent longitudinal alignment and segmentation for serial image computing," *NeuroImage*, vol. 30, no. 2, pp. 388–399, 2006.

[25] D. Shen and C. Davatzikos, "HAMMER: Hierarchical attribute matching mechanism for elastic registration," *IEEE Transactions on Medical Imaging*, vol. 21, no. 11, pp. 1421–1439, 2002.

[26] T. A. Glass, "Conjugating the "tenses" of function: discordance among hypothetical, experimental, and enacted function in older adults," *Gerontologist*, vol. 38, no. 1, pp. 101–112, 1998.

[27] S. M. Resnick, D. L. Pham, M. A. Kraut, A. B. Zonderman, and C. Davatzikos, "Longitudinal magnetic resonance imaging studies of older adults: a shrinking brain," *Journal of Neuroscience*, vol. 23, no. 8, pp. 3295–3301, 2003.

[28] C. D. Smith, H. Chebrolu, D. R. Wekstein, F. A. Schmitt, and W. R. Markesbery, "Age and gender effects on human brain anatomy: a voxel-based morphometric study in healthy elderly," *Neurobiology of Aging*, vol. 28, no. 7, pp. 1075–1087, 2007.

[29] R. D. Terry, R. DeTeresa, and L. A. Hansen, "Neocortical cell counts in normal human adult aging," *Annals of Neurology*, vol. 21, no. 6, pp. 530–539, 1987.

[30] E. Masliah, M. Mallory, L. Hansen, R. DeTeresa, and R. D. Terry, "Quantitative synaptic alterations in the human neocortex during normal aging," *Neurology*, vol. 43, no. 1, pp. 192–197, 1993.

[31] G. L. Wenk, "Neuropathologic changes in Alzheimer's disease," *Journal of Clinical Psychiatry*, vol. 64, supplement 9, pp. 7–10, 2003.

[32] N. Scarmeas and Y. Stern, "Cognitive reserve and lifestyle," *Journal of Clinical and Experimental Neuropsychology*, vol. 25, no. 5, pp. 625–633, 2003.

[33] B. Draganski and A. May, "Training-induced structural changes in the adult human brain," *Behavioural Brain Research*, vol. 192, no. 1, pp. 137–142, 2008.

[34] E. Gould, A. J. Reeves, M. S. A. Graziano, and C. G. Gross, "Neurogenesis in the neocortex of adult primates," *Science*, vol. 286, no. 5439, pp. 548–552, 1999.

[35] H. Van Praag, G. Kempermann, and F. H. Gage, "Neural Consequences of environmental enrichment," *Nature Reviews Neuroscience*, vol. 1, no. 3, pp. 191–198, 2000.

[36] C. T. Siwak-Tapp, E. Head, B. A. Muggenburg, N. W. Milgram, and C. W. Cotman, "Region specific neuron loss in the aged canine hippocampus is reduced by enrichment," *Neurobiology of Aging*, vol. 29, no. 1, pp. 39–50, 2008.

[37] E. R. Kandel, J. H. Schwartz, and T. M. Jessell, *Principles of Neural Science*, Appleton & Lange, East Norwalk, Conn, USA, 3rd edition, 1991.

[38] T. L. Jernigan, S. L. Archibald, C. Fennema-Notestine et al., "Effects of age on tissues and regions of the cerebrum and cerebellum," *Neurobiology of Aging*, vol. 22, no. 4, pp. 581–594, 2001.

[39] R. I. Scahill, C. Frost, R. Jenkins, J. L. Whitwell, M. N. Rossor, and N. C. Fox, "A longitudinal study of brain volume changes in normal aging using serial registered magnetic resonance imaging," *Archives of Neurology*, vol. 60, no. 7, pp. 989–994, 2003.

[40] C. D. Good, I. S. Johnsrude, J. Ashburner, R. N. A. Henson, K. J. Friston, and R. S. J. Frackowiak, "A voxel-based morphometric study of ageing in 465 normal adult human brains," *NeuroImage*, vol. 14, no. 1 I, pp. 21–36, 2001.

[41] J. S. Saczynski, L. A. Pfeifer, K. Masaki et al., "The effect of social engagement on incident dementia and hippocampal volume: the Honolulu-Asia aging study," *Alzheimer's & Dementia*, vol. 1, no. 1, supplement, p. S27, 2005.

[42] R. Cabeza, N. D. Anderson, J. K. Locantore, and A. R. McIntosh, "Aging gracefully: compensatory brain activity in high-performing older adults," *NeuroImage*, vol. 17, no. 3, pp. 1394–1402, 2002.

[43] D. W. Desmond, J. T. Moroney, M. Sano, and Y. Stern, "Mortality in patients with dementia after ischemic stroke," *Neurology*, vol. 59, no. 4, pp. 537–543, 2002.

5

Psychological Impacts among Older and Younger People Living with HIV/AIDS in Nanning, China

Hongjie Liu,[1] Xin He,[1] Judith A. Levy,[2] Yongfang Xu,[3] Chunpeng Zang,[1] and Xinqin Lin[3]

[1] *Department of Epidemiology and Biostatistics, School of Public Health, University of Maryland, College Park, MD 20742, USA*
[2] *Health Policy and Administration, School of Public Health, University of Illinois, Chicago, IL 60612, USA*
[3] *Nanning Center for Disease Control and Prevention, Nanning 530023, China*

Correspondence should be addressed to Hongjie Liu; hliu1210@umd.edu

Academic Editor: Holly M. Brown-Borg

Objectives. The HIV epidemic has drastically increased among older adults in China, yet little research has examined the psychological impacts among older and younger people living with HIV/AIDS (PLWHAs). This study examined and compared self-efficacy, depression, well-being, and quality of life among older and younger PLWHAs in China. *Method.* A two-stage sampling procedure was used to recruit a final sample of 148 participants. Older adults were defined as age 50 and older. *Result.* Compared to younger PLWHAs aged 18–49 years old, older PLWHAs reported lower levels of well-being (7.6 versus 11.4), higher levels of depression (18.6 versus 15.8), and poorer quality of life. Self-efficacy was similar among older (23.9) and younger (24.6) PLWHAs. A higher level of depression among older PLWHAs was associated with much lower levels of subjective well-being and quality of life (physical health and psychological health). *Conclusion.* The findings suggest that older PLWHAs face psychological problems and mental health challenges beyond those experienced by younger PLWHAs. Intervention programs dedicated to improving mental health and quality of life are greatly needed for HIV infected older adults.

1. Introduction

According to a recent report by the Chinese Ministry of Health, the proportion of people age 50 or older living with HIV/AIDS (PLWHAs) among the total reported HIV cases in China increased 11-fold from 1.9% in 2000 to 21.1% in 2011 [1]. In some geographic areas of the country, the HIV prevalence among older adults has rapidly increased. For example, from 2007 to 2011, the proportion of older PLWHAs among the total reported HIV cases increased from 16.5% to 42.7% in Nanning, one of the HIV epicenters in China [2].

The aging of the AIDS epidemic is occurring globally, not just in China. By 2015, about half of PLWHAs in the United States will be 50 years of age or older [3], with comparable trends reported in Sub-Saharan Africa [4] and Australia [5]. As effective antiretroviral therapy (ART) becomes increasingly available throughout parts of the world, many PLWHAs who were infected as young or middle-aged adults now survive into older age. Additionally, growing older does not necessarily prevent these individuals from engaging in risky behaviors and contracting the virus.

Living with HIV/AIDS can be extremely challenging at any age, but older PLWHAs have to contend with the physical declines of an aging body. As both aging and HIV infection can work separately or interactively to reduce human immune response, older PLWHAs are particularly susceptible to AIDS related or non-AIDS related chronic diseases [6]. While ART has led to a marked reduction in the incidence of AIDS-defining illnesses, a variety of HIV associated non-AIDS (HANA) conditions are becoming increasingly commonplace in individuals with long standing HIV infection [7]. These conditions include cardiovascular disease, lung disease, infection-related and non-infection-related cancers, neuropsychiatric disorders, liver cirrhosis, and renal disease. As reported by Negin et al. [8], HIV-infected older adults in South Africa have high rates of chronic diseases, compared with those aged 18–49 years old.

In addition, the interaction of aging processes and AIDS-associated conditions can create considerable psychosocial challenges for older PLWHAs. Social relationships may become strained or disrupted due to HIV's association with stigmatizing behaviors and also through social discrimination [9, 10]. Acquiring and living with HIV can lead to psychological difficulties and reduced mental health, including decreased self-efficacy, depression, impaired well-being, and poor quality of life. Age-related reductions in immune response, impaired physical function, and reduced social support can contribute to or exacerbate existing psychological and mental problems [11]. Compared to their younger counterparts, older PLWHAs may experience greater difficulty coping with HIV-driven psychological challenges and mental health due to the correlates of advancing age.

Despite the rapidly increasing number of older adults living with the virus globally, little research to date has compared psychosocial health of older PLWHAs to younger PLWHAs [9, 12]. Moreover, almost nothing is known about how HIV may affect the psychosocial functioning and the well-being of older PLWHAs in China and other Asian countries. The scant findings that are available for China report that older PLWHAs often worry that disclosing their positive status will lead to social isolation and rejection [13], especially if the source of infection is through paid sex or illicit drug use [14]. Older adults also tend to internalize feelings of worthlessness and self-blame for becoming infected [13].

To understand the psychological challenges that older adults confront living with HIV and also to obtain baseline data for further research, we conducted a study of older PLWHAs in China. Consistent with other HIV research [7], we defined older PLWHAs as men and women at age 50 and older. Younger PLWHAs were defined as 18–49 years old. The objectives of this study were to examine the patterns of psychological challenges faced by older PLWHAs in China and to compare their levels of self-efficacy, depression, psychosocial well-being, and quality of life to younger PLWHAs.

2. Methods

The study protocol and consent procedures were reviewed and approved by the Institutional Review Boards of Virginia Commonwealth University and Guangxi Center for Disease Control and Prevention. In accordance with the approved protocol, written informed consent was obtained from all study participants prior to data collection.

2.1. Study Sites and Subjects. The cross-sectional study was conducted in Nanning, the capital city of the Guangxi Province. In 2011, Guangxi ranked second among China's 31 provinces for reported number of HIV infections. Although about 30% of all PLWHAs (including both younger and older ones) in Nanning acquired HIV through heterosexual intercourses and 45% through needle-sharing, the dominant HIV transmission mode among older adults was heterosexual (90%) [2].

A two-stage sampling approach was used to recruit eligible subjects [15]. Eligibility criteria included PLWHAs who were at least 18 years old and able to participate in a face-to-face interview. For the first stage, we purposely selected three study sites that provided HIV care and treatment services for the majority of PLWHAs in the city: an infectious disease hospital that was designated to provide care and treatment for PLWHAs, a methadone maintenance treatment (MMT) clinic run by Nanning Center for Disease and Control, and a healthcare center run by PLWHA volunteers. During the second stage, based on a list of PLWHAs in each site, all eligible subjects were invited to participate in the study during the study period. HIV status was confirmed by surveillance data provided by the Nanning Center for Disease Control and Prevention.

2.2. Measures. In addition to collecting basic demographic information, we administered four well-validated scales to assess quality of life, general self-efficacy, subjective well-being, and depression. The demographic items and scales initially were drafted in English and then translated into Chinese by three research team members who were fluent in both languages. The Chinese version of the measurement items was then distributed to research team members for further review and word-modified to assure that the measures were appropriate within a Chinese context. The four scales are as follows.

The Chinese version of the World Health Organization Quality of Life Assessment (WHOQOL-BREF) was used to measure the level of quality of life [16, 17]. The WHOQOL-BREF consists of 26 items that measure four QOL-domains: physical health (pain, energy, sleep, mobility, activities, medication, and work), psychological health (positive and negative feelings, cognitions, self-esteem, body image, and spirituality), social relationships (personal relationships, social support, and sexual activities), and environmental aspects (safety and security, home environment, finances, health and care, information, leisure, physical environment, and transport). Interviewees responded to these items on a five-point Likert scale. The four-domain scores indicated an individual's perception of quality of life in each particular domain. Domain scores were scaled in a positive direction (i.e., higher scores indicate better quality of life). Cronbach's reliability alpha of the measurement domains was between 0.43 and 0.85 (0.79 in physical health, 0.76 in psychological health, 0.43 in social relations, and 0.85 in environment) in older PLWHAs and 0.64–0.84 in younger PLWHAs (0.83 in physical health, 0.84 in psychological health, 0.64 in social relations, and 0.83 in environment). The domain score was calculated as the mean score of items within each domain.

The general self-efficacy scale is a 10-item scale used to measure perceived self-efficacy [18]. Sample items included, "I can always manage to solve difficult problems if I try hard enough" and "I can solve most problems if I invest the necessary effort." Participants responded on a four-point scale ranging from "not at all true (1)" to "exactly true (4)." Cronbach's alpha was 0.87 in older PLWHAs and 0.84 in younger PLWHAs. A composite score was calculated by totaling the responding value of the 10 items. The composite scores ranged from 1 to 40 with higher scores indicating higher self-efficacy.

The WHO well-being index was used to measure the level of subjective well-being [19]. This index consisted of five measurement items on a six-point scale ranging from "at no time (0)" to "all of the time (5)." Sample items included, "I have felt cheerful and in good spirits" and "My daily life has been filled with things that interest me." Cronbach's alpha was 0.95 in older PLWHAs and 0.92 in younger PLWHAs. A composite score was calculated by totaling the value of the five items. Higher scores represent better well-being.

Center for Epidemiologic Studies Depression Scale (CES-D) is a 10-item scale designed to measure depressive symptoms experienced in the past week [20]. Responses ranged from 0 to 3: 0 = rarely or none of the time (less than 1 day); 1 = some or a little of the time (1-2 days); 2 = occasionally or a moderate amount of the time (3-4 days); and 3 = most or all of the time (5–7 days). The CES-D total score was calculated by adding the scores for all 10 items ranging from 0 to 30. Cronbach's alpha was 0.78 in older PLWHAs and 0.82 in younger PLWHAs. Higher scores indicate greater depression.

The above measurement scales have been used successfully in other studies with Chinese populations [16, 18, 21, 22]. In addition, HIV knowledge regarding transmission and prevention of HIV/AIDS was measured by 11 true/false/unsure questions. One point was given for a correct answer, with a possible score ranging from 0 to 11 points.

2.3. Data Analysis. Chi-square tests were used to determine statistical differences in demographic variables (i.e., gender, education, and marital status) between older and younger PLWHAs. Pearson's correlation coefficients were calculated to measure bivariate correlations. The comparisons of psychosocial and mental health between older and younger PLWHAs were conducted using Student's t tests, given that the normality assumption was not violated; otherwise, a logarithmic transformation was applied to remove skewness. General linear models were used to estimate and compare adjusted means of HIV knowledge, self-efficacy, depression, well-being, and quality of life after accounting for gender, education, marital status, current ART treatment, and self-reported years since HIV diagnosis. SAS Version 9.3 (SAS Inc., Cary, NC) was used to perform all the analyses.

3. Results

3.1. Demographic Characteristics of the Two Groups. A total of 170 PLWHAs were invited to participate in the study. Of these, 20 PLWHAs declined participation due to unavailability (n = 18) or failure to provide information on key measures (n = 2), resulting in a total of 148 PLWHAs (31 older PLWHAs and 117 younger PLWHAs). The mean age of older PHWHAs was 58.4 years old (range: 50–80 years old) and 36.0 (range: 20–49) for younger PLWHAs. Across both age categories of PLWHAs, length of time between HIV diagnosis and the interview ranged from 1 month to 13.5 years, with a median of 18 months (12 months among older PLWHAs and 19 months among younger PLWHAs). China's Comprehensive AIDS Response Program (China CARES) is the single largest AIDS project in the world, covering 83.3 million people in 127 program sites in 28 provinces [23]. Under this program, forty-eight percent of older PLWHAs (15/31) and 56% of younger PLWHAs (65/117) received ART. Compared to the younger PLWHAs, older PLWHAs were more likely to be married (87% versus 66%). No statistically significant differences were found for the variables: gender, education, number of years after HIV diagnosis, and being on ART among older and younger PLWHAs (Table 1).

Table 1: Demographic characteristics of two subsamples.

	Older PLWHAs* number (%)	Younger PLWHAs* number (%)	P value
Gender			0.53
Female	8 (25.8)	37 (31.6)	
Male	23 (74.2)	80 (68.4)	
Education			0.06
No school or primary school	12 (38.7)	26 (22.2)	
Middle school or above	19 (61.3)	91 (77.8)	
Marital status			0.02
Unmarried	4 (12.9)	40 (34.2)	
Married	27 (87.1)	77 (65.8)	
Years after HIV diagnosis			0.19
<1	15 (48.4)	42 (35.9)	
1-2	12 (38.7)	42 (35.9)	
≥3	4 (12.9)	33 (28.2)	
Being on ART			0.48
Yes	15 (48.4)	65 (55.6)	
No	16 (51.6)	52 (44.4)	

*People living with HIV/AIDS.

3.2. Comparisons of Psychosocial and Mental Health between Older and Younger PLWHA. Using a cut-off score of 10 or more to classify participants as having depressive symptoms [24, 25], the prevalence of depressive symptom was 74.2% (23/31) among older PLWHAs and 48.7% (57/117) in younger PLWHAs (χ^2 = 6.40, P = 0.01). Compared to younger PLWHAs, older PLWHAs reported lower levels of well-being (7.6 versus 11.4) and higher levels of depression (18.6 versus 15.8). There were no significant differences in self-efficacy (23.9 versus 24.6) and HIV knowledge (9.3 versus 10.3) between older and younger PLWHAs, respectively.

Three out of four quality of life domains (physical health, psychological, and social relationships) were significantly lower among older PLWHAs when compared to younger PLWHAs (Table 2). Both groups, however, scored nearly the same in environmental quality of life (9.8 versus 10.2; P = 0.32) (Table 2). Among older PLWHAs, depression was negatively associated with well-being and quality of life in two domains: physical and psychological health. Subjective well-being was positively related to quality of life in all four domains. Perceived general self-efficacy was not statistically

TABLE 2: Distributions of HIV knowledge, self-efficacy, well-being, depression and quality of life.

	Crude mean (SD)			Adjusted mean[2]		
	Older PLWHAs	Younger PLWHAs	*P* value	Older PLWHAs	Younger PLWHAs	*P* value
HIV knowledge[1]	8.5 (3.9)	10.1 (2.3)	0.20	9.3	10.3	0.07
Self-efficacy[1]	24.6 (3.4)	25.3 (3.4)	0.34	23.9	24.6	0.31
Depression	13.6 (5.6)	10.8 (6.5)	0.03	18.6	15.8	0.03
Well-being	7.8 (5.6)	11.7 (6.3)	<0.01	7.6	11.4	<0.01
Quality of life:						
Physical health	10.4 (2.8)	12.2 (2.9)	<0.01	10.3	11.9	<0.01
Psychological[1]	10.1 (2.4)	11.4 (2.8)	0.02	9.5	10.9	0.01
Social relationships	12.0 (2.5)	13.0 (2.6)	0.05	11.8	12.9	0.05
Environment[1]	10.5 (2.7)	10.8 (2.4)	0.41	9.8	10.2	0.32

[1]Logarithmic transformation was applied.
[2]Adjusted for gender, education, and marital status, being on ART, and years after HIV diagnosis.

TABLE 3: Correlations of self-efficacy, depression, well-being, and quality of life among older PLWHAs.

	Depression	Well-being	Physical	Psychological	Social	Environment
Self-efficacy	0.18	−0.28	−0.13	0.16	0.26	0.23
Depression		−0.55**	−0.59**	−0.63**	−0.05	−0.13
Well-being			0.76**	0.68**	0.36*	0.37*
Quality of life:						
Physical health				0.77**	0.35*	0.39*
Psychological					0.42**	0.53**
Social relationships						0.43*
Environment						1.00

*$P \leq 0.05$.
**$P \leq 0.01$.

associated with depression, well-being, and quality of life (Table 3).

4. Discussion

Although the demographic profile of the HIV epidemic in China is rapidly aging, this is the first study, to our knowledge, to examine psychological and mental health status among older PLWHAs. Our findings show that when compared to younger PLWHAs, older PLWHAs exhibited significantly greater symptoms of depression, poorer well-being, and poorer quality of life in three domains: physical health, psychological health, and social relationships. We also found that a higher level of depression among older PLWHAs was associated with much lower levels of subjective well-being and quality of life (physical health and psychological domain).

Overall participants in our study were found to experience symptoms of clinical depression irrespective of age. This finding is consistent with reports from USA showing depression rates for HIV-positive adults to be twice that of the general population [26]. Older PLWHAs, however, reported greater levels of depression than younger counterparts. As a psychosocial burden, depression likely adds formidable challenges for older PLWHAs to cope with HIV and seek social support. Given these obstacles, it is not surprising that PLWHAs exhibited depressive symptoms in our sample. Moreover, the level of depression reported in this study was much greater among older adults than typically found in research in China on depression unrelated to HIV. For example, in a study of depression among the general Chinese elderly population [25], the mean level of depression measured by the same CES-D scale was between 7.3 and 8.3 and the depression prevalence was between 17 and 22%, compared with the mean level of 10.8–13.6 and prevalence of 48.7–74.2% in our sample. Similarly, the quality of life experienced by PLWHAs in this study also was lower than Chinese general population studies tend to report. For example in a study of Chinese adults, Skevington et al. reported mean scores of 15.8 in physical health, 14.3 in psychological health, 13.7 in social relationships, and 13.2 in the environmental domain [16].

Our data also show that older PLWHAs in this study had poorer quality of life than adult PLWHAs reported in other studies. Shan et al. reported that the physical, psychological, social, and environmental domain scores were 12.9, 12.4, 14.0, and 12.5, respectively, among adult PLWHAs aged between 29 and 60 years old [27]. In addition to the age effects of having a somewhat younger sample, this difference could be due to different stages of disease progression, effects of antiretroviral treatment, or other psychosocial factors. Although AIDS-defining illnesses can be reduced from ART, the likelihood of developing HIV-associated non-AIDS conditions such as cardiovascular disease, lung disease, and cancers can increase with age. The interaction of advancing age, chronic diseases conditions, and psychological problems will continue to affect older PLWHAs' aging process, quality of life, and well-being if no effective intervention exists in this vulnerable population.

In contrast to our expectation, the level of general self-efficacy among older and younger PLWHAs is comparable to the level reported from other studies among Chinese general populations. In a study of 1,003 participants in Hong Kong [28], the mean self-efficacy score was 25.3 among participants aged less than 40 years old, 25.9 among those aged 40–59, and 25.8 among those who were 60 years old and older. In another study, the mean score was 25.5 among Chinese college students [29]. Individuals with adequate self-efficacy are more likely to build resilience to life adversity such as those encountered living with HIV [29].

Despite experiences of significant adversity, individuals with strong resilience may have positive adaptation or coping skills [30]. Resilience as an adaptive process is posited to be important to successful aging [31–33]. The relationships among self-efficacy, resilience, and successful aging are seen as a dynamic process and not a static trait; therefore, it is important to examine the processes by which burdensome and adverse situations may lead to positive adaptations [34]. While resilience has been found to influence quality of life and successful health management among HIV-positive older adults in USA [35], few, if any, empirical studies have longitudinally investigated the dynamic development of resilience and its impact on aging with HIV in China or Asia in general.

Several limitations to this study should be noted. First, due to the nature of a preliminary study with a small sample size, we could not fully investigate and address potential psychosocial factors contributing to depression and quality of life through more complex and in-depth data analysis. Large-scale studies are needed to examine the interaction effects of aging in tandem with psychological and mental health factors among older PLWHAs. Second, the single study site with an intentionally chosen convenience sample may limit the generalizability of our findings. Third, the study relied on self-reported data and consequently may be subject to both recall and social desirability bias. Also, previous studies have found gender differences in reported quality of life in older adults. Due to the small sample size, we could not investigate these differences.

Despite these limitations, our study provides preliminary information regarding the extent to which older PLWHAs in China confront psychological challenges. The findings demonstrate that older PLWHAs reported lower well-being and experienced greater depressive symptoms and poorer quality of life when compared to younger PLWHAs. When coupled with the normal processes of aging and AIDS-associated conditions, the psychosocial and mental health challenges faced by older PLWHAs may go well beyond those of their younger HIV-infected counterparts. Because it was a preliminary study, factors determining the impaired psychological and physical functions and their consequences were not fully investigated. Further research with a larger sample of older PLWHAs is needed to confirm our findings and to understand how aging can accelerate disease progression and affect the psychosocial and mental well-being of older adults living with HIV.

Conflict of Interests

The authors declare that there is no conflict of interests regarding the publication of this paper.

Acknowledgments

The authors are grateful to the staff from Nanning Center for Disease and Control for participation in the study and to all the participants who gave so willingly their time to provide the study data. This study was conducted when Dr. Hongjie Liu worked at Virginia Commonwealth University School of Medicine. This work was partially supported by a research Grant (R01 HD068305-01) from the NIH-NICHD and a research Grant from the Virginia Commonwealth University School of Medicine. The Chicago Developmental Center for AIDS Research provided additional assistance (P30 AI 082151).

References

[1] China Ministry of Health, *China AIDS Response Progress Report*, China Ministry of Health, Beijing, China, 2012, http://www.unaids.org/en/dataanalysis/knowyourresponse/countryprogressreports/2012countries/ce_CN_Narrative_Report[1].pdf.

[2] H. Liu, X. Lin, Y. Xu, S. Chen, J. Shi, and D. Morisky, "Emerging HIV epidemic among older adults in Nanning, China," *AIDS Patient Care and STDs*, vol. 26, no. 10, pp. 565–567, 2012.

[3] R. B. Effros, C. V. Fletcher, K. Gebo et al., "Workshop on HIV infection and aging: what is known and future research directions," *Clinical Infectious Diseases*, vol. 47, no. 4, pp. 542–553, 2008.

[4] E. Bendavid, N. Ford, and E. J. Mills, "HIV and Africa's elderly: the problems and possibilities," *AIDS*, vol. 26, no. 1, pp. S85–S91, 2012.

[5] J. Jansson and D. P. Wilson, "Projected demographic profile of people living with hiv in australia: planning for an older generation," *PLoS ONE*, vol. 7, no. 8, Article ID e38334, 2012.

[6] S. Cahill and R. Valadéz, "Growing older with HIV/AIDS: new public health challenges," *American Journal of Public Health*, vol. 103, no. 3, pp. e7–e15, 2013.

[7] K. P. High, M. Brennan-Ing, D. B. Clifford et al., "HIV and aging: state of knowledge and areas of critical need for research. A report to the NIH office of AIDS research by the HIV and aging working group," *Journal of Acquired Immune Deficiency Syndromes*, vol. 60, supplement 1, pp. S1–S18, 2012.

[8] J. Negin, A. Martiniuk, R. G. Cumming et al., "Prevalence of HIV and chronic comorbidities among older adults," *AIDS*, vol. 26, supplement 1, no. 1, pp. S55–S63, 2012.

[9] J. A. Levy, D. Holmes, and M. Smith, "Conceptual and methodological issues in research on age and aging," *Journal of Acquired Immune Deficiency Syndromes*, vol. 33, supplement 2, pp. S206–S217, 2003.

[10] J. J. Schensul, J. A. Levy, and W. B. Disch, "Individual, contextual, and social network factors affecting exposure to HIV/AIDS

risk among older residents living in low-income senior housing complexes," *Journal of Acquired Immune Deficiency Syndromes*, vol. 33, supplement 2, pp. S138–S152, 2003.

[11] J. E. Nichols, D. C. Speer, B. J. Watson, T. L. Vergon, C. M. Vallee, and J. M. Meah, *Aging with HIV: psycological, social, and health issues*, Academic Press, San Diego, Calif, USA, 2002.

[12] A. Sankar, A. Nevedal, S. Neufeld, R. Berry, and M. Luborsky, "What do we know about older adults and HIV? a review of social and behavioral literature," *AIDS Care*, vol. 23, no. 10, pp. 1187–1207, 2011.

[13] Y. J. Zhang, Y. G. Fan, S. Y. Dai et al., "HIV/AIDS stigma among older PLWHA in south rural China," *International Journal of Nursing Practice*, 2014.

[14] X. Li, H. Wang, A. Williams, and G. He, "Stigma reported by people living with HIV in South Central China," *Journal of the Association of Nurses in AIDS Care*, vol. 20, no. 1, pp. 22–30, 2009.

[15] H. Liu, Y. Xu, X. Lin, J. Shi, and S. Chen, "Associations between perceived HIV stigma and quality of life at the dyadic lvel: the actor-partner interdependence model," *PLoS ONE*, vol. 8, no. 2, Article ID e55680, 2013.

[16] S. M. Skevington, M. Lotfy, and K. A. O'Connell, "The World Health Organization's WHOQOL-BREF quality of life assessment: psychometric properties and results of the international field trial a Report from the WHOQOL Group," *Quality of Life Research*, vol. 13, no. 2, pp. 299–310, 2004.

[17] WHOQOL Group, *The World Health Organization Quality of Life (WHOQOL)-BREF*, WHO, Geneva, Switzerland, 2004 (Chinese).

[18] J. X. Zhang and R. Schwarzer, "Measuring optimistic self-beliefs: a Chinese adaptation of the general self-efficacy scale," *Psychologia*, vol. 38, no. 3, pp. 174–181, 1995.

[19] P. Bech, L. R. Olsen, M. Kjoller, and N. K. Rasmussen, "Measuring well-being rather than the absence of distress symptoms: a comparison of the SF-36 mental health subscale and the WHO-five well-being scale," *International Journal of Methods in Psychiatric Research*, vol. 12, no. 2, pp. 85–91, 2003.

[20] F. J. Kohout, L. F. Berkman, D. A. Evans, and J. Cornoni-Huntley, "Two shorter forms of the CES-D depression symptoms index," *Journal of Aging and Health*, vol. 5, no. 2, pp. 179–193, 1993.

[21] H. Chen and A. C. Mui, "Factorial validity of the Center for Epidemiologic Studies Depression Scale short form in older population in China," *International Psychogeriatrics*, vol. 26, no. 1, pp. 49–57, 2014.

[22] E. Volinn, B. Yang, J. He et al., "West china hospital set of measures in Chinese to evaluate back pain treatment," *Pain Medicine*, vol. 11, no. 5, pp. 637–647, 2010.

[23] Z. Wu, Y. Wang, R. Detels, and M. J. Rotheram-Borus, "China AIDS policy implementation: reversing the HIV/AIDS epidemic by 2015," *International Journal of Epidemiology*, vol. 39, supplement 2, pp. iil–ii3, 2010.

[24] E. M. Andresen, J. A. Malmgren, W. B. Carter, and D. L. Patrick, "Screening for depression in well older adults: evaluation of a short form of the CES-D (Center for Epidemiologic Studies Depression Scale)," *The American Journal of Preventive Medicine*, vol. 10, no. 2, pp. 77–84, 1994.

[25] K. W. Boey, "Cross-validation of a short form of the CES-D in Chinese elderly," *International Journal of Geriatric Psychiatry*, vol. 14, no. 8, pp. 608–617, 1999.

[26] B. D. Kennard, L. T. Brown, L. Hawkins et al., "Development and implementation of health and wellness CBT for individuals with depression and HIV," *Cognitive and Behavioral Practice*, vol. 21, no. 2, pp. 237–246, 2013.

[27] D. Shan, Z. Ge, S. Ming et al., "Quality of life and related factors among HIV-positive spouses from serodiscordant couples under antiretroviral therapy in Henan Province, China," *PLoS ONE*, vol. 6, no. 6, Article ID e21839, 2011.

[28] D. S. Leung and B. C. P. Liu, "Lifelong education, quality of life and self-efficacy of Chinese older adults," *Educational Gerontology*, vol. 37, no. 11, pp. 967–981, 2011.

[29] M. Li, R. Eschenauer, and Y. Yang, "Influence of efficacy and resilience on problem solving in the United States, Taiwan, and China," *Journal of Multicultural Counseling and Development*, vol. 41, no. 3, pp. 144–157, 2013.

[30] S. S. Luthar and D. Cicchetti, "The construct of resilience: implications for interventions and social policies," *Development and Psychopathology*, vol. 12, no. 4, pp. 857–885, 2000.

[31] A. J. Lamond, C. A. Depp, M. Allison et al., "Measurement and predictors of resilience among community-dwelling older women," *Journal of Psychiatric Research*, vol. 43, no. 2, pp. 148–154, 2008.

[32] D. V. Jeste, G. N. Savla, W. K. Thompson et al., "Association between older age and more successful aging: critical role of resilience and depression," *The American Journal of Psychiatry*, vol. 170, no. 2, pp. 188–196, 2013.

[33] P. B. Baltes, "On the incomplete architecture of human ontogeny: selection, optimization, and compensation as foundation of developmental theory," *The American Psychologist*, vol. 52, no. 4, pp. 366–380, 1997.

[34] R. S. Allen, P. P. Haley, G. M. Harris, S. N. Fowler, and R. Pruthi, "Resilience: definitions, ambiguities, and applications," in *Resilience in Aging: Concepts, Research, and Outcomes*, B. Resnick, L. P. Gwyther, and K. A. Roberto, Eds., pp. 1–13, Springer, New York, NY, USA, 2011.

[35] C. A. Emlet, S. Tozay, and V. H. Raveis, ""I'm not going to die from the AIDS": resilience in aging with HIV disease," *Gerontologist*, vol. 51, no. 1, pp. 101–111, 2011.

6

Sedentary Behavior and Physical Activity Are Independent Predictors of Successful Aging in Middle-Aged and Older Adults

Shilpa Dogra[1] and Liza Stathokostas[2]

[1] *School of Recreation Management and Kinesiology, Acadia University, Wolfville, NS, Canada B4P 2R6*
[2] *Centre for Activity and Aging, University of Western Ontario, London, ON, Canada N6G 2M3*

Correspondence should be addressed to Shilpa Dogra, shilpa.dogra@acadiau.ca

Academic Editor: Roger A. Fielding

Background. Sedentary behavior is emerging as an important risk factor for poor health. Physical activity has proven to be important in determining overall successful aging (SA) among older adults; however, no data exists on the influence of sedentary behavior on SA. The purpose of this analysis was to determine whether there is an association between sedentary behavior and successful aging, independent of physical activity levels. *Methods.* 9,478 older (M = 4,245; F = 5,233) and 10,060 middle-aged (M = 4.621; F = 5,439) adults from the Healthy Aging cycle of the Canadian Community Health Survey were analyzed. Multivariate logistic regressions were conducted with SA and its three components as outcomes while physical activity and sedentary behavior were entered as main exposures. *Results.* Among older adults, compared to those who were sedentary (4 hours or more/day), those who were moderately (2–4 hours/day) and least sedentary (<2 hours/day) were 38% (OR: 1.38; CI: 1.12–1.69) and 43% (OR: 1.43; CI: 1.23–1.67) more likely to age successfully, respectively. Among middle-aged adults, those who were least sedentary were 43% (OR: 1.43; CI: 1.25–1.63) more likely to age successfully. *Conclusions.* These novel findings suggest that sedentary activities are significantly associated with lower odds of SA among middle-aged and older adults, potentially in a dose-dependent manner.

1. Introduction

Recent research suggests that despite meeting the minimum physical activity recommendations, sitting for prolonged periods (i.e., sedentary behavior) can compromise the health of adults [1]. Literature has established that a physically inactive lifestyle and low levels of cardiorespiratory fitness lead to an increase in the risk of developing numerous chronic diseases as well as all-cause mortality [2]. Interestingly, sedentary behavior is emerging as a potentially important independent contributor to the relationship between lifestyle and health [3, 4].

Sedentary behavior is defined as any waking behavior characterized by an energy expenditure ≤1.5 METs and a sitting or reclining posture [5]. Accumulating evidence shows that, independent of physical activity levels, sedentary time is associated with an increased risk of cardiometabolic disease and all-cause mortality in children and adults [6–8]. Similar evidence is emerging for the older adult population. Katzmarzyk et al. [8] reported that all-cause death rates increased across daily sitting time categories in a dose-response manner in groups of adults under the age of 59 years and over 60 years. It has also been demonstrated that individuals greater than 60 years of age with metabolic syndrome spend a greater percentage of waking hours in sedentary time versus those with no metabolic disease [3]. Unfortunately, according to the 2007 Canadian Community Health Survey (CCHS), television viewing time increases steadily with age such that 36% of those aged from 55 to 64, 47% of adults from 65 to 74 years and 52% of adults 75 years and older spend 15 or more hours per week viewing television [6].

Beyond the influence on health, sedentary behavior may also influence overall successful aging (SA); a term used to represent the physical, psychological, and social success with which adults age. The relationship between physical activity and SA is already well established [9]. Unfortunately, there is limited data on the relationship between sedentary behavior and SA or the components of SA. There is also a dearth of data available on SA and physical activity in middle-aged adults. This information is critical as lifestyle behaviors have been shown to persist once they are developed [10–13]. For example, using a modified Rowe and Kahn [14] definition of SA, Sun et al. [15] showed that participants of the Nurse's Health Study surviving to age 70 who had higher levels of midlife physical activity had higher odds of "successful survival." Similarly, in a 17-year longitudinal study, Britton et al. [11] found early-life exercise (mean age 44 years) to be a predictor of SA (free from major disease, good physical and mental function). No data exists on the relationship between overall SA and sedentary behavior in middle-aged adults.

Recent reports indicate that 69% of waking hours of middle-aged and older adults are spent performing sedentary activities [16]. Given the strong relationship between physical activity and SA, an investigation between sedentary behavior and SA is warranted in this population. Clearly, if sedentary behavior is related to SA, middle-aged and older adult populations are at high risk of poor physical, psychological, and social health. The purpose of the present study therefore was to determine whether there is an association between sedentary behavior and SA, independent of physical activity, in a Canadian population of middle-aged and older adults.

2. Methods

2.1. Sample. The Healthy Aging cycle of the Canadian Community Health Survey (CCHS-HA) was used for the current analysis. The objective of the CCHS-HA is to provide information on SA, examine healthy aging from a multidisciplinary approach, examine the effects of lifestyle on age, and better understand the aging process in those aged 45 years and older. All data contained in this survey were self-reported and all participants provided informed consent prior to participation. The total sample size of the CCHS-HA is 30,865. For purposes of the current analysis the sample was restricted to those who had complete data for all variables of interest as outlined below ($n = 19{,}538$). Detailed information on data collection methods and data weighting can be found in the CCHS user guide [17].

2.2. Main Outcome. SA variables were created for all three components of SA, that is, physical, psychological, and sociological. Young et al. [18] recently outlined the required variables to assess each of the components of SA based on Rowe and Kahn's model of SA [14]. Each SA component for the current analysis was based on this outline within the limitations of the database.

2.2.1. Physical Component of SA. The physical component of SA generally includes both the presence of chronic disease and functional impairments; however, Strawbridge et al. [19] showed that SA is not dependent on the presence or absence of disease and that many older adults were being misclassified based on this variable. Recent evidence using data in the CCHS indicates that self-perceived health is a better indicator of physical activity levels than the presence of chronic disease [20]. As such, the current analysis limited the definition of physical SA to those with functional impairment only. Participants were classified as having no mobility problems, having a problem but not requiring any aids, requiring mechanical support, or requiring help from others or cannot walk as per their responses to five separate questions in the CCHS-HA. Those in the first two groups were categorized as aging successfully and those in the latter two groups were categorized as aging poorly.

2.2.2. Psychological Component of SA. As per Young et al. [18] the psychological component should include data on cognitive function, emotional vitality, and depression. The CCHS-HA collected data on all three of these variables. Using two questions participants were classified into one of six categories for cognitive function: (1) able to remember most things, think clearly, and solve day-to-day problems, (2) able to remember most things but have a little difficulty when trying to think and solve day-to-day problems, (3) somewhat forgetful but able to think clearly and solve day-to-day problems, (4) somewhat forgetful and have a little difficulty when trying to think or solve day-to-day problems, (5) very forgetful and have great difficulty when trying to think or solve day-to-day problems, or (6) unable to remember anything at all and unable to think or solve day-to-day problems. Emotional vitality was based on a single question which classified participants as either (1) happy and interested in life, (2) somewhat happy, (3) somewhat unhappy, (4) very unhappy, or (5) so unhappy that life is not worthwhile. Finally, depression was assessed using a single question on the presence or absence of depression. Those in the first three categories of cognitive function and the first 2 categories of emotional vitality who did not have depression were classified as aging successfully in the psychological domain; all other were classified as aging poorly.

2.2.3. Sociological Component of SA. Engagement with life, social support, and spirituality are the main variables used to assess the sociological component of SA. Unfortunately there were no data pertaining to spirituality in the CCHS-HA. Two variables were used to classify participants as aging successfully and aging poorly, sense of belonging to the local community and the loneliness scale. Sense of belonging was a single question that classified participants as very strong, somewhat strong, somewhat weak, or very weak. The loneliness scale was based on three items: lack of companionship, feeling left out, and feeling isolated. Participants responded with either hardly ever, sometimes, or often. These scores were summed to create the loneliness scale. Those who had a strong sense of belonging and a loneliness scale score of ≤ 6 were classified as aging successfully, all other were classified as aging poorly.

2.2.4. Overall SA. Those who were classified as aging successfully in the physical, psychological, and sociological domains were classified as aging successfully. All other were classified as aging poorly.

2.3. Main Exposures

2.3.1. Physical Activity. Unlike the other CCHS cycles, the CCHS-HA does not contain data on energy expenditure. The PA variable for the current analysis was therefore based on the number of hours the participant walked each week. Participants who spent 1 hour or more/day walking were classified as active, those who spent 30–60 minutes/day walking were classified as moderately active and those who spent <30 minutes/day walking were classified as inactive.

2.3.2. Sedentary Behavior. The number of hours spent sitting per day were used to classify participants as sedentary (4 hours or more/day), moderately sedentary (2–4 hours/day), or least sedentary (<2 hours/day).

2.4. Covariates. Middle-aged adults were those between the ages of 45 and 64 years, and older adults were those between the ages of 65 years and more. The CCHS-HA public access file does not contain age as a continuous variable for maintenance of confidentiality; therefore these data are presented in categories. Participants were classified as male or female based on self-reported biological sex. Marital status was categorized as either married/common-law, widowed/separated/divorced, or single/never married. Income was used as a proxy for socioeconomic status and was categorized as <20,000, $20–39,000, $40–59,000, $60–79,000, or >$80,000. These covariates were chosen based on previous literature [8, 19]. Marital status was additionally included as it is related to SA in older adults [20].

2.5. Statistical Analysis. Pearson chi-square analyses and standardized adjusted residuals that denote deviations from a normal distribution were [21] calculated to determine differences in all sample characteristics with the exception of age. Bivariate associations between each SA outcome and physical activity or sedentary behavior were conducted using logistic regression analysis for each sex and age group. Multivariate logistic regressions controlling for age, marital status, and income were conducted for each SA outcome with both physical activity and sedentary behavior entered in the model. These models were created for each sex and age group (middle-aged and older adults). All analyses were conducted using SPSS version 17.0 with statistical significance set at alpha < 0.05. In order to compensate for the deliberate over-sampling of particular groups, population weights supplied by Statistics Canada were applied to the entire dataset to ensure accurate population estimates. To estimate variance, the sample population weights were rescaled, standardized, and reapplied to the dataset.

3. Results

Sample characteristics are described in Table 1. Overall there were significant differences between older and middle-aged adults for all covariates investigated. Interestingly there were no differences between overall SA between age groups, nor were there for the psychological component of SA for either of both sexes combined or for females.

Bivariate associations (Table 2) indicated a consistent trend for both physical activity and sedentary behavior such that those who were active and moderately active were significantly more likely to be aging successfully compared to those who were inactive. Similarly, those who were moderately sedentary and least sedentary were significantly more likely to be aging successfully compared to those who were sedentary. This trend was true for both sexes combined and for males and females separately. Additionally, in most cases there was a dose-response relationship such that those who were active or least sedentary had greater odds of SA than those who were moderately active or moderately sedentary, respectively.

Regressions adjusted for age, income, and marital status showed similar trends as bivariate regression (Table 3). Compared to inactive older adults, moderately active and active older adults were 41% (OR: 1.41; CI: 1.19–1.67) and 42% (OR: 1.42; CI: 1.20–1.69) more likely to be aging successfully overall, respectively. Similarly, compared to sedentary older adults, moderately sedentary and least sedentary older adults were 38% (OR: 1.38; CI: 1.12–1.69) and 43% (OR: 1.43; CI: 1.23–1.67) more likely to be aging successfully overall, respectively. This was similar to the results seen in middle-aged adults except that moderately sedentary adults were not more likely to be aging successfully overall compared to sedentary adults (OR: 1.08; CI: 0.96–1.21).

4. Discussion

Using a sample of middle-aged and older adults from the CCHS-HA, we analyzed the relationship of SA with physical activity and sedentary behavior. Similar to previous research, we found that physical activity is strongly related to SA and each of its components. The novel findings of this study pertain to the association between sedentary behavior and SA. Our primary finding is that sedentary behavior is associated with SA such that those who spend less time in sedentary activities are more likely to age successfully, regardless of their physical activity levels. Our secondary finding is that the relationship between the physical component of SA with physical activity and sedentary behavior was stronger and occurred in a dose-response manner. Finally, for the psychological and sociological components of SA, it seems that sedentary behavior lasting <2 hours/day is required for SA. The present study is one of the first to highlight the adverse role of sedentary behavior in SA. These findings have implications for the development of sedentary guidelines for middle-aged and older adults.

Our finding that there is a strong association between physical activity and SA was as expected based on research pertaining to physical activity and SA. A direct association between SA and physical activity was noted by Baker et al. [9] using data from the CCHS (cycle 2.1, $n = 12{,}042$). They reported that only 11% of Canadians were aging successfully and that older adults who were physically active were 2.26 (estimate = 0.817, CI: 0.703–0.931) times more likely to

Table 1: Characteristics of the sample by age group and sex.

			Older adults			Middle-aged adults		
			Both sexes	Males	Females	Both sexes	Males	Females
n (unweighted sample size)			9,478	4,245	5,233	10,060	4,621	5,439
Age	65–69 y	45–49 y	26.9	30.1	24.5	26.6	25.1	28.0
	70–74 y	50–54 y	19.8	21.2	18.6	30.8	34.3	27.5
	75–79 y	55–59 y	17.2	16.9	17.4	22.2	20.9	23.4
	80–84 y	60–64 y	12.8	9.9	15.0	20.4	19.6	21.0
	>80 y		23.3	21.8	24.4			
Income	>$20,000		24.1	13.7	32.2	8.3*	7.1*	9.5*
	$20,000–39,000		37.8	37.9	37.7	13.4*	11.3*	15.4*
	$40,000–59,000		18.3	21.3	15.9	17.2	15.5*	18.9*
	$60,000–79,000		8.9	11.1	7.2	18.6*	18.6*	18.7*
	>$80,000		10.9	16.0	7.0	42.4*	47.5*	37.5*
Marital status	Married/common law		48.7	67.0	34.4	74.9*	78.3*	71.8*
	Widowed		38.0	19.7	52.3	3.5*	1.5*	5.3*
	Separated/divorced		8.4	8.0	8.7	12.7*	10.6*	14.6*
	Single/never married		4.9	5.2	4.6	8.9*	9.6*	8.3*
Physical activity levels	Active		33.3	36.4	30.9	39.3*	42.7*	36.2*
	Moderately active		35.3	35.6	35.2	37.9*	35.7	40.1*
	Inactive		31.3	28.0	33.9	22.7*	21.6*	23.8*
Sedentary behaviour	Least sedentary		14.9	15.7	14.3	25.2*	25.6*	24.9*
	Moderately sedentary		33.8	34.4	33.3	34.0	33.2	34.7
	Sedentary		51.3	49.9	52.4	40.8*	41.2*	40.4*
Overall SA			56.8	58.0	55.8	56.9	58.1	55.6
Physical SA			87.6	90.4	85.5	98.4*	98.8*	98.1*
Psychological SA			85.3	84.9	85.7	86.6	89.2*	84.1
Sociological SA			70.5	70.8	70.2	63.2*	63.3*	63.2*

* significant differences between older and middle-aged adults within sex category.
n: sample size; SA: successful aging.
All data are weighted unless otherwise stated.
All data are a percent of the sample.

age successfully compared to those who were physically inactive. In a follow-up study, Meisner et al. [21] showed that physical activity influences each component of SA, such that greater levels of physical inactivity were associated with an increased likelihood of reporting disease and disablement, low functional capacities, and being socially disengaged with life. While the results of these two studies imply that sedentary behavior would be associated with SA, no specific analyses to this effect were conducted. A study published by Ko et al. [22] showed that engaging in a greater number of activities (physical and nonphysical in nature) was significantly associated with several indicators of SA. Therefore this study shows that those who did not engage in activities (i.e., sedentary individuals) were less likely to age successfully. This is in direct line with the findings of our study.

Physical activity is an established determinant of SA [23]. Moreover, the master athlete has been suggested as a model of SA given that this group of middle-aged and older adults is healthier and has a better quality of life than age-matched peers [24]. It is not surprising then that the strongest association in our study was found between sedentary behavior and the physical component of SA, that is, functional limitations. Several studies have shown that functional dependence is more likely to develop in older adults who are not physically active, or who were not physically active in middle age. Patel et al. [25] found that sedentary behavior in middle age had a significant impact on functional autonomy in older age using a population-based study. Similarly, Huang et al. [26] showed that middle-aged adults who were physically active and fit were less likely to have functional impairments in older age. These studies support our findings that middle-aged and older adults who were physically active and not sedentary were most likely to be aging successfully in the physical domain, that is, to maintain functional autonomy.

In addition to a strong association between the physical component of SA and sedentary behavior, we also noted a dose-response relationship, that is, less time spent in sedentary activities was associated with higher odds of SA. In a recent review conducted on physical activity and functional limitations, a similar dose-response relationship was displayed such that those with higher levels of physical activity were less likely to develop functional limitations as compared to a sedentary group [27]. Spirduso and Cronin

TABLE 2: Bivariate associations of successful aging with physical activity and sedentary behaviour.

		Older adults						Middle-aged adults					
Overall SA		Both sexes		Males		Females		Both sexes		Males		Females	
		OR	CI	OR	CI	OR	CI	OR	CI	OR	CI	OR	CI
Physical activity	Inactive	1.00	Ref.	1.00	Ref.	1.00	Ref.	1.00	Ref.	1.00	Ref.	1.00	Ref.
	Moderately active	1.60	1.36–1.89	1.34	1.08–1.57	1.39	1.16–1.67	1.37	1.20–1.56	1.34	1.08–1.57	1.39	1.16–1.67
	Active	1.69	1.43–1.99	1.30	1.08–1.57	1.58	1.31–1.90	1.44	1.27–1.65	1.30	1.08–1.57	1.58	1.31–1.90
Sedentary behaviour	Sedentary	1.00	Ref.	1.00	Ref.	1.00	Ref.	1.00	Ref.	1.00	Ref.	1.00	Ref.
	Moderately sedentary	1.58	1.36–1.84	0.91	0.77–1.07	1.31	1.11–1.54	1.09	0.97–1.23	0.91	0.77–1.07	1.31	1.11–1.54
	Least sedentary	1.60	1.31–1.95	1.22	1.02–1.46	1.63	1.36–1.94	1.41	1.24–1.61	1.22	1.02–1.46	1.63	1.36–1.94
		Older adults						Middle-aged adults					
Physical SA		Both sexes		Males		Females		Both sexes		Males		Females	
		OR	CI	OR	CI	OR	CI	OR	CI	OR	CI	OR	CI
Physical activity	Inactive	1.00	Ref.	1.00	Ref.	1.00	Ref.	1.00	Ref.	1.00	Ref.	1.00	Ref.
	Moderately active	2.64	1.66–4.17	3.22	1.51–6.84	2.34	1.30–4.19	2.64	1.66–4.17	3.22	1.51–6.84	2.34	1.30–4.19
	Active	4.03	2.4–6.78	5.81	2.44–13.86	3.07	1.60–5.90	4.03	2.4–6.78	5.81	2.44–13.86	3.07	1.60–5.90
Sedentary behaviour	Sedentary	1.00	Ref.	1.00	Ref.	1.00	Ref.	1.00	Ref.	1.00	Ref.	1.00	Ref.
	Moderately sedentary	1.91	1.20–3.05	2.83	1.19–6.73	1.61	0.92–2.82	1.91	1.20–3.05	2.83	1.19–6.73	1.61	0.92–2.82
	Least sedentary	2.61	1.45–4.68	1.90	0.83–4.34	3.44	1.48–7.97	2.61	1.45–4.68	1.90	0.83–4.34	3.44	1.48–7.97
		Older adults						Middle-aged adults					
Psychological SA		Both sexes		Males		Females		Both sexes		Males		Females	
		OR	CI	OR	CI	OR	CI	OR	CI	OR	CI	OR	CI
Physical activity	Inactive	1.00	Ref.	1.00	Ref.	1.00	Ref.	1.00	Ref.	1.00	Ref.	1.00	Ref.
	Moderately active	1.47	1.23–1.75	1.30	0.98–1.72	1.59	1.27–200	1.47	1.23–1.75	1.30	0.98–1.72	1.59	1.27–200
	Active	2.18	1.81–2.63	2.13	1.58–2.86	2.13	1.66–2.72	2.18	1.81–2.63	2.13	1.58–2.86	2.13	1.66–2.72
Sedentary behaviour	Sedentary	1.00	Ref.	1.00	Ref.	1.00	Ref.	1.00	Ref.	1.00	Ref.	1.00	Ref.
	Moderately sedentary	1.08	0.92–1.27	0.90	0.69–1.97	1.24	1.00–1.53	1.08	0.92–1.27	0.90	0.69–1.97	1.24	1.00–1.53
	Least sedentary	1.53	1.26–1.86	1.44	1.06–1.97	1.59	1.24–2.05	1.53	1.26–1.86	1.44	1.06–1.97	1.59	1.24–2.05
		Older adults						Middle-aged adults					
Sociological SA		Both sexes		Males		Females		Both sexes		Males		Females	
		OR	CI	OR	CI	OR	CI	OR	CI	OR	CI	OR	CI
Physical activity	Inactive	1.00	Ref.	1.00	Ref.	1.00	Ref.	1.00	Ref.	1.00	Ref.	1.00	Ref.
	Moderately active	1.32	1.15–1.51	1.19	0.98–1.46	1.44	1.20–1.73	1.32	1.15–1.51	1.19	0.98–1.46	1.44	1.20–1.73
	Active	1.32	1.15–1.51	1.14	0.94–1.38	1.51	1.25–1.83	1.32	1.15–1.51	1.14	0.94–1.38	1.51	1.25–1.83
Sedentary behaviour	Sedentary	1.00	Ref.	1.00	Ref.	1.00	Ref.	1.00	Ref.	1.00	Ref.	1.00	Ref.
	Moderately sedentary	1.03	0.92–1.16	0.89	0.75–1.05	1.19	1.01–1.41	1.03	0.92–1.16	0.89	0.75–1.05	1.19	1.01–1.41
	Least sedentary	1.37	1.20–1.56	1.25	1.03–1.51	1.50	1.24–1.80	1.37	1.20–1.56	1.25	1.03–1.51	1.50	1.24–1.80

SA: successful aging; OR: odds ratio; CI: confidence interval.

TABLE 3: Adjusted regressions of successful aging with physical activity and sedentary behaviour.

Overall SA		Older adults						Middle-aged adults					
		Both sexes		Males		Females		Both sexes		Males		Females	
		OR	CI	OR	CI	OR	CI	OR	CI	OR	CI	OR	CI
Physical activity	Inactive	1.00	Ref.	1.00	Ref.	1.00	Ref.	1.00	Ref.	1.00	Ref.	1.00	Ref.
	Moderately active	1.41*	1.19–1.67	1.62*	1.24–2.10	1.27*	1.02–1.58	1.35*	1.18–1.54	1.36*	1.11–1.66	1.33*	1.10–1.59
	Active	1.42*	1.20–1.69	1.57*	1.21–2.05	1.33*	1.06–1.68	1.45*	1.27–1.66	1.35*	1.12–1.64	1.54*	1.28–1.86
Sedentary behaviour	Sedentary	1.00	Ref.	1.00	Ref.	1.00	Ref.	1.00	Ref.	1.00	Ref.	1.00	Ref.
	Moderately sedentary	1.38*	1.12–1.69	1.36*	1.08–1.72	1.49*	1.22–1.83	1.08	0.96–1.21	0.90	0.76–1.07	1.27*	1.08–1.50
	Least sedentary	1.43*	1.23–1.67	1.20	0.88–1.62	1.56*	1.18–2.07	1.43*	1.25–1.63	1.23*	1.01–1.48	1.65*	1.37–1.98
Physical SA		Older adults						Middle-aged adults					
		Both sexes		Males		Females		Both sexes		Males		Females	
		OR	CI	OR	CI	OR	CI	OR	CI	OR	CI	OR	CI
Physical activity	Inactive	1.00	Ref.	1.00	Ref.	1.00	Ref.	1.00	Ref.	1.00	Ref.	1.00	Ref.
	Moderately active	1.62*	1.26–1.08	1.65*	1.09–2.51	1.61*	1.18–2.21	2.46*	1.53–3.94	2.90*	1.34–6.30	2.24*	1.35–7.55
	Active	1.80*	1.37–2.37	1.96*	1.25–3.07	1.75*	1.24–2.48	3.87*	2.28–6.58	5.63*	2.33–13.63	3.18*	1.62–6.22
Sedentary behaviour	Sedentary	1.00	Ref.	1.00	Ref.	1.00	Ref.	1.00	Ref.	1.00	Ref.	1.00	Ref.
	Moderately sedentary	1.75*	1.37–2.24	1.85*	1.22–2.79	1.69*	1.24–2.31	1.68*	1.04–2.72	2.28	0.93–5.56	1.50	0.84–2.66
	Least sedentary	2.44*	1.64–3.65	2.48*	1.28–4.79	2.45*	1.47–4.07	2.15*	1.18–3.92	1.27*	0.54–3.02	3.20*	1.62–6.22
Psychological SA		Older adults						Middle-aged adults					
		Both sexes		Males		Females		Both sexes		Males		Females	
		OR	CI	OR	CI	OR	CI	OR	CI	OR	CI	OR	CI
Physical activity	Inactive	1.00	Ref.	1.00	Ref.	1.00	Ref.	1.00	Ref.	1.00	Ref.	1.00	Ref.
	Moderately active	1.53*	1.22–1.91	1.96*	1.40–2.76	1.26	0.93–1.70	1.40*	1.17–1.68	1.27	0.95–1.71	1.46*	1.15–1.85
	Active	1.74*	1.37–2.21	2.47*	1.73–3.54	1.33	0.96–1.83	2.16*	1.78–2.63	2.29*	1.69–3.12	2.03*	1.58–2.62
Sedentary behaviour	Sedentary	1.00	Ref.	1.00	Ref.	1.00	Ref.	1.00	Ref.	1.00	Ref.	1.00	Ref.
	Moderately sedentary	1.08	0.82–1.44	1.03	0.75–1.42	1.40*	1.05–1.88	1.02	0.86–1.21	0.82	0.62–1.07	1.15	0.92–1.44
	Least sedentary	1.21	0.98–1.50	0.89	0.59–1.35	1.28	0.86–1.91	1.51*	1.23–1.85	1.30*	0.94–1.80	1.60*	1.23–2.08
Sociological SA		Older adults						Middle-aged adults					
		Both sexes		Males		Females		Both sexes		Males		Females	
		OR	CI	OR	CI	OR	CI	OR	CI	OR	CI	OR	CI
Physical activity	Inactive	1.00	Ref.	1.00	Ref.	1.00	Ref.	1.00	Ref.	1.00	Ref.	1.00	Ref.
	Moderately active	1.19*	1.00–1.43	1.30	0.98–1.72	1.11	0.88–1.40	1.30*	1.14–1.49	1.21	0.99–1.48	1.39*	1.15–1.67
	Active	1.21*	1.01–1.46	1.23	0.93–1.63	1.21	0.94–1.55	1.33*	1.16–1.52	1.17	0.96–1.43	1.49*	1.23–1.80
Sedentary behaviour	Sedentary	1.00	Ref.	1.00	Ref.	1.00	Ref.	1.00	Ref.	1.00	Ref.	1.00	Ref.
	Moderately sedentary	1.32*	1.12–1.56	1.17	0.85–1.62	1.30*	1.04–1.61	1.03	0.91–1.16	0.90	0.76–1.08	1.17	0.99–1.38
	Least sedentary	1.25*	1.00–1.55	1.35*	1.05–1.74	1.32	0.98–1.78	1.39*	1.22–1.59	1.28*	1.05–1.55	1.52*	1.26–1.84

SA: successful aging; OR: odds ratio; CI: confidence interval.
Adjusted for age, marital status, and income.

[28] conducted a review on the effect of the exercise dose response on SA using functional autonomy as a main outcome. The authors found that long-term physical activity was closely related to delaying disability and independent living in older adults. They also found that evidence for a dose response or a "threshold" between physical activity and physical functioning exists. It is difficult to assess a true dose response in the current analysis given the categorical nature of the variables in the data set. Whether there is indeed a threshold or a dose-response relationship should be determined in the future in order to develop optimal sedentary guidelines.

The possibility of a threshold for sedentary behavior was also observed for the psychological and sociological components of SA. Among older adults, the psychological component was not influenced by sedentary behavior whereas the sociological component was only influenced by sedentary behavior lasting less than two hours. Among the middle-aged adults, only those who were sedentary for less than two hours per day were more likely to age successfully, that is, those engaging in sedentary activities for 2–4 hours per day were not more likely to age successfully in these domains than those sedentary for 4 hours or more per day. In other words, less than two hours of sedentary activity per day may serve as a minimum duration (threshold) that must be achieved in order to age successfully in these two domains. This idea of a dose-dependent relationship or a threshold has been assessed in studies using physical inactivity and the psychological component of SA. Pietrelli et al. [29] found a dose-dependent effect of exercise on cognitive function and anxiety in an animal study using aerobic exercise in middle-aged and older rats. In the area of depression, a recent randomized control trial among adults aged 18–70 with depression found that the group who was assigned a higher dose of exercise had greater benefit than a group assigned a lower dose of exercise; however, both had clinically meaningful improvements with exercise participation [30]. There are also cross-sectional studies on the relationship between sedentary behavior and depression or hopelessness that support our findings. de Wit et al. [31] found that those who had depression and anxiety disorders were more likely to engage in sedentary activities such as television watching and computer use in a sample of adults aged 18–65. Similarly, among a group of middle-aged men, a negative association between engaging in physical activity and developing hopelessness was found such that those who engaged in higher volumes of physical activity were less likely to develop feelings of hopelessness [32]. With regards to the sociological component of SA, factors such as satisfaction with life [33], sense of belonging to community [34], and loneliness [35] are associated with physical inactivity, but again, little data exist on sedentary behavior. Future research should assess the dose-response relationship between sedentary activity and each component of SA. Furthermore, a consensus on the definition of SA should be reached.

4.1. Limitations. The current analysis has two limitations that are noteworthy. First, the CCHS-HA uses self-reported data; as such it is difficult to truly know how much time participants were spending in sedentary activities or being physically active. Therefore some participants may have been misclassified. Social desirability would dictate that physical activity was overreported and sedentary behavior was underreported. Given the broad categories used in the current analysis, it is less likely that such misclassification occurred. Second, the CCHS is a cross-sectional data set, so reverse causality cannot be ruled out. In other words, it cannot be said with certainty that sedentary behavior is causing poor outcomes as it is possible that poor outcomes are leading to sedentary lifestyles.

In conclusion, using a large database of middle-aged and older adults we found that similar to previous research, physical activity is strongly associated with SA. The novel finding of the current study is that sedentary behavior is significantly associated with lower odds of SA independent of physical activity levels, that is, sedentary behavior and physical activity may be independent risk factors for poor health among aging populations. We also found evidence for a dose-dependent relationship between sedentary behavior and each of the components of SA. Results of the present analysis are novel and have implications for the development of sedentary guidelines for middle-aged and older adults.

References

[1] N. Owen, G. N. Healy, C. E. Matthews, and D. W. Dunstan, "Too much sitting: the population health science of sedentary behavior," *Exercise and Sport Sciences Reviews*, vol. 38, no. 3, pp. 105–113, 2010.

[2] S. N. Blair and W. L. Haskell, "Objectively measured physical activity and mortality in older adults," *Journal of the American Medical Association*, vol. 296, no. 2, pp. 216–218, 2006.

[3] A. Bankoski, T. B. Harris, J. J. McClain et al., "Sedentary activity associated with metabolic syndrome independent of physical activity," *Diabetes Care*, vol. 34, no. 2, pp. 497–503, 2011.

[4] S. Lord, S. F. M. Chastin, L. McInnes, L. Little, P. Briggs, and L. Rochester, "Exploring patterns of daily physical and sedentary behaviour in community-dwelling older adults," *Age and Ageing*, vol. 40, no. 2, pp. 205–210, 2011.

[5] *Sedentary Behavior Research Network*, Sedentary Behavior Research Network, 2012.

[6] M. Shields and M. S. Tremblay, "Screen time among Canadian adults: a profile," *Health Reports*, vol. 19, no. 2, pp. 31–43, 2008.

[7] E. S. Ford, H. W. Kohl, A. H. Mokdad, and U. A. Ajani, "Sedentary behavior, physical activity, and the metabolic syndrome among U.S. adults," *Obesity Research*, vol. 13, no. 3, pp. 608–614, 2005.

[8] P. T. Katzmarzyk, T. S. Church, C. L. Craig, and C. Bouchard, "Sitting time and mortality from all causes, cardiovascular disease, and cancer," *Medicine and Science in Sports and Exercise*, vol. 41, no. 5, pp. 998–1005, 2009.

[9] J. Baker, B. A. Meisner, A. J. Logan, A. M. Kungl, and P. Weir, "Physical activity and successful aging in canadian older adults," *Journal of Aging and Physical Activity*, vol. 17, no. 2, pp. 223–235, 2009.

[10] B. J. Willcox, Q. He, R. Chen et al., "Midlife risk factors and healthy survival in men," *Journal of the American Medical Association*, vol. 296, no. 19, pp. 2343–2350, 2006.

[11] A. Britton, M. Shipley, A. Singh-Manoux, and M. G. Marmot, "Successful aging: the contribution of early-life and midlife risk factors," *Journal of the American Geriatrics Society*, vol. 56, no. 6, pp. 1098–1105, 2008.

[12] K. G. Arbeev, S. V. Ukraintseva, I. Akushevich et al., "Age trajectories of physiological indices in relation to healthy life course," *Mechanisms of Ageing and Development*, vol. 132, no. 3, pp. 93–102, 2011.

[13] P. K. Myint, R. D. Smith, R. N. Luben et al., "Lifestyle behaviors and quality-adjusted life years in middle and older age," *Age and Ageing*, vol. 40, pp. 589–595, 2011.

[14] J. W. Rowe and R. L. Kahn, "Human aging: usual and successful," *Science*, vol. 237, no. 4811, pp. 143–149, 1987.

[15] Q. Sun, M. K. Townsend, O. I. Okereke, O. H. Franco, F. B. Hu, and F. Grodstein, "Physical activity at midlife in relation to successful survival in women at age 70 years or older," *Archives of Internal Medicine*, vol. 170, no. 2, pp. 194–201, 2010.

[16] R. C. Colley, D. Garriguet, I. Janssen, C. L. Craig, J. Clarke, and M. S. Tremblay, "Physical activity of Canadian children and youth: accelerometer results from the 2007 to 2009 Canadian Health Measures Survey.," *Health Reports*, vol. 22, no. 1, pp. 15–23, 2011.

[17] *Statistics Canada*, Canadian Community Health Survey Healthy Aging, 2011.

[18] Y. Young, K. D. Frick, and E. A. Phelan, "Can successful aging and chronic illness coexist in the same individual? A multidimensional concept of successful aging," *Journal of the American Medical Directors Association*, vol. 10, no. 2, pp. 87–92, 2009.

[19] W. J. Strawbridge, M. I. Wallhagen, and R. D. Cohen, "Successful aging and well-being: self-rated compared with Rowe and Kahn," *Gerontologist*, vol. 42, no. 6, pp. 727–733, 2002.

[20] S. Dogra, "Better self-perceived health is associated with lower odds of physical inactivity in older adults with chronic disease," *Journal of Aging and Physical Activity*, vol. 19, no. 4, pp. 322–335, 2011.

[21] B. A. Meisner, S. Dogra, A. J. Logan, J. Baker, and P. L. Weir, "Do or decline? Comparing the effects of physical inactivity on biopsychosocial components of successful aging," *Journal of Health Psychology*, vol. 15, no. 5, pp. 688–696, 2010.

[22] K. J. Ko, C. A. Berg, J. Butner, B. N. Uchino, and T. W. Smith, "Profiles of successful aging in middle-aged and older adult married couples," *Psychology and Aging*, vol. 22, no. 4, pp. 705–718, 2007.

[23] E. Palmore, "Predictors of successful aging," *Gerontologist*, vol. 19, no. 5, part 1, pp. 427–431, 1979.

[24] S. A. Hawkins, R. A. Wiswell, and T. J. Marcell, "Exercise and the master athlete- a model of successful aging?" *Journals of Gerontology A*, vol. 58, no. 11, pp. 1009–1011, 2003.

[25] K. V. Patel, A. K. Coppin, T. M. Manini et al., "Midlife physical activity and mobility in older age. The InCHIANTI Study," *American Journal of Preventive Medicine*, vol. 31, no. 3, pp. 217–224, 2006.

[26] Y. Huang, C. A. Macera, S. N. Blair, P. A. Brill, H. W. Kohl, and J. J. Kronenfeld, "Physical fitness, physical activity, and functional limitation in adults aged 40 and older," *Medicine and Science in Sports and Exercise*, vol. 30, no. 9, pp. 1430–1435, 1998.

[27] D. H. Paterson and D. E. R. Warburton, "Physical activity and functional limitations in older adults: a systematic review related to Canada's Physical Activity Guidelines," *International Journal of Behavioral Nutrition and Physical Activity*, vol. 11, no. 7, article 38, 2010.

[28] W. W. Spirduso and D. L. Cronin, "Exercise dose-response effects on quality of life and independent living in older adults," *Medicine and Science in Sports and Exercise*, vol. 33, no. 6, pp. S598–S608, 2001.

[29] A. Pietrelli, J. Lopez-Costa, R. Goni, A. Brusco, and N. Basso, "Aerobic exercise prevents age-dependent cogntive decline and reduces anxiety-related behaviors in middle-aged and old rats," *Neuroscience*, vol. 202, pp. 252–266, 2012.

[30] M. H. Trivedi, T. L. Greer, T. S. Church et al., "Exercise as an augmentation treatment for nonremitted major depressive disorder: a randomized, parallel dose comparison," *Journal of Clinical Psychiatry*, vol. 72, no. 5, pp. 677–684, 2011.

[31] L. de Wit, A. van Straten, F. Lamers, P. Cuijpers, and B. Penninx, "Are sedentary television watching and computer use behaviors associated with anxiety and depressive disorders?" *Psychiatry Research*, vol. 186, no. 2-3, pp. 239–243, 2011.

[32] M. Valtonen, D. E. Laaksonen, J. Laukkanen et al., "Sedentary lifestyle and emergence of hopelessness in middle-aged men," *European Journal of Cardiovascular Prevention and Rehabilitation*, vol. 17, no. 5, pp. 524–529, 2010.

[33] A. M. Ni Mhaolain, D. Gallagher, H. O'Connell et al., "Subjective well-being amongst community-dwelling elders: what determines satisfaction with life?" *International Psychogeriatrics*, vol. 24, no. 2, pp. 316–323, 2012.

[34] A. F. Young, A. Russell, and J. R. Powers, "The sense of belonging to a neighbourhood: can it be measured and is it related to health and well being in older women?" *Social Science and Medicine*, vol. 59, no. 12, pp. 2627–2637, 2004.

[35] L. C. Hawkley, R. A. Thisted, and J. T. Cacioppo, "Loneliness predicts reduced physical activity: cross-sectional & longitudinal analyses," *Health Psychology*, vol. 28, no. 3, pp. 354–363, 2009.

7

The Use of Session RPE to Monitor the Intensity of Weight Training in Older Women: Acute Responses to Eccentric, Concentric, and Dynamic Exercises

Sandro S. Ferreira,[1] Kleverton Krinski,[2] Ragami C. Alves,[1] Mariana L. Benites,[1] Paulo E. Redkva,[1] Hassan M. Elsangedy,[3] Cosme F. Buzzachera,[4] Tácito P. Souza-Junior,[1] and Sergio G. da Silva[1]

[1] *Department of Physical Education, Federal University of Parana, Caixa Postal 92, JD Botânico, 80215-370 Curitiba, PR, Brazil*
[2] *Federal University of Sao Francisco Valley, 56304205 Petrolina, PE, Brazil*
[3] *Center for Health Sciences, Federal University of Rio Grande do Norte, Caixa Postal 3000, Lagoa Nova, 59078970 Natal, RN, Brazil*
[4] *University Norte of Parana, Caixa Postal 675, JD Piza, 86041-100 Londrina, PR, Brazil*

Correspondence should be addressed to Sergio G. da Silva; sergiogregorio@ufpr.br

Academic Editor: Holly M. Brown-Borg

The rating of perceived exertion (RPE) is ability to detect and interpret organic sensations while performing exercises. This method has been used to measure the level of effort that is felt during weight-training at a given intensity. The purpose of this investigation was to compare session RPE values with those of traditional RPE measurements for different weight-training muscle actions, performed together or separately. Fourteen women with no former weight-training experience were recruited for the investigation. All participants completed five sessions of exercise: familiarization, maximum force, concentric-only (CONC-only), eccentric-only (ECC-only), and dynamic (DYN = CONC + ECC). The traditional RPE method was measured after each series of exercises, and the session RPE was measured 30 min after the end of the training session. The statistical analyses used were the paired t-test, one-way analysis of variance, and repeated measures analysis of variance. Significant differences between traditional RPE and session RPE for DYN, CONC, and ECC exercises were not found. This investigation demonstrated that session RPE is similar to traditional RPE in terms of weight-training involving concentric, eccentric, or dynamic muscle exercises, and that it can be used to prescribe and monitor weight-training sessions in older subjects.

1. Introduction

Weight training has been commonly recommended for elderly subjects [1, 2]. Based on this premise, it is important to consider that weight training is conducted by eccentric, concentric, and isometric muscle actions, which can be performed together or separately [3, 4]. Thus, an action involving the generation of tension in the muscle, without external changes in the muscle length or joint angle with movement, is characterized as isometric action (ISOM). On the other hand, muscular tension related to decreases in the muscle length and joint angle is called concentric action (CONC), and when the generation of force causes stretching of the muscle length and angle joint, it is known as eccentric action (ECC) [5]. Most weight training programs primarily include dynamic exercises with both CON and ECC muscle actions, whereas ISOM actions play a secondary role [3].

Over the past decades, several investigations have demonstrated that a routine of weight training involving ECC and CONC muscle actions, in a combined or isolated manner, contributes to improved cardiovascular health, muscle strength, and functional capacity in the elderly [6, 7]. However, the benefits derived from these muscle actions are dependent on correct application and intensity control, including the numbers of sets and repetitions, rest intervals between sets, resistance used (load), and execution of velocity [3, 4]. Thus, adjustment and manipulation of each of these variables provide intensity capable of inducing a muscle response according to individual needs [8]. In this sense, developing strategies to measure the intensity utilized for weight training represents a considerable challenge.

Previous studies have used the rating of perceived exertion (RPE) as a method to measure the level of effort that is felt during weight training at a given intensity [9, 10]. The rating of perceived exertion (RPE) can be defined as the ability to detect and interpret organic sensations while performing exercises [11]. In fact, the recent guidelines proposed by the American College of Sports Medicine for physical activity and public health in older adults have suggested scales of perceived exertion of 0–10 for measuring exertion during weight training [12].Thus, the traditional method of measuring RPE is commonly used immediately after the execution of each exercise, reflecting various measurement points according to the amount of exercise performed. To facilitate the measurement and quantification of exercise intensity, Foster et al. [13] developed the method of subjective perception of exertion during a training session (session RPE), used to monitor various exercise types, particularly weight training. This method is based on a simple question that the subject responds to 30 min after the end of the training session: "What level of exertion did you feel in your body during the training session?" This reflects the feeling of global exertion experienced during the entire session.

A number of studies [9, 14, 15] have shown that a single session RPE may accurately reflect the intensity of a weight training session. In addition, this method allows an easy and reliable resistance training program manipulation required for continual increases in strength, including all workout stages in a single measure for the individual after each exercise session [9, 14]. In addition, it allows greater training synchronicity between a training regimen prescribed by a trainer and the actual intensity at which the subjects train. However, no study has investigated the application of session RPE in older individuals for different muscle actions used in weight training. Consequently, a better understanding of the session RPE in older individuals can provide valuable insight to health care professionals for prescribing weight training comprising different muscle actions. Therefore, the aim of this study was to compare values between session RPE and traditional measurement of RPE for different muscle actions performed together or separately in weight training.

2. Methodology

2.1. Subjects. A convenience sample of 14 older women met the inclusion criteria and gave their written consent to participate in this study. All were classified as either physically active (regular exercise ≥ 3 days·week^{-1}) or as having no former weight training experience. The inclusion criteria were (a) between the ages of 60 and 75 years; (b) ability to take part in regular physical exercise; (c) negative responses to all questions in the Physical Activity Readiness Questionnaire (PAR-Q); (d) a body mass index (BMI) between 18.5 and 30 kg·m^{-2}; and (e) a personal statement of not having smoked in the last 12 months. Criteria for exclusion included the presence of cardiovascular, metabolic, or orthopedic disease or any other contraindications as determined by a medical history from the previous 12 months. The study was approved by the Research Ethics Committee of the Department of Health Sciences at the Federal University of Paraná (UFPR) in Curitiba, Brazil.

2.2. Experimental Design. The experimental design of this study can be classified ascross-sectional [16]. All subjects completed five sessions of exercise: (a) sample screening and familiarization, (b) determination of 1RM (Repetition Maximum), and (c) three sessions of weight training conducted on different days, with 24–48 h between sessions, with the orders counterbalanced. Each session involved a different protocol: (1) ECC-only exercise, which consisted only of stretching of the muscle length and angle joint; (2) CONC-only exercise, which consisted of only the shortening phase of the muscle and angle joint; (3) DYN = CONC + ECC, which consisted of both a lengthening and shortening phase. The RPE and session RPE were recorded during each experimental session. Thus, the independent variable was muscle action (ECC-only, CONC-only, and DYN), whereas the dependent variables were RPE in-task and session RPE to the task. Subjects were advised not to consume alcohol, caffeine, or practice vigorous physical activity 24 h prior to each test.

2.3. Familiarization Session. To facilitate the elderly's understanding of the experimental procedures, subjects performed a familiarization session. Instructions were provided on the correct execution and proper form of the prescribed exercises, mainly regarding the appropriate posture, utilization of constant range of motion, and movement speed. In addition, information concerning the use of the OMNI Resistance Exercise Scale (OMNI-RES), which ranges from 0 to 10, was provided to the subjects [17] with the following specific instructions: "Please use this scale to translate into numbers your perception of exertion while exercising. The numbers on the scale represent a range of feelings from extremely easy 0 (low anchor) to extremely hard 10 (higher anchor). To help you select a number that corresponds to your perceptions regarding the exercise, consider the following: when the exercise seems extremely easy respond with a 0; on the other hand, when the exercise seems extremely hard, respond with a 10." Thus, subjects were instructed to use their memory of the least and greatest effort experienced while lifting weights to establish a visual-cognitive link with low and high perceptual anchors of the OMNI-RES, respectively. Furthermore, each subject was asked to select a load (light, moderate, or high) based on perceived exertion ratings on the OMNI-RES scale (0–10) with respect to all of the exercises (chest press, leg extension, lat pulldown, leg curl, and lateral shoulder raise).

2.4. Determination of 1RM. The 1RM testing session began with a specific warm-up, consisting of five to eight repetitions of each exercise using a self-selected, light weight. After this initial procedure, subjects were requested to take 5 min for passive recovery. Determination of the 1RM load was executed over a maximum of four attempts for each exercise, with 3 min of rest. Therefore, in each attempt, weight was successively added until only one repetition (completed with good form) was successfully lifted or until the participant indicated that he could not lift any more weight. Thus, the 1RM test was performed with each resistance exercise (chest press, leg extension, lat pulldown, leg curl, and lateral shoulder raise). To reduce the possible cumulative effect of fatigue on 1RM performance, the exercise order was alternated between upper and lower body exercises to allow greater recovery. All subjects were familiarized with the experimental procedures and were subjected to different exercise intensities (low, moderate, and high) for all the previously mentioned exercises. Consequently, this facilitated estimation of the initial loads and subsequent increments on 1RM tests.

2.5. Weight Training Sessions. All subjects completed three sessions of weight training, which were conducted on different days and with the orders counterbalanced. Thus, each weight training session was categorized according to the type of muscle action (CONC-only, ECC-only, and DYN). To guarantee the correct execution of the exercise and load application, each weight training session and each exercise were supervised by two experienced fitness instructors. In addition, during the CONC-only and ECC-only weight training sessions, subjects received help from two instructors, which allowed for these exercises to be performed in an isolated manner. Therefore, during the CONC-only session, subjects lifted the weight for complete execution of each movement (shortening of muscle length and angle joint), whereas two fitness instructors reduced the weight during the eccentric phase with the help of hands. On the other hand, during the ECC-only session, two fitness instructors lifted the weight for each repetition, and then the subject used strength to lower the weight (stretching of muscle length and angle joint). During the DYN session, both muscle actions (ECC and CONC) were performed without the help of instructors, only supervision to verify the correct execution of the exercise.

The weight training sessions (CONC-only, ECC-only, and DYN) consisted of uniarticular and multiarticular exercises, free weights and machines (Nakagym, São Paulo, Brazil), for large and small muscle groups, based on three sets of 8 to 10 repetitions each. Thus, all weight training sessions adopted the following exercises: chest press, leg extension, lat pulldown, leg curl, and lateral shoulder raise, with the order alternating between upper and lower body exercises. All exercises were performed on machines with the exception of the lateral shoulder raise, which used free weights. The intensity of each weight training session was classified as follows: CONC-only (70% 1RM); ECC-only (90% 1RM); and DYN (70% 1RM). According to Hortobagyi and Katch [18], 90% 1RM with the eccentric action is equivalent to 70% 1RM with the concentric force. The execution speed of the exercises was controlled by verbal commands from the evaluator, such that the subject maintained a concentric to eccentric phase ratio of 2 : 2 s, in accordance with the procedures suggested by Kraemer and Ratamess [3].

2.6. Rating Perception of Exertion. The RPE was used after each series of exercises (traditional measurement). Session RPE was measured 30 min after the end of the training session following procedures described by Foster et al. [13]. The subject was presented with the OMNI-RES scale and asked to answer the following question: "What level of exertion did you feel in your body during the training session?" Subjects were instructed to consider only the overall perception of exertion. While the subjects were waiting, they were allowed to drink water as they wished, but they were not allowed to perform other tasks, such as eating or showering.

2.7. Statistical Analysis. To characterize those taking part in the study, descriptive statistics using means ± standard deviations (SD) were performed on the data collected. A paired t-test was used to measure differences between the traditional RPE and session RPE means. To compare perceptual responses between training sessions for the mean RPE and session RPE, one-way analysis of variance (ANOVA) was used. To analyze perceptual responses during the exercise session, repeated measures ANOVA was used. Because violations in the assumption of sphericity appeared, such were addressed using Greenhouse-Geisser corrections. The significance level adopted for the analysis was $P < 0.05$. Data were analyzed statistically using SPSS software (version 17.0).

3. Results

The corresponding age, anthropometric measurement, and 1RM percentage values for DYN, CONC, and ECC are shown in Table 1 as means ± standard deviations (SD).

Figure 1 shows the perceptual responses of the muscle exercises expressed as means ± SD. Significant differences between traditional RPE and session RPE for DYN ($P = 0.626$), CONC ($P = 0.084$), and ECC ($P = 0.983$) were not found. Significant differences were also not detected between mean RPE ($F_{(2,26)} = 0.412$, $P = 0.667$, $n_p^2 = 0.031$) and session RPE ($F_{(3.619,26)} = 1.698$, $P = 0.203$, $n_p^2 = 0.116$) for the training sessions analyzed. For the perceptual responses during the session, differences were only observed in eccentric action ($F_{(3.389,26)} = 4.921$, $P = 0.004$, $n_p^2 = 0.275$).

4. Discussion

The benefits of weight training on neuromuscular aging have been widely presented in the literature, in theoretical and practical studies [19, 20]. However, in practice, few people adhere to a regular training program in order to obtain these benefits [21]. The high intensity of weight training programs during the early stages is one of the factors hindering the subjects' adherence to regular exercise [21]. This fact may

Table 1: Anthropometric variables, 1RM tests, and training loads.

Variables	Average ± SD	Variables	1RM	70%	90%
Age (year)	68.5 ± 4.6	Chess press (kg)	22.23 ± 6.2	16.7 ± 5.6	21.1 ± 7.2
Weight (kg)	63.0 ± 12.0	Leg extension (kg)	59.62 ± 14.7	40.8 ± 9.5	51.5 ± 12.2
Height (cm)	154 ± 0.06	Lat pulldown (kg)	35.85 ± 6.6	25.4 ± 4.5	32.3 ± 5.8
BMI (kg·m^{-2})	26.1 ± 3.5	Leg curl (kg)	23.31 ± 9.6	17.2 ± 6.7	20.8 ± 7.5
		Lateral shoulder raise (kg)	4.08 ± 0.7	2.7 ± 0.6	3.2 ± 0.7

BMI: body mass index; data are expressed as means ± SD.

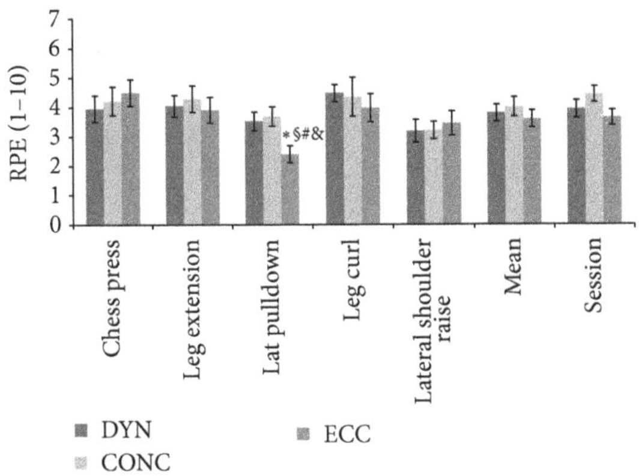

Figure 1: Significant differences: (*) Chess Press × Lat pulldown; (§) Leg Extension × Lat pulldown; (#) Mean × Lat pulldown; (&) Session × Lat pulldown.

contribute to high RPE and influence the decision of subjects to keep up regular exercise [22].

Session RPE is a modification of the traditional RPE scale. The difficulty of using conventional methods, such as measurements of heart rate, percentage of maximum oxygen consumption, and lactate threshold during weight training, has motivated researchers to use session RPE to facilitate and quantify the measurement of perceptual responses to exercise using weights [15]. The study by Day et al. [9] measured the session RPE during low, moderate, and high intensity weight training and the required reliability of the method in adult subjects. With the same perspective, other studies used the session RPE for exercising with weights.

In overweight and obese children, McGuigan et al. [23] identified no significant difference between the session RPE and traditional RPE. Sweet et al. [15] found consistent results between the session RPE used for aerobic exercise and that used for weight training. Pritchett et al. [24] studied high resistance (90% RM) and moderate (60% RM) exercise intensity in adult men and found differences between the mean RPE and session RPE for low intensity exercise. However, the authors suggested that the protocol used (multiple sets until exhaustion) may have been primarily responsible for the difference.

The investigations performed so far consider the session RPE to be a useful and important tool for exercise with weights [15, 25]. However, no studies in older populations or on different muscle actions were performed. Therefore, the aim of this study was to compare session RPE and traditional RPE measurement values for different muscle actions performed together or separately for weight training conducted in elderly women.

The results of this study detected no differences between traditional RPE and session RPE for DYN ($P = 0.626$), CONC ($P = 0.084$), and EXC ($P = 0.983$) sessions, corroborating data from previous research using dynamic actions [9, 25]. These findings agree with previous investigations, which showed similarity between traditional RPE and session RPE.

After analyzing the results of the traditional RPE and comparing them with the mean final and session RPE, differences were found only for the lat pulldown exercise session. It is speculated that the higher absolute overload for eccentric action (90% 1RM) and the characteristics of the lat pulldown exercise used to assign overhead, compared with other exercises that sustain overhead, were the factors driving this significant difference. However, no studies have observed similar responses.

The prescription of each CONC, EXC, and DIN exercise session was conducted according to the American College of Sports Medicine's model of weight training progression for elderly subjects [2, 26, 27]. Although the overhead used is equivalent to 70% of the maximum strength, the perceptual responses obtained were approximately 4 on the OMNI scale, which represents a somewhat easy perceived exertion. According to the authors [28, 29], during weight training, the percentage of overhead used in the exercises (% 1RM) did not directly reflect the effort of the subjects in the exercises, because variables such as number of repetitions, execution time of the exercises, and rest intervals between sets influenced the interpretation of this effort.

No differences in RPE (mean final or session) were observed among the different muscle action responses. This result should be considered when prescribing training for elderly subjects, because the eccentric activity can promote increased strength and muscle mass with less of a response in heart rate, systolic blood pressure, diastolic blood pressure, and double product, compared with concentric and dynamic exercise [30–33].

5. Conclusion

This research showed that perceptual responses observed using the session RPE method were similar to those using the traditional RPE method in weight training involving concentric, eccentric, and dynamic muscle actions. This result enables the use of a method with easy application and low financial cost for monitoring the intensity of exercises in older subjects.

In weight training for elderly beginners, the session RPE can assist in prescribing exercise to avoid high intensities that promote cardiovascular overload and muscle damage and dispel the subject to regular exercise and low intensities do not provide inadequate physiological stimuli to the proposed objectives. However, a limitation of this study was the lack of an additional training session, involving the same variables, to test the reliability of the method in elderly subjects.

Conflict of Interests

The authors declare that there is no conflict of interests regarding the publication of this paper.

References

[1] American College of Sports Medicine, W. J. Chodzko-Zajko, D. N. Proctor et al., "American College of Sports Medicine position stand. Exercise and physical activity for older adults," *Medicine & Science in Sports & Exercise*, vol. 41, no. 7, pp. 1510–1530, 2009.

[2] ACSM, "American College of Sports Medicine. Position stand on exercise and physical activity for older adults," *Medicine & Science in Sports & Exercise*, vol. 30, no. 6, pp. 992–1008, 1998.

[3] W. J. Kraemer and N. A. Ratamess, "Fundamentals of resistance training: progression and exercise prescription," *Medicine & Science in Sports & Exercise*, vol. 36, no. 4, pp. 674–688, 2004.

[4] S. P. Bird, K. M. Tarpenning, and F. E. Marino, "Designing resistance training programmes to enhance muscular fitness: a review of the acute programme variables," *Sports Medicine*, vol. 35, no. 10, pp. 841–851, 2005.

[5] W. J. Evans, "Effects of exercise on senescent muscle," *Clinical Orthopaedics and Related Research*, no. 403, supplement, pp. S211–S220, 2002.

[6] K. Krinski, H. M. Elsangedy, I. A. Soares, C. F. Buzzachera, W. de Campos, and S. G. da Silva, "Efeitos cardiovasculares agudos do exercício resistido em idosas hipertensas," *Acta Scientiarum Health Science*, vol. 30, no. 2, pp. 107–112, 2008.

[7] C. F. Buzzachera, H. M. Elsangedy, K. Krinski, H. Colombo, W. de Campos, and S. G. da Silva, "Efeitos do treinamento de força com pesos livres sobre os componentes da aptidão funcional em mulheres idosas," *Revista da Educação Física/UEM*, vol. 19, no. 2, pp. 195–203, 2008.

[8] A. Costa and C. Fernandes, "Utilização da percepção subjectiva do esforço para monitorização da intensidade do treino de força em idosos," *Motricidade*, vol. 3, no. 2, pp. 37–46, 2007.

[9] M. L. Day, M. R. McGuigan, G. Brice, and C. Foster, "Monitoring exercise intensity during resistance training using the session RPE scale," *Journal of Strength and Conditioning Research*, vol. 18, no. 2, pp. 353–358, 2004.

[10] B. C. Focht, "Perceived exertion and training load during self-selected and imposed-intensity resistance exercise in untrained women," *Journal of Strength and Conditioning Research*, vol. 21, no. 1, pp. 183–187, 2007.

[11] B. J. Noble and R. J. Robertson, *Perceived Exertion*, Human Kinetics Books, Champaign, Ill, USA, 1996.

[12] ACSM, American College of Sports Medicine, *ACSM's Guidelines for Exercise Testing and Prescription*, Lippincott Williams & Wilkins, Philadelphia, Pa, USA, 8th edition, 2010.

[13] C. Foster, J. A. Florhaug, J. Franklin et al., "A new approach to monitoring exercise training," *Journal of Strength and Conditioning Research*, vol. 15, no. 1, pp. 109–115, 2001.

[14] A. D. Egan, J. B. Winchester, C. Foster, and M. R. McGuigan, "Using session RPE to monitor different methods of resistance exercise," *Journal of Sports Science and Medicine*, vol. 5, pp. 289–295, 2006.

[15] T. W. Sweet, C. Foster, M. R. McGuigan, and G. Brice, "Quantitation of resistance training using the session rating of perceived exertion method," *Journal of Strength and Conditioning Research*, vol. 18, no. 4, pp. 796–802, 2004.

[16] J. Thomas, J. Nelson, and S. Silverman, Eds., *Research Methods in Physical Activity*, vol. 5, Human Kinetics, Champaign, Ill, USA, 2005.

[17] R. J. Robertson, F. L. Goss, J. Rutkowski et al., "Concurrent validation of the OMNI perceived exertion scale for resistance exercise," *Medicine & Science in Sports & Exercise*, vol. 35, no. 2, pp. 333–341, 2003.

[18] T. Hortobagyi and F. I. Katch, "Role of concentric force in limiting improvement in muscular strength," *Journal of Applied Physiology*, vol. 68, no. 2, pp. 650–658, 1990.

[19] R. Seguin and M. E. Nelson, "The benefits of strength training for older adults," *American Journal of Preventive Medicine*, vol. 25, no. 3, supplement 2, pp. 141–149, 2003.

[20] D. H. Paterson, G. R. Jones, and C. L. Rice, "Ageing and physical activity: evidence to develop exercise recommendations for older adults," *Canadian Journal of Public Health*, vol. 98, supplement 2, pp. S69–S108, 2007.

[21] R. K. Dishman, R. P. Farquhar, and K. J. Cureton, "Responses to preferred intensities of exertion in men differing in activity levels," *Medicine & Science in Sports & Exercise*, vol. 26, no. 6, pp. 783–790, 1994.

[22] W. S. Bibeau, J. B. Moore, N. G. Mitchell, T. Vargas-Tonsing, and J. B. Bartholomew, "Effects of acute resistance training of different intensities and rest periods on anxiety and affect," *Journal of Strength and Conditioning Research*, vol. 24, no. 8, pp. 2184–2191, 2010.

[23] M. R. McGuigan, A. Al Dayel, D. Tod, C. Foster, R. U. Newton, and S. Pettigrew, "Use of session rating of perceived exertion for monitoring resistance exercise in children who are overweight or obese," *Pediatric Exercise Science*, vol. 20, no. 3, pp. 333–341, 2008.

[24] R. C. Pritchett, J. M. Green, P. J. Wickwire, and M. S. Kovacs, "Acute and session RPE responses during resistance training: bouts to failure at 60% and 90% of 1RM," *South African Journal of Sports Medicine*, vol. 21, no. 1, 2009.

[25] F. Singh, C. Foster, D. Tod, and M. R. McGuigan, "Monitoring different types of resistance training using session rating of perceived exertion," *International Journal of Sports Physiology and Performance*, vol. 2, no. 1, pp. 34–45, 2007.

[26] J. E. Donnelly, S. N. Blair, J. M. Jakicic, M. M. Manore, J. W. Rankin, and B. K. Smith, "Appropriate physical activity intervention strategies for weight loss and prevention of weight regain for adults," *Medicine & Science in Sports & Exercise*, vol. 41, no. 2, pp. 459–471, 2009.

[27] C. E. Garber, B. Blissmer, M. R. Deschenes et al., "Quantity and quality of exercise for developing and maintaining cardiorespiratory, musculoskeletal, and neuromotor fitness in apparently healthy adults: guidance for prescribing exercise," *Medicine & Science in Sports & Exercise*, vol. 43, no. 7, pp. 1334–1359, 2011.

[28] A. D. Egan, J. B. Winchester, C. Foster, and M. R. McGuigan, "Using session RPE to monitor different methods of resistance

exercise," *Journal of Sports Science and Medicine*, vol. 5, pp. 289–295, 2006.

[29] K. M. Genner and M. Weston, "A comparison of workload quantification methods in relation to physiological responses to resistance exercise," *Journal of Strength and Conditioning Research*, 2014.

[30] T. Hortobagyi, "The positives of negatives: clinical implications of eccentric resistance exercise in old adults," *The Journals of Gerontology A: Biological Sciences and Medical Sciences*, vol. 58, no. 5, pp. M417–M418, 2003.

[31] N. D. Reeves, C. N. Maganaris, S. Longo, and M. V. Narici, "Differential adaptations to eccentric versus conventional resistance training in older humans," *Experimental Physiology*, vol. 94, no. 7, pp. 825–833, 2009.

[32] T. Hortobágyi and P. de Vita, "Favorable neuromuscular and cardiovascular responses to 7 days of exercise with an eccentric overload in elderly women," *Journals of Gerontology A: Biological Sciences and Medical Sciences*, vol. 55, no. 8, pp. B401–B410, 2000.

[33] M. Roig, K. O'Brien, G. Kirk et al., "The effects of eccentric versus concentric resistance training on muscle strength and mass in healthy adults: a systematic review with meta-analysis," *British Journal of Sports Medicine*, vol. 43, no. 8, pp. 556–568, 2009.

8

Intramuscular Olanzapine in the Management of Behavioral and Psychological Symptoms in Hospitalized Older Adults

Silvia Duong,[1,2] Kam-Tong Yeung,[1] and Feng Chang[1,3]

[1]*North York General Hospital, 4001 Leslie Street, Toronto, ON, Canada M2K 1E1*
[2]*Herzl CRIU Walk-In Centre, Jewish General Hospital, 5858 Côte-des-Neiges, Suite 500, Montreal, QC, Canada H3S 1Z1*
[3]*School of Pharmacy, University of Waterloo, 200 University Avenue West, Waterloo, ON, Canada N2L 3G1*

Correspondence should be addressed to Feng Chang; feng.chang@uwaterloo.ca

Academic Editor: F. R. Ferraro

Background. While behavioral and psychological symptoms are frequent in hospitalized older adults with dementia or delirium, data supporting the off-label use of intramuscular atypical antipsychotics remain scarce. We examined the use of short-acting intramuscular (IM) olanzapine in hospitalized older adults to manage behavioral and psychological symptoms. *Methods.* A retrospective observational study of inpatients 65 years or older with at least one order for olanzapine IM during admission in urban Ontario Canada was conducted. Patient demographics, prescriptions for olanzapine IM, reason for administration, perceived effectiveness, adverse events, concurrently prescribed psychotropics, comorbidities, and patient discharge destination were recorded. *Results.* Among 82 patients aged 65–96 years (mean ± SD 79.3 ± 7.7) 85 cases were identified. Cognitive impairment or dementia affected 63.5% and 50.6% had comorbidities. Olanzapine IM was ordered 102 times and 34 patients (41%) received at least one dose. The intended efficacy was achieved in 79.4% of 78 cases of 124 doses given (62.9%). Fourteen (41%) patients who received doses experienced adverse events, with sedation and hypotension being the most common. *Conclusions.* Olanzapine IM appears effective in hospitalized older adults but is associated with potential adverse events. Structured monitoring and documentation are needed to ensure safe use in this high-risk population.

1. Introduction

Behavioral and psychological symptoms, such as agitation, aggression, wandering, delusions, and hallucinations, are often observed in older patients with dementia or delirium. Dementia is estimated to affect 7% of Canadians over the age of 60 and 55% of these patients are over the age of 80 [1]. Since the proportion of the population that is over the age of 80 is projected to continue to rise over the next 30 years, the number of people affected by dementia is expected to increase [1, 2]. Ninety percent of afflicted people experience neuropsychiatric or behavioral symptoms during the course of the disease [3]. Furthermore, dementia is associated with increased risk of developing delirium in hospitalized older patients: 10–15% of hospitalized seniors are admitted to hospital with delirium and 15–25% will develop delirium following admission [1]. Thus, the aging of the population also predicts that an increased number of elderly patients will exhibit behavioral and psychological symptoms.

The current evidence supporting drug treatment of behavioral and psychological symptoms in the elderly is scarce. Antipsychotics and benzodiazepines have been proposed as treatment options for the acute management of delirium [4]. Pharmacotherapy options for behavioral and psychological symptoms of dementia include antipsychotics, anticonvulsants, antidepressants, and anxiolytics. While oral therapy is the preferred route of administration in the management of behavioral and psychological symptoms due to its convenience, intramuscular formulations are often required when a patient refuses to take oral medications, is unable to swallow, or is too agitated to comply. The fast onset of parenteral administration also reduces the risk of potential harm to both the patient and others. As a result, clinicians commonly use intramuscular formulations of first-generation antipsychotics, benzodiazepines, or a combination of both for this purpose especially when no intravenous access is available. However, the potential for adverse events remains of concern especially in the more vulnerable and susceptible elderly population. Sedation, confusion, and respiratory depression are associated with benzodiazepines. First-generation antipsychotics may cause acute dystonia, extrapyramidal symptoms (EPS), neuroleptic malignant syndrome, and electrocardiographic abnormalities including QTc interval prolongation. Since they are associated with a lower risk of EPS, atypical or second-generation antipsychotics have become attractive alternatives over first-generation antipsychotics: a recent survey study reports that 86.3% of US nursing home residents receive atypical antipsychotics for off-label indications [5].

Short-acting olanzapine IM (Zyprexa Intramuscular) is currently approved for the treatment of acute agitation associated with schizophrenia and bipolar mania in many countries including Canada and the United States [6]. In adults, olanzapine IM has been shown to be efficacious in the management of agitation associated with schizophrenia, borderline personality disorder, bipolar disorder, and drug- and alcohol-using patients [7–12]. However, the use of olanzapine IM for the acute management of behavioral and psychological symptoms observed in older adults with dementia or delirium remains off-label to date. One published randomized controlled trial (RCT) reports similar efficacy between olanzapine IM and lorazepam IM in reducing agitation in patients with dementia [13]. No study has yet compared olanzapine IM with the combination of haloperidol and lorazepam. With the scarcity of data directing care, research is needed to better understand how olanzapine IM is being used in the management of acute behavioral and psychological symptoms in this patient population. This study has three main objectives: (1) to describe the patient characteristics of hospitalized older adults who receive a prescription for olanzapine IM, (2) to identify prescribing patterns of olanzapine IM in this population, and (3) to report documentation practices related to efficacy and adverse drug events associated with olanzapine IM use.

2. Methods

A retrospective descriptive study was carried out at a general tertiary care hospital in Toronto, Canada. The hospital had approximately 300 beds including an acute psychiatric inpatient unit, acute geriatric medicine, intensive care (ICU), internal medicine and surgical units, and emergency. Using the Inpatient Pharmacy Services database (PharmNet), the investigators identified all patients prescribed olanzapine IM between September 1, 2008, and March 1, 2010. Patients were included if they were at least 65 years of age and had at least one order for olanzapine IM during their hospital stay. The medical records of all cases were retrospectively reviewed and analyzed.

While all cases that were prescribed olanzapine are included in this review, we analyzed only those who actually received a minimum of one dose of olanzapine. The records of the remaining patients who were prescribed olanzapine but did not actually receive any are included separately for completeness.

Data collected included demographic characteristics, the prescribing patterns of olanzapine IM (indication, dose, frequency, and duration of therapy), relevant concurrently prescribed psychotropic medications (other prescribed antipsychotics, benzodiazepines, antidepressants, antidementia medications, mood stabilizers, pain medications, and other sedative-hypnotics) ordered within 24 hours of the initial prescription for olanzapine IM, comorbidities, and patient discharge destination. All comorbidities that could potentially contribute to patients' behavioral and psychological symptoms were recorded. These included cognitive impairment or dementia, delirium, psychiatric disorders (schizophrenia, bipolar affective disorder, and depression), neurological disorder (stroke and Parkinson's disease), insomnia, pain, and acute infection. Any unlisted potential factors were included if deemed applicable by consensus among investigators. The documented reason of administration and any findings on the effectiveness after dose were also noted. Subjective assessments based on clinician documentation were categorized as "achieved effect," "partial effect" (adjunct therapy or repeated dose was required), "no effect," or "not documented." Documentation for adverse events associated with olanzapine IM including hypotension, falls, decreased level of consciousness, EPS, weakness, sedation, and potential events such as infections was reviewed. All monitoring for vital signs (temperature, heart rate, blood pressure, respiration rate, and oxygen saturation) within six hours after dose was also included. The duration of therapy was determined by counting the number of days with an active order for olanzapine IM according to Physician's Order Sheet and the Medication Administration Record.

A standardized data abstraction form in Microsoft Excel was used and pilot-tested. Data were managed with Excel for descriptive analysis. This study was conducted with approval from the North York General Hospital Research Ethics Board.

3. Results

A total of 87 cases met the inclusion criteria; however, two charts were neither available nor accessible at the time of the data collection. Eighty-five cases were found among 82 older inpatients (two patients were readmitted once ($n = 1$) or twice ($n = 1$) during the course of the study and ordered olanzapine IM during each admission). Most cases (52; 61.2%) were admitted to the psychiatric ward while 31 (36.4%) were from internal medicine. Other cases came from surgical, transitional, and intensive care units (2.4%). Of the 85 cases, 51 (60%) had an order for olanzapine IM but did not require any doses, while 34 (40%) received at least one dose. There were slightly more women (52.9%) than men (47.1%). The age ranged from 65 to 96 years (mean ± SD age, 79.3 ± 7.7 years). Two patients who were prescribed olanzapine, but who did not receive any, passed away during admission due to sepsis and sepsis-related complications. Detailed demographic data and clinical characteristics of both those who did and did not receive olanzapine are presented in Table 1. Most suffered from cognitive impairment or dementia (63.5%) and about half (50.6%) had two or more comorbidities. In terms of concurrent pharmacotherapy, most cases were prescribed another antipsychotic (83.4%) and other psychotropic medications (75.3%), with olanzapine oral (41%), risperidone (40%), and quetiapine (22%) most commonly prescribed.

During the study period, 102 orders for olanzapine IM were written for these 85 cases, mostly initiated by a psychiatrist (82.4%) for the following two indications: agitation as assessed and documented by a clinician and/or patient's refusal or inability to receive oral antipsychotics (Table 2). The prescribed dose of olanzapine IM ranged from 2.5 mg to 10 mg per injection (mean ± SD, 5.51 ± 1.91 mg). All prescriptions were written on an "if needed" (PRN) basis with the frequency of administration varying from every 1 hour to every 12 hours. Three (2.9%) orders had a frequency of every 1 hour. A maximum daily dose (5–20 mg/day) was prespecified in 25.5% of the orders only.

Among the 34 cases who received at least one dose of olanzapine IM, the most common reasons for administering included patient's refusal or inability to take oral antipsychotics (33.9%), agitation and patient's refusal/inability to take oral medication (33.9%), and aggression and patient's refusal/inability to take oral medications (22.6%). Patients received 1 to 3 doses (dosage varying between 2.5 mg and 10 mg) per day and 1 to 24 doses throughout admission (3.3 ± 4.5 doses). The total dose administered during admission varied between 2.5 and 120 mg (12.1 ± 20.1 mg). In 46 (37.1%) of 124 administered doses, the effectiveness was not documented in the patients' chart. For the remaining 78 doses, 68 (87%) achieved the intended or partial effect. Five (6.4%) had no effect and five (6.4%) were undetermined. Doses of 2.5 mg and 5 mg were sufficient in achieving effectiveness in 82.1% and 80% of cases, respectively.

Fourteen of the 34 cases (41.2%) documented experiencing at least one adverse event associated with the administration of olanzapine IM. Sedation and hypotension were the most commonly reported (Table 3). Four patients (11.8%) experienced a fall within a period of 24 hours after dose and 11 patients suffered from an infection after receiving at least one dose (six cases of a urinary tract infection, three cases of pneumonia, and one case each of cellulitis and *Clostridium difficile*-associated infection). Monitoring for patient's vital signs within six hours after dose was completed in about one-third of cases.

4. Discussion

To our knowledge, this is the first study to report the clinical use of short-acting olanzapine IM for its off-label use in the management of behavioral and psychological symptoms in hospitalized older adults. In our center, olanzapine IM was commonly prescribed to manage acute agitation and aggression related to dementia, delirium, or psychiatric disorders. It was also used as an alternative when patients refused or were unable to take oral antipsychotics. In a double-blind, placebo-controlled study of 272 patients (mean age 77) with Alzheimer's disease, vascular or mixed dementia, Meehan and colleagues demonstrated that 5 mg of olanzapine IM had similar efficacy to 1 mg of lorazepam IM in reducing agitation [13]. In contrast to this previous study, 50% of the older inpatients in our present study suffered from two or more comorbidities that can cause acute behavioral and/or psychological symptoms. Furthermore, most patients received concurrent oral antipsychotics or other psychotropic medications.

Currently, olanzapine is the only intramuscular short-acting second-generation antipsychotic formulation available on the Canadian market. In the USA, intramuscular formulations for ziprasidone and aripiprazole are short-acting alternatives for the management of acute agitation. In the older population, ziprasidone has been reported to be effective in short-term treatment of acute psychosis or agitation, offering similar effectiveness as conventional therapy (haloperidol with or without lorazepam) [14, 15]. A recent double-blind randomized placebo-controlled study in a long-term care setting demonstrated that aripiprazole is effective in the management of agitation associated with Alzheimer's, vascular or mixed dementia [16]. Furthermore, in a randomized controlled trial, Baldaçara and colleagues compared the effectiveness of intramuscular olanzapine, ziprasidone, haloperidol plus promethazine, haloperidol plus midazolam, and haloperidol alone for the treatment of patients (mean age 32.2 years) with agitation and aggressive behavior in the emergency rooms for psychiatric patients [17]. The authors concluded that all were effective in controlling agitation/aggressive behaviors associated with psychotic or bipolar disorder over a period of 12 hours. Among the different study groups, they noted that patients receiving olanzapine had better agitation control, experienced less excessive sedation, and were less likely to require physical restraint. Since the efficacy and safety of two second-generation intramuscular antipsychotics in management of acute agitation in the elderly have never been directly compared, it is impossible to conclude whether a particular agent is preferred in the geriatric population.

In our study, the 2.5 mg and 5 mg doses of olanzapine IM appeared to achieve efficacy in about 80% of the documented cases. Breier and colleagues reported that 2.5 mg of olanzapine IM was less efficacious than haloperidol IM 7.5 mg and higher doses of olanzapine IM (5 mg, 7.5 mg, and 10 mg) in the management of acute agitation in adult patients (mean age 36.3 years, range from 18 to 73 years) with schizophrenia [7]. Response rates ranged from 50% to 80% with olanzapine 2.5 mg to 10 mg. Conversely, Meehan and colleagues reported that olanzapine IM 2.5 mg and 5 mg were superior to placebo and offered similar efficacy as lorazepam IM 1 mg in alleviating acute agitation in patients with dementia [11]. An initial treatment dose of 2.5 mg/day has also been previously proposed in older patients with Alzheimer's disease [13]. Our data suggested that olanzapine IM 2.5 mg offered similar efficacy as 5 mg in these older patients. Prescribers may consider initiating therapy at the lower dose of 2.5 mg and provide a second dose to be given at least two hours after if needed [13]. The Zyprexa IM product

TABLE 1: Baseline demographic characteristics of older patients prescribed olanzapine.

	Received olanzapine $N = 34$	No olanzapine $N = 51$	All cases $N = 85$
Age, mean (years)	79.6	79.0	79.3
Female	19 (55.9%)	26 (51%)	45 (52.9%)
Admission from			
Home	18 (52.9%)	41 (80.4%)	59 (69.4%)
Another hospital	4 (11.8%)	2 (3.9%)	6 (7.1%)
Retirement/LTC facilities	12 (35.3%)	8 (15.7%)	20 (23.5%)
Discharge destination			
Home	10 (29.4%)	20 (39.2%)	30 (35.3%)
Another institution	6 (17.6%)	6 (11.8%)	12 (14.1%)
Retirement/LTC facilities	18 (53.0%)	23 (45.1%)	41 (48.2%)
Death	0	2 (3.9%)	2 (2.4%)
Types of patients			
Psychiatry	22 (64.7%)	29 (56.9%)	51 (60.0%)
General medicine	12 (35.3%)	21 (41.2%)	31 (36.4%)
Surgery	0	2 (3.9%)	2 (2.4%)
Intensive care unit	0	1 (2.0%)	1 (1.2%)
Comorbidities			
Cognitive impairment/dementia	21 (61.8%)	33 (64.7%)	54 (63.5%)
Delirium	9 (26.5%)	16 (31.4%)	25 (29.4%)
Psychiatric disorders	19 (55.9%)	24 (47.1%)	43 (50.6%)
Neurological disorder	5 (14.7%)	6 (11.8%)	11 (12.9%)
Insomnia	3 (8.8%)	5 (9.8%)	8 (9.4%)
Pain	0	1 (1.9%)	1 (1.2%)
Acute infection	7 (20.6%)	13 (25.5%)	20 (23.5%)
Other	6 (17.6%)	5 (9.8%)	11 (12.9%)
Number of comorbidities			
1	17 (50.0%)	25 (49.0%)	42 (49.4%)
2	11 (32.3%)	10 (19.6%)	21 (24.7%)
3	2 (5.9%)	10 (19.6%)	12 (14.1%)
≥4	4 (11.8%)	6 (11.8%)	10 (11.8%)
Concurrent psychotropic medications			
Other antipsychotics	29 (85.3%)	41 (80.4%)	70 (83.4%)
Benzodiazepines	11 (32.4%)	10 (19.6%)	21 (24.7%)
Antidepressants	18 (52.9%)	18 (35.3%)	36 (42.4%)
Antidementia medications	7 (20.6%)	14 (27.4%)	21 (24.7%)
Mood stabilizer	4 (11.8%)	4 (7.8%)	8 (9.4%)
Pain medications	0	1 (1.96%)	1 (1.2%)
Other sedatives	0	2 (3.9%)	2 (2.4%)
Number of psychotropic medications (nonantipsychotics)			
0	8 (23.5%)	13 (25.5%)	21 (24.7%)
1	9 (26.5%)	20 (39.2%)	29 (34.1%)
2	14 (41.2%)	17 (33.3%)	31 (36.4%)
3	1 (2.9%)	1 (2.0%)	2 (2.4%)
4	2 (5.9%)	0	2 (2.4%)

*LTC: long-term care.

Table 2: Prescribing patterns of olanzapine IM.

	Received olanzapine $N = 46$	Received no olanzapine $N = 56$	All prescriptions $N = 102$
Indication(s) of therapy		Number (%)	
Refusal/unable to take oral meds	9 (19.6%)	7 (12.5%)	16 (15.7%)
Agitation	3 (6.5%)	3 (5.3%)	6 (5.9%)
Others	2 (4.3%)	1 (1.8%)	3 (2.9%)
Combination of indications			
Agitation and/or refusal/unable	12 (26.1%)	22 (39.3%)	34 (33.3%)
Agitation, refusal/unable, and/or aggression	9 (19.6%)	12 (21.4%)	21 (20.6%)
Agitation and/or aggression	4 (8.7%)	8 (14.3%)	12 (11.8%)
Psychosis and/or agitation	1 (2.2%)	2 (3.6%)	3 (2.9%)
Psychosis, agitation, and/or aggression	3 (6.5%)	0 (0.0%)	3 (2.9%)
Psychosis, agitation, and/or refusal/unable	2 (4.3%)	0 (0.0%)	2 (2.0%)
Agitation and/or others	1 (2.2%)	0 (0.0%)	1 (1.0%)
Aggression and/or refusal/unable	0 (0.0%)	1 (1.8%)	1 (1.0%)
Duration of therapy (days)			
Mean ± SD	26.7 ± 39.6	14.1 ± 13.0	19.2 ± 27.80
Range	5–250	1–60	1–250

Table 3: Documented adverse events and monitoring among cases that received olanzapine IM.

Adverse event	Number (%)
Sedation	7 (20.6%)
Orthostatic hypotension	5 (14.7%)
Falls	4 (11.8%)
Decreased level of consciousness	4 (11.8%)
Extrapyramidal symptoms	3 (8.8%)
Weakness	1 (2.9%)
Monitoring of vital signs (within 6 hrs)	
Complete monitoring	42 (33.9%)
Incomplete monitoring	10 (8.1%)
No monitoring documented	58 (46.8%)
Patient refuses to comply	14 (11.2%)

monograph recommends a maximum daily dose of 20 mg [6]. Since renal and hepatic impairments are common in the elderly, a more conservative maximum daily dose of 10 mg may be considered for hospitalized elderly patients.

In terms of adverse events, previous studies reported high prevalence of sedation and orthostatic hypotension with the use of olanzapine IM [7, 13]. Importantly, older adults also experience decreased level of consciousness and increased risk of falls. Close monitoring of vitals, level of consciousness, and gait stability are recommended to detect and, hopefully, prevent adverse events. Marder and colleagues identified that the most common postmarketing adverse events associated with olanzapine IM included pyrexia, hypotension, syncope, neuroleptic malignant syndrome, somnolence, cardiac arrest, rise in the serum creatine phosphokinase (CPK), and falls [18]. Adverse events were frequently reported in patients with comorbid conditions and those receiving concomitant treatment with benzodiazepine (39%) and other antipsychotic agents (54%) [18]. Therefore, in the susceptible older population, clinicians should attempt to reduce the risk of potential adverse events by exercising caution when prescribing olanzapine IM concomitantly with other psychotropic medications. In our study, a significant portion of patients did not have documentation relevant to efficacy or safety. The development of an appropriately structured postdose monitoring protocol that includes neurological assessment, mobility assessment, fall prevention strategies, and swallowing assessment would ensure safer use. Vital signs should be taken within six hours after a given dose if clinically feasible.

As with any retrospective study, our data are limited by the availability and accuracy of medical records. The lack of documentation in 37.1% of administered doses of olanzapine reduces the ability to draw firm conclusions about the safety and effectiveness of its use in this vulnerable population. A comparator group would have permitted us to more accurately assess the efficacy and risk of adverse events associated with olanzapine IM. Also, our data are reflective of one site only and practice may differ in other settings. However, this study does provide a glimpse into the clinical use of olanzapine IM among hospitalized older adults in naturalistic acute care practice.

Results can be used to direct future prospective studies comparing management strategies. In these future studies, it is recommended that agitation be measured objectively rather than subjectively, so that multisite comparisons can be made. Examples of agitation measurement tools used with people with dementia include the Agitated Behavior Scale (ABS), the Pittsburgh Agitation Scale, and the Cohen-Mansfield Agitation Inventory. Consistent use of such a tool will enable a thorough assessment of benefit versus risk. Future studies focusing on surgical and ICU patient populations can further understanding for the dosing approach required by medically compromised patients.

5. Conclusions

Olanzapine IM appears to be commonly prescribed for behavioral and psychological symptoms in older patients in the acute care setting. The use of olanzapine IM appears effective; however, its administration is associated with a significant risk of potentially related adverse events. A structured approach to monitoring and documentation will be needed to ensure safe use.

Conflict of Interests

The authors have no financial or other conflict of interests regarding this paper. The sponsor had no involvement in the study design, methods, participant identification, data collection, data analysis, or preparation of the paper.

Authors' Contribution

Study concept and design are done by Feng Chang and Kam-Tong Yeung. All authors contributed to the data acquisition and analysis and paper preparation.

Acknowledgments

The authors acknowledge and thank the physicians and staff at North York General Hospital for their generous input into the project and assistance during data collection. They also thank the inpatient pharmacy department for assistance with patient identification. This work was funded by the Iris and Dalton Bales Research Endowment Fund administered through the North York General Hospital Foundation.

References

[1] Alzheimer Society, *Rising Tide: The Impact of Dementia on Canadian Society*, Alzheimer Society, 2010, http://www.alzheimer.ca/~/media/Files/national/Advocacy/ASC_Rising_Tide_Full_Report_e.pdf.

[2] International Psychogeriatric Association, *The IPA Complete Guides to Behavioral and Psychological Symptoms of Dementia (BPSD)*, 2012, http://www.ipa-online.org/members/pdfs/____IPA_BPSD_Nurses_Guide_Interior_Online.pdf.

[3] N. Herrmann, S. Gauthier, and P. G. Lysy, "Clinical practice guidelines for severe Alzheimer's disease," *Alzheimer's & Dementia*, vol. 3, no. 4, pp. 385–397, 2007.

[4] D. Hogan, L. Gage, V. Bruto et al., "National guidelines for seniors'mental health: the assessment and treatment of delirium," *Canadian Journal of Geriatrics*, vol. 9, supplement 2, pp. S42–S51, 2006, http://www.ccsmh.ca/pdf/final%20supplement.pdf.

[5] P. Kamble, J. Sherer, H. Chen, and R. Aparasu, "Off-label use of second-generation antipsychotic agents among elderly nursing home residents," *Psychiatric Services*, vol. 61, no. 2, pp. 130–136, 2010.

[6] Eli Lilly Canada, *Product Monograph Zyprexa Intramuscular*, Eli Lilly Canada, 2011.

[7] A. Breier, K. Meehan, M. Birkett et al., "A double-blind, placebo-controlled dose-response comparison of intramuscular olanzapine and haloperidol in the treatment of acute agitation in schizophrenia," *Archives of General Psychiatry*, vol. 59, no. 5, pp. 441–448, 2002.

[8] P. Wright, M. Birkett, S. R. David et al., "Double-blind, placebo-controlled comparison of intramuscular olanzapine and intramuscular haloperidol in the treatment of acute agitation in schizophrenia," *American Journal of Psychiatry*, vol. 158, no. 7, pp. 1149–1151, 2001.

[9] P. Wright, S. R. Lindborg, M. Birkett et al., "Intramuscular olanzapine and intramuscular haloperidol in acute schizophrenia: antipsychotic efficacy and extrapyramidal safety during the first 24 hours of treatment," *Canadian Journal of Psychiatry*, vol. 48, no. 11, pp. 716–721, 2003.

[10] C. Damsa, E. Adam, F. de Gregorio et al., "Intramuscular olanzapine in patients with borderline personality disorder: an observational study in an emergency room," *General Hospital Psychiatry*, vol. 29, no. 1, pp. 51–53, 2007.

[11] K. Meehan, F. Zhang, S. David et al., "A double-blind, randomized comparison of the efficacy and safety of intramuscular injections of olanzapine, lorazepam, or placebo in treating acutely agitated patients diagnosed with bipolar mania," *Journal of Clinical Psychopharmacology*, vol. 21, no. 4, pp. 389–397, 2001.

[12] K. MacDonald, M. P. Wilson, A. Minassian et al., "A retrospective analysis of intramuscular haloperidol and intramuscular olanzapine in the treatment of agitation in drug- and alcohol-using patients," *General Hospital Psychiatry*, vol. 32, no. 4, pp. 443–445, 2010.

[13] K. M. Meehan, H. Wang, S. R. David et al., "Comparison of rapidly acting intramuscular olanzapine, lorazepam, and placebo: a double-blind, randomized study in acutely agitated patients with dementia," *Neuropsychopharmacology*, vol. 26, no. 4, pp. 494–504, 2002.

[14] A. R. Rais, K. Williams, T. Rais, T. Singh, and M. Tamburrino, "Use of intramuscular ziprasidone for the control of acute psychosis or agitation in an inpatient geriatric population: an open-label study," *Psychiatry*, vol. 7, no. 1, pp. 17–24, 2010.

[15] I. Kohen, H. Preval, R. Southard, and A. Francis, "Naturalistic study of intramuscular ziprasidone versus conventional agents in agitated elderly patients: retrospective findings from a psychiatric emergency service," *American Journal Geriatric Pharmacotherapy*, vol. 3, no. 4, pp. 240–245, 2005.

[16] S. A. Rappaport, R. N. Marcus, G. Manos, R. D. McQuade, and D. A. Oren, "A randomized, double-blind, placebo-controlled tolerability study of intramuscular aripiprazole in acutely agitated patients with Alzheimer's, vascular, or mixed dementia," *Journal of the American Medical Directors Association*, vol. 10, no. 1, pp. 21–27, 2009.

[17] L. Baldaçara, M. Sanches, D. C. Cordeiro, and A. P. Jackoswski, "Rapid tranquilization for agitated patients in emergency psychiatric rooms: a randomized trial of olanzapine, ziprasidone, haloperidol plus promethazine, haloperidol plus midazolam and haloperidol alone," *Revista Brasileira de Psiquiatria*, vol. 33, no. 1, pp. 30–39, 2011.

[18] S. R. Marder, S. Sorsaburu, E. Dunayevich et al., "Case reports of postmarketing adverse event experiences with olanzapine intramuscular treatment in patients with agitation," *Journal of Clinical Psychiatry*, vol. 71, no. 4, pp. 433–441, 2010.

9

Response to Acute Psychophysical Stress and 24-Hour Glycemic Control in Healthy Older People

Loretta DiPietro,[1,2,3] Catherine W. Yeckel,[1,2] and Andrei Gribok[4]

[1] *The John B. Pierce Laboratory, Yale School of Medicine, New Haven, CT 06519, USA*
[2] *Department of Epidemiology and Public Health, Yale School of Medicine, New Haven, CT 06519, USA*
[3] *The Department of Exercise Science, School of Public Health and Health Services, The George Washington University, 817 23rd Street, NW, Washington, DC 20052, USA*
[4] *Beltsville Human Nutrition Research Center, The United States Department of Agriculture, Beltsville, MD 20705, USA*

Correspondence should be addressed to Loretta DiPietro, ldp1@gwu.edu

Academic Editor: Hiroshi Nose

We examined the relation between stress reactivity and 24 h glycemic control in 17 inactive, healthy older people (≥60 years) under both a novel psychophysical stress and a seated control condition. Plasma cortisol was measured over the course of the stress and recovery periods. Glycemic control was determined over the subsequent 3 h from an oral glucose tolerance test (OGTT) and over 24 h *via* continuous glucose monitoring (CGM). We observed significant ($P < 0.05$) elevations in perceived stress, cardiovascular activity, and peak cortisol response at 30 min (10.6 ± 3.1 versus $8.6 \pm 2.6\,\mu g \cdot dL^{-1}$, resp.) during the stress compared with the control condition; however, 3 h OGTT glucose and insulin responses were similar between conditions. The CGM data suggested a 30–40 min postchallenge delay in peak glucose response and attenuated glucose clearance over the 6 h following the stress condition, but these alterations were not statistically significant. Healthy older people may demonstrate minimal disruption in metabolic resiliency following everyday psychological stress.

1. Introduction

"Stress" is a common and adaptive component of our interaction with the environment [1], and *allostasis* refers to the body's ability to reestablish stability (i.e., homeostasis) when confronted by various environmental challenges through the activation of neural, neuroendocrine, and neuroendocrine-immune responses [2]. There is some evidence from animal models that aging *per se* alters allostatic ability, although the data in humans are inconclusive [3]. Nonetheless, older age is characterized by diminished physical capabilities (e.g., vision, strength, and reaction time), which may make normal everyday experiences and challenges (like driving an automobile or crossing the street) more stressful [4]. Thus, older people may have more frequent exposures to stressful situations, along with a compromised ability to respond appropriately to them. There are significant individual differences in how individuals cope with environmental challenges, however, and this may be due to the interaction of heredity, development, education, and life experiences [5, 6]. Furthermore, there is substantial heterogeneity with regard to patterns of aging [7] such that some older people appear more resilient than others to the physiological consequences of various environmental challenges. Resiliency to psychophysical stress therefore may be considered an important indicator of successful aging.

To date, much of the experimental study of stress reactivity and health has focused on cardiovascular function. Despite the epidemiologic data describing the association between adverse psychosocial factors and poor diabetes control [6], the harmful effect of acute psychological stress on metabolic control is often difficult to demonstrate experimentally [8, 9]. Moreover, the studies that have investigated the role of stress response in glycemic control have included primarily younger people [8, 10], or those with already established type 1 or type 2 diabetes [9], have used specific tasks or responses to natural disasters [11] that are not usually encountered on a daily basis by older people, and have only considered glycemic responses over 2-3 hours. The purpose of this study was to examine the relation between stress reactivity and glycemic control over 24 h in healthy older people, using a common "everyday life" stress challenge. We hypothesized that (1) older subjects would demonstrate elevated cardiovascular and hormonal responses to this challenge compared with a control condition and (2) an exaggerated stress response would result in significantly disrupted glycemic control in the short term (i.e., 3 h) but not over 24 hours. Due to the robust health status of this study sample, we proposed that alterations in metabolic control in the short term would be normalized over the remainder of the day. To our knowledge, these hypotheses have not been tested before in healthy people of any age using continuous glucose monitoring.

2. Methods

2.1. Study Subjects. Older (≥60 years) volunteers ($N = 6$ men and 11 women) were recruited by advertisement from community senior centers throughout the greater New Haven County. Eligible subjects were nonsmoking, and not taking beta-blockers, glucose-lowering medication, antidepressants, or reporting an alcohol intake >2 drinks/day. To eliminate the confounding influence of cardiovascular fitness on stress reactivity and on glycemic control, all subjects were reported to be inactive (<2 days/week of moderate-intensity physical activity lasting more than 10 min duration). Interested subjects first were administered a cognitive function screening using the nine-item Short Portable Mental Status Questionnaire [12]. All persons achieving a score of 5 or fewer correct answers on the SPMSQ were excluded from further study. Interested subjects meeting the cognitive function criterion then were given a screening oral glucose tolerance test (OGTT (75 g load)) to rule out undiagnosed type 2 diabetes. Those with a fasting plasma glucose concentration $\geq 110\,\mathrm{mg\cdot dL^{-1}}$, a 2 h postchallenge measurement $\geq 140\,\mathrm{mg\cdot dL^{-1}}$ or at least one other postchallenge $\geq 180\,\mathrm{mg\cdot dL^{-1}}$ were excluded from further study. Eligible volunteers had all details of the study explained to them and signed a form indicating their informed consent. All protocols were approved by the Human Investigations Committee of the Yale School of Medicine.

2.2. Study Protocol. Each study subject underwent two separate study conditions: (1) the actual psychophysical stress challenge and (2) a seated control condition. The two conditions were randomly ordered and spaced approximately 2–4 weeks apart. Because depression may influence the relation between stress response and insulin sensitivity, subjects were administered the Center for Epidemiologic Studies-Depression (CES-D) [13] scale (a 20-item measure of the frequency of depressive symptoms over the past week) one week prior to their first study. The Perceived Stress Scale (PSS) [14] (a 10-item measure of perceived psychological stress over the previous month) was also administered at this time.

On the day of testing, subjects arrived at the Hospital Research Unit (HRU) of the Yale Center for Clinical Investigation (YCCI) at 8:00 AM in the fasted state. We chose to apply the stress stimulus in the fasted (rather than postprandial) state to avoid an anticipated wide range of postmeal glucose excursions in these older people, which could potentially mask any stress-related effects on glycemic control. Subjects were weighed and the abdominal circumference [15] was measured. Subjects then sat in a semirecumbent position for the placement of a catheter in an antecubital vein. A blood sample was drawn (15 cc) for the determination of basal glucose, insulin, and cortisol. At approximately 8:30 AM, the probe of the continuous glucose monitoring system (CGM) (MiniMed, Sylmar, CA, USA) was inserted subcutaneously in the abdominal wall and the CGM was calibrated while subjects sat quietly in the recumbent position for a 60 min equilibration period. Following the equilibration period, a baseline blood sample was drawn for the study substrates and stress hormones of interest. At about 9:30 AM, subjects then either sat quietly for 30 min reading or listening to music (seated control) or were given instructions about the tasks involved in the psychophysical challenge. Following the 30 min psychophysical challenge (or seated control condition), subjects sat quietly for another 30 min recovery period. Blood samples were taken every 15 min over the experimental (or control) and the recovery periods, and heart rate and blood pressure were measured continuously *via* an automated device (Colin Medical Instruments, Komaki, Japan), with recordings every 5 min. Interstitial glucose concentrations were also measured continuously during this time using CGM. Following the recovery period (~10:30 AM), subjects were allowed to void and were moved from the testing chair to an adjacent bed in order to perform the 3 h OGTT. Following the OGTT (~1:30 PM), subjects were fed a standardized lunch (60% carbohydrate; 20% protein; ~32 $\mathrm{kcal\cdot kg\ body\ weight^{-1}/day}$), instructed on the home use of CGM and provided with a standardized evening meal before being released from the HRU. Subjects were instructed to rest quietly for the remainder of the afternoon and evening, to eat their evening meal at ~6:00 PM, and to retire by 10:00 PM. On the following morning, subjects were visited at home in order to obtain fasting blood samples of glucose and cortisol, as well as to remove the glucose sensor probe.

2.3. Psychophysical Stress Challenge. The automated psychophysical test (APT) (National Public Services Research Center, 1996) [16, 17] is a computerized series of *timed performance measures* such as simple reaction time, choice reaction, visual tracking, static and dynamic acuity, and information processing. The APT contains a battery of items that tests specific automobile driving-related perceptual and cognitive abilities developed by the National Public Services Research Institute. As we employed these driving-related tasks solely to elicit a stress response, we did not actually score their performance. Subjects were told, however, that we were testing their driving performance as part of a study on psychophysical abilities in older age and diabetes risk. To enhance the social evaluation component of the psychophysical challenge, performance was "monitored" with a shame video camera. Immediately after the challenge (or control), subjects rated their *level of perceived threat* using 8 visual analog (100 mm) scales.

2.4. Oral Glucose Tolerance Test. To measure transient disruptions in glycemic control following the stress challenge, a 75 g OGTT was performed according to the American Diabetes Association guidelines [18]. Blood samples (5 cc each) were collected before (−15, 0 min) and following (5, 10, 20, 30, 45, 60, 90, 120, 150, and 180 min) glucose ingestion for the determination of glucose and insulin concentrations. The OGTT was terminated when the glucose value for a given subject returned to be within 10 $mg \cdot dL^{-1}$ of baseline; otherwise subjects were monitored over 3 hours.

2.5. Continuous Glucose Monitoring. Whole-day interstitial glucose profiles were collected over 24 hours using the CGMS. The device provided glucose pattern and trend data up to 288 times per day over 24 h [19, 20] by measuring interstitial glucose and converting it at a glucose oxidase interface to hydrogen peroxide, which was then oxidized to produce an amperometric signal [19]. This signal is proportional to the interstitial glucose concentration and is stored in the monitor. The stored amperometric data then were transferred and converted to glucose concentrations after data collection was completed using an infrared link to a personal computer and the data analyzed using the CGM systems solution software (version 3.0B). Four to six actual blood glucose values (obtained *via* glucometer (Medtronics, Sylmar, CA, USA)) were entered into the monitor in order to calibrate the interstitial readings. In addition to continuous readings, a number of summary data over a 24 h period were generated by CGM: (1) averaged premeal; (2) averaged 2 h postprandial; (3) 24 h averaged glucose concentrations.

2.6. Ratings of Perceived Stress and Threat. Upon completion of the psychophysical challenge, subjects rated their level of perceived stress and threat to social self using 8 visual analog (100 mm) scales [3]. These scales assessed: (1) how difficult the challenge was; (2) how confident they were in their performance; (3) how much they were personally involved in the challenge; (4) how controllable the situation was; (5) how threatening the situation was; (6) how much stress they were experiencing due to failure; (7) how much stress they were feeling due to time constraints; (8) how content they were with their performance. At one end of the scale was the rating of "not at all" (0 mm) and at the other (100 mm), the rating "extremely."

2.7. Stress Hormone and Substrate Analysis. All blood samples were analyzed in the core laboratory of the YCCI. Plasma *cortisol* concentrations were determined by radioimmunoassay (Diagnostic Products Corporation, Los Angeles, CA, USA). Plasma *glucose* was analyzed by the glucose oxidase method (YSI 2300, Yellow Springs Instruments, Yellow Springs, OH, USA). Plasma immunoreactive *insulin* concentrations were determined with a double antibody radioimmunoassay (Diagnostic, Webster, TX, USA).

2.8. Statistical Analysis. Univariate statistics ($\chi \pm$ SD) were first generated on all study variables for descriptive purposes. Total area and incremental area under the cortisol, as well as under the OGTT glucose and insulin curves (AUC), were determined by the trapezoidal method. In addition, we considered peak cortisol response, as well as the basal cortisol concentrations taken in the morning before and the morning after the psychological challenge to use in combination with the cortisol response curve as an additional indicator of integrated stress response. Mean differences in the physiological response variables between the two conditions were tested using paired *t*-tests. The relation between stress response and disrupted glycemic control (AUC and CGM summary variables) was determined using analysis of variance (ANOVA) for repeated measures. The original CGM data then were transferred into StatLab and were smoothed using cubic splines with an empirically selected smoothing parameter. Individual and pooled CGM data curves were examined by study condition to determine the degree of variability of response between the two conditions. Statistical significance was set at an alpha level of 0.05.

3. Results

The age of the study sample was 72 ± 9 years, with a range from 60 to 88 years. On average, subjects were overweight (27 ± 4 $kg \cdot m^{-2}$), but were normotensive (127 ± 10/73 ± 10 mmHg) and had normal glucose tolerance based on 2 h postchallenge blood glucose concentrations from the screening OGTT (130 ± 22 $mg \cdot dL^{-1}$). In addition, scores of depressive symptoms (9 ± 4) and perceived stress (12 ± 6) were within normative values for that age group (12,13). Not surprisingly, subject perception of the difficulty (56.8 ± 18.6 versus 3.7 ± 4.2 mm), threat (34.3 ± 30.3 versus 4.8 ± 5.7 mm), time stress (61.8 ± 39.4 versus 16.4 ± 28.0 mm), and failure stress (61.7 ± 34.3 versus 5.0 ± 5.8 mm) were significantly greater following the psychophysical challenge, compared with the control condition ($P < 0.01$). These perceptual data were corroborated by significant differences in cardiovascular responses in both systolic and diastolic blood pressure and heart rate between the two conditions ($P < 0.01$; Figure 1).

Average cortisol AUC response over the experimental and recovery period was not significantly higher during the stress relative to the control condition, with the exception of peak response at 30 min (10.6 ± 3.1 versus 8.6 ± 2.6 $\mu g \cdot dL^{-1}$, resp.; $P < 0.05$). When the data were stratified by median age, however, peak cortisol response from the stress condition was significantly amplified in subjects <70 years ($n = 9$) but reversed in those ≥70 years ($n = 8$) (Figure 2). For example, during the stress condition, 30 min cortisol concentrations increased from baseline by 22% ($P < 0.05$) in the younger subjects, but *decreased* by 7% in those aged 70 years and older. This variation in cortisol response was attributable to a significantly higher basal level in those ≥70 years, compared with their younger counterparts ($P < 0.05$).

The OGTT-derived glucose and insulin response curves following the stress and control conditions are shown in Figure 3. Although clearly elevated and indicative of

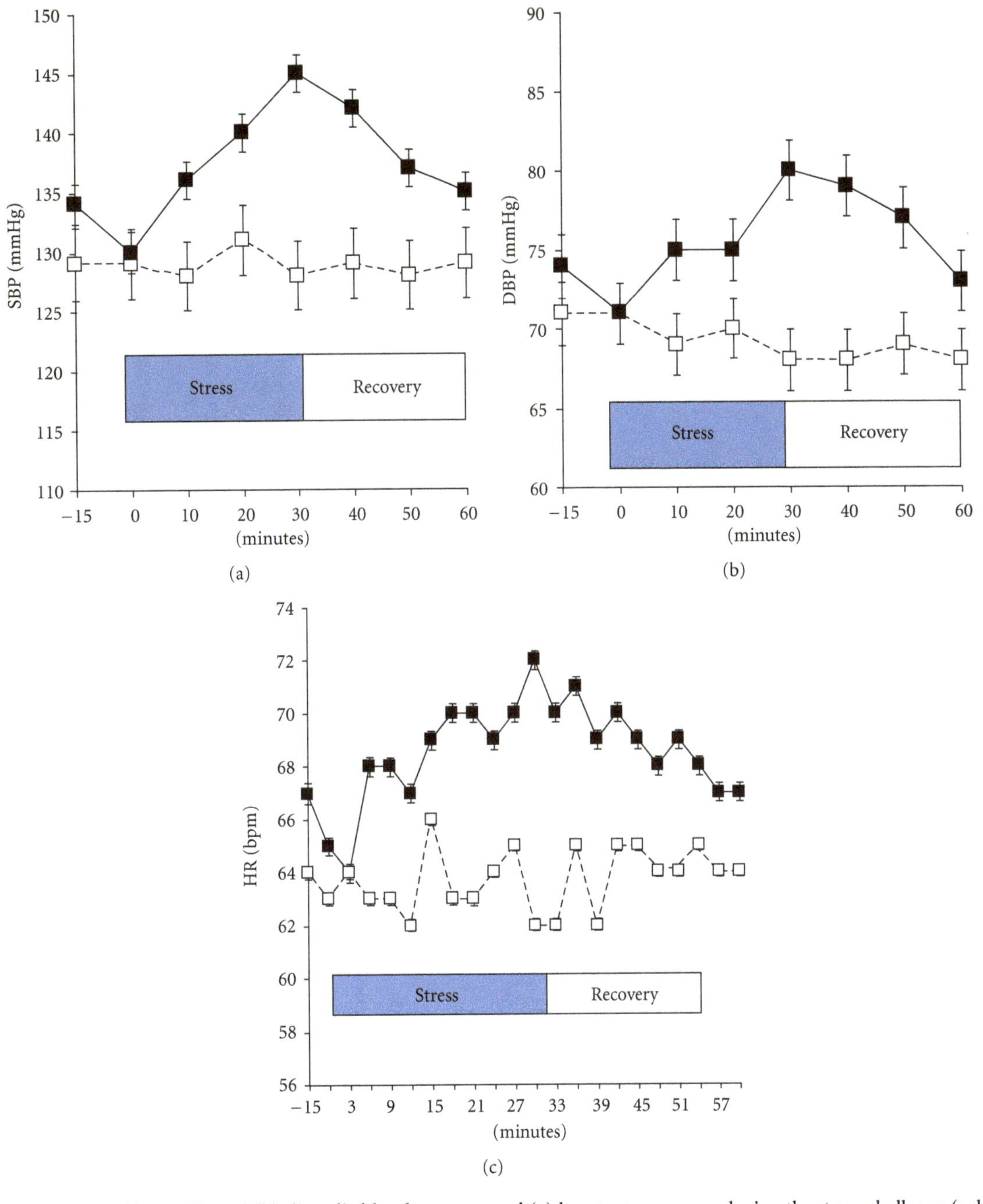

FIGURE 1: Differences in (a) systolic and (b) diastolic blood pressure and (c) heart rate response during the stress challenge (solid line) and control (broken line) condition. Data are mean ± se; $N = 17$.

impaired glycemic control, the curves are quite similar for the two conditions, with the exception of the peak glucose response shifting from 60 to 90 min and the peak insulin response shifting from 90 to 120 min following the stress condition. These findings were unaltered after stratifying the data by age group (<70/≥70 yrs). Of note in this figure, however, is the average 2 h glucose concentration from the screening OGTT, which is significantly lower (130 ± 22 mg·dL^{-1}; $P < 0.05$) than 2 h values following either the stress (182 ± 43 mg·dL^{-1}) or control (174 ± 60 mg·dL^{-1}) conditions. Glucose curves obtained *via* CGM over 24 h are displayed for each condition in Figure 4 and suggest a rightward shift and a 30–40 min delay in peak postchallenge glucose response following the stress condition, with glucose levels elevated relative to the control condition for as long as 6 hours afterward. We observed no difference, however, in averaged 24 h glucose concentrations (111.7 ± 12.3 versus 114.0 ± 24.0 mg·dL^{-1}), or averaged prelunch concentrations (130.7 ± 43.9 versus 129.7 ± 47.0 mg·dL^{-1}) between the two conditions, although averaged 2 h postlunch glucose concentrations (measured at approximately 4 PM) were slightly higher following the stress compared with the control

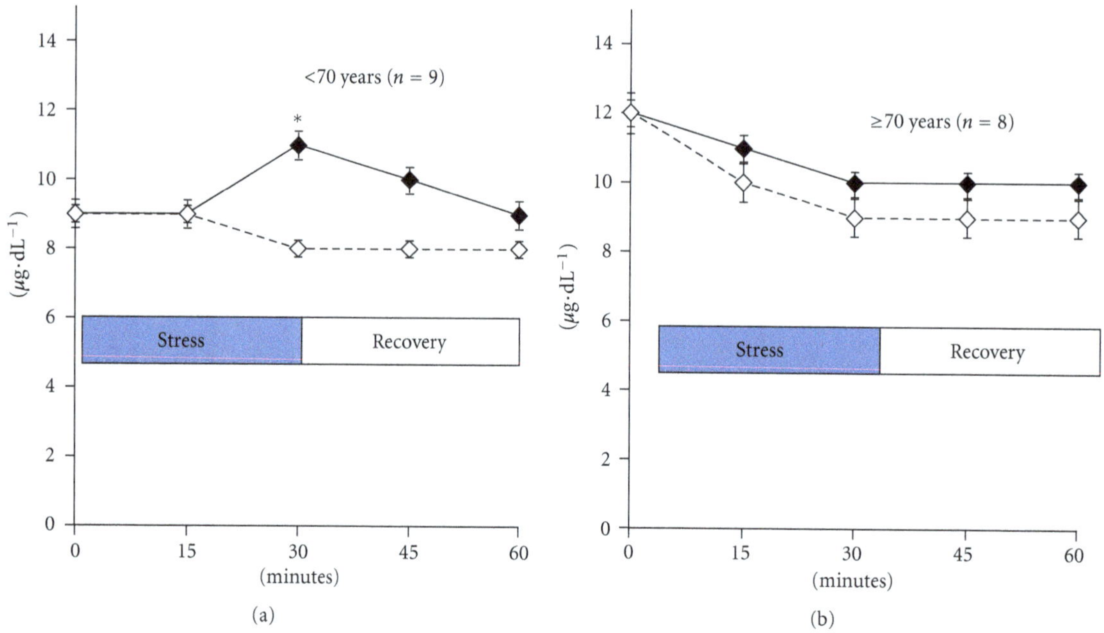

FIGURE 2: Cortisol responses between the stress condition (solid line) and the control (broken line) condition by age group. Age groups are based on the median cut point of the distribution. Data are mean ± se; $N = 17$; $^*P < 0.05$.

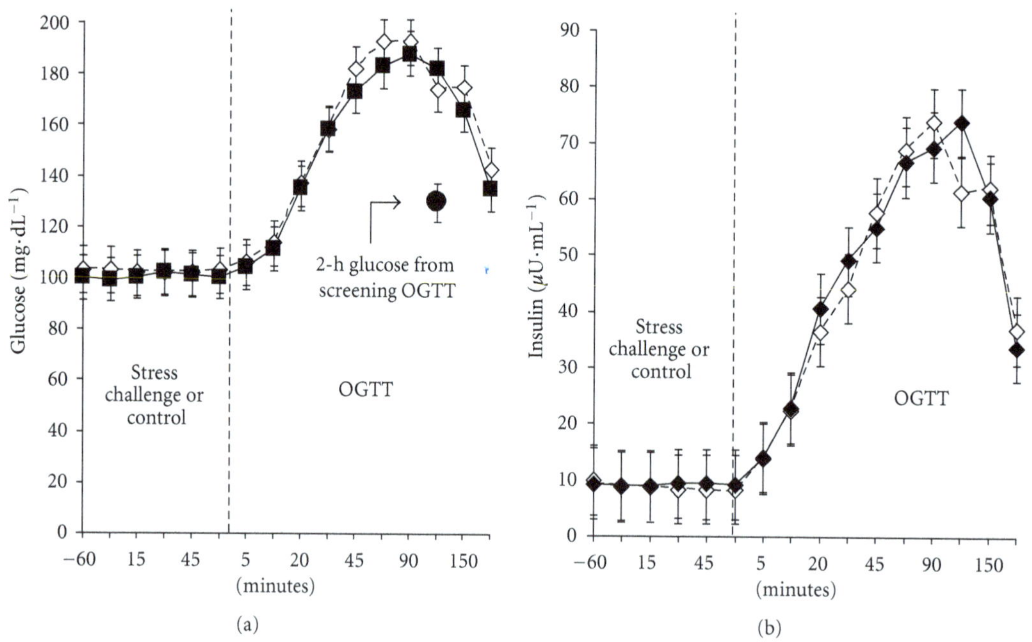

FIGURE 3: Glucose and insulin responses over the experimental period and the OGTT between the stress (solid line) and control (broken line) conditions. Data are mean ± se; $N = 17$. To convert to the International System of Units (mmol), multiply glucose values by 0.055.

condition (106.6 ± 22.3 versus $96.9 \pm 12.3\,\text{mg}\cdot\text{dL}^{-1}$, resp.; $P < 0.07$). Variability of glycemic response appeared greater following the stress, compared with the control condition; however, differences in the estimates of mean skewness (0.70 ± 0.51 versus 0.57 ± 0.56, resp.) and kurtosis (3.38 ± 0.91 versus 3.04 ± 1.22, resp.) were not statistically significant.

4. Discussion

Adaptation to stress frequently involves the activation of the hypothalamic pituitary adrenal (HPA) axis in order to mobilize energy stores. Although the anti-insulin and gluconeogenetic actions of cortisol appear consistent with this

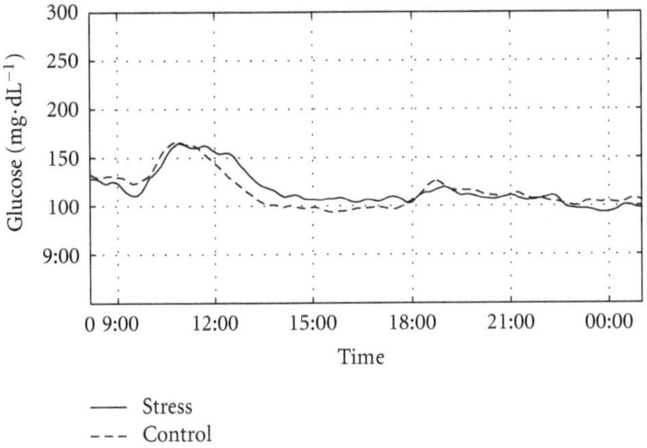

FIGURE 4: Glucose response curves obtained over 24 h *via* CGMS following the stress (solid line) or control (broken line) conditions. Data are mean values; Time = time of day; $N = 17$. To convert to the International System of Units (mmol), multiply glucose values by 0.055.

notion, there is limited experimental evidence to support this idea [8]. We observed significant evidence of perceived stress and cardiovascular engagement to a 30 min psychophysical stressor among healthy older people, although HPA response appeared somewhat blunted relative to responses observed in other studies of older people [21, 22]. We did observe that our oldest study subjects (i.e., ≥70 years) had significantly greater basal cortisol concentrations compared with younger (<70 years) subjects, which is consistent with what has been proposed by Seeman and Robbins [23] and perhaps reflects the allostatic burden of aging, as the perceived stress scores were significantly higher in the oldest subjects compared with the younger subjects (14.4 ± 5.2 versus 9.5 ± 5.8; $P < 0.05$). Contrary to what we hypothesized, 3 h post-OGTT glucose and insulin concentrations were elevated equally under both conditions, suggesting little effect of the stress challenge *per se* on short-term glycemic control in those both older and younger than 70 years. Moreover, the CGM data provided evidence that tight glucose homeostasis may be only minimally altered following a stressful episode in healthy older people. Any subtle differences in glycemic control apparent up to 6 h after challenge had completely dissipated by 24 h, and CGMS data averaged over 24 h indicated no differences in overall response following the stress and control conditions. Whether these findings are indicative of heightened resiliency in successful (relative to normal) aging, of normal aging-specific homeostatic control, or of methodological differences between our study and others is not clear.

In general, studies that applied stressors during the fasted state observed significantly blunted cortisol and negligible glycemic responses [8, 9] compared with stress applied in the postprandial state [8, 9, 24], suggesting that ready access to energy is necessary for the permissive effects of HPA reactivity on glycemic control. We applied the psychophysical stress in the fasted state (thinking that prevailing glucose stores would be ample in this older population and wishing to avoid large postmeal glucose excursions), which more than likely explains the blunted cortisol response and minimal stress effects on 3 h postchallenge metabolic control.

Interestingly, 2 h postchallenge glycemic responses to the OGTT (measured at ~12:30 PM) were markedly elevated in both the stress and control conditions, compared with the early morning screening OGTT (182 ± 43 versus 174 ± 60 versus 130 ± 22 mg·dL^{-1}, resp., for the stress, control, and screening conditions). These previously reported late-morning exaggerated glycemic excursions [25] may be attributed to the diurnal drop in insulin secretion reported in older people at this time of day [26] and more than likely prevented any further stress-related disruption. However, there is also other evidence that a stress challenge does not increase overall glycemic response, but rather shifts the peak response to the right, suggesting a stress-related *delay* in glucose absorption by the gut [23]. Our postchallenge glucose and CGM response curves are consistent with this delayed absorption phenomenon, as are the prevailing insulin concentrations from the OGTT, as the peak insulin response shifted from 90 min to 120 min. Nonetheless, if we consider the OGTT as the trigger for setting the stress-induced allostatic control response in motion, we observed only slight alterations with this control following the stress compared with the control condition—evidenced by the small lag in peak glucose response at 30–40 min after challenge, the slower rate of glucose clearance over the subsequent 6 hours (but not beyond), and the slightly greater individual variability in glycemic control. Consistent with HPA reactivity studies performed in the postprandial state [8, 9, 24], greater fuel availability 2 h following refeeding may have contributed to greater averaged postlunch glucose concentrations following the stress relative to the control condition, despite the fact that prelunch values were similar. These subtle differences would not have been detected without the use of CGM over 24 h.

The issue of selective survival is an important consideration when performing challenge studies in people who are in their 8th and 9th decades of life. Indeed, one hallmark of successful aging is a greater physiological resiliency to various environmental perturbations compared with people who have not survived to that age or who could not meet inclusion criteria for the study. Thus, although we used a stressor that mimics challenges often encountered daily in real life, it may not have been of sufficient intensity or duration for such a robust older population. This issue of an insufficient stimulus may be particularly problematic given the degree of inter- and intraindividual variability in physiological response to stress that was evident in our data and those of others [21, 27]. Also, the stress challenge was applied in the morning, when glucose concentrations were at their lowest. Had we performed the stress challenge in the later afternoon, when cortisol concentrations reach their daily nadir, we likely would have observed a greater relative increase in HPA response as others have [21, 22]. However, due to a possible diurnal drop in insulin secretion in the late afternoon, glucose responses under both conditions would have been exaggerated even more than we observed, thereby further masking any stress-induced effects.

In conclusion, the true nature of the relationship between stress and glucose homeostasis remains elusive and may be influenced by a number of individual, environmental, or temporal conditions. Our use of CGM allowed us to unmask some subtle short-term stress-related disruptions, but these alterations dissipated over 24 h in this healthy sample. On the other hand, given the number of environmental (e.g., driving, shopping) and psychological stressors encountered daily among the general population of older people, these findings may have greater relevance for less robust people with already-existing impairments in glucose control or with diabetes.

Acknowledgments

The authors thank the nursing and technical staffs of the Hospital Research Unit of the Yale Center for Clinical Investigations for their technical expertise and the study subjects for their commitment to this research. This paper was made possible by the CTSA Grant no. UL1 RR024139 from the National Center for Research Resources (NCRR), a component of the National Institutes of Health (NIH), and NIH Roadmap for Medical Research. Its contents are solely the responsibility of the authors and do not necessarily represent the official view of NCRR or NIH. This work was supported by Grant NIH/NIA R21 AG.027470 (LDP).

References

[1] K. E. Habib, P. W. Gold, and G. P. Chrousos, "Neuroendocrinology of stress," *Endocrinology and Metabolism Clinics of North America*, vol. 30, no. 3, pp. 695–728, 2001.

[2] P. Sterling and J. Eyer, "Allostasis: a new paradigm to explain arousal pathology," in *Handbook of Life Stress, Cognition, and Health*, S. Fisher and J. Reason, Eds., pp. 629–649, John Wiley & Sons, New York, NY, USA, 1988.

[3] B. M. Kudielka, A. K. Schmidt-Reinwald, D. H. Hellhammer, T. Schürmeyer, and C. Kirschbaum, "Psychosocial stress and HPA functioning: no evidence for a reduced resilience in healthy elderly men," *Stress*, vol. 3, no. 3, pp. 229–240, 2000.

[4] W. W. Spirduso, "Aging and motor control," in *Prospectives in Exercise Science and Sports Medicine*, D. R. Lamb, C. V. Gisolfi, and E. R. Nadel, Eds., vol. 8 of *Exercise in Older Adults*, pp. 53–114, Cooper Publishing, Carmel, Indiana, 1995.

[5] B. McEwen, T. E. Seeman, and The Allostatic Load Working Group, "Allostatic load and allostasis," MacArthur Research Network on Socioeconomic Status and Health, The John D. and Catherine T. MacArthur Foundation, 1999, http://www.macses.ucsf.edu/research/allostatic/.

[6] Y. Chida and M. Hamer, "An association of adverse psychosocial factors with diabetes mellitus: a meta-analytic review of longitudinal cohort studies," *Diabetologia*, vol. 51, no. 12, pp. 2168–2178, 2008.

[7] J. W. Rowe and R. L. Kahn, "Human aging: usual and successful," *Science*, vol. 237, no. 4811, pp. 143–149, 1987.

[8] C. Kirschbaum, E. G. Bono, N. Rohleder et al., "Effects of fasting and glucose load on free cortisol responses to stress and nicotine," *Journal of Clinical Endocrinology and Metabolism*, vol. 82, no. 4, pp. 1101–1105, 1997.

[9] P. Wiesli, C. Schmid, O. Kerwer et al., "Acute psychological stress affects glucose concentrations in patients with type 1 diabetes following food intake but not in the fasting state," *Diabetes Care*, vol. 28, no. 8, pp. 1910–1915, 2005.

[10] G. Seematter, E. Guenat, P. Schneiter, C. Cayeux, E. Jéquier, and L. Tappy, "Effects of mental stress on insulin-mediated glucose metabolism and energy expenditure in lean and obese women," *American Journal of Physiology*, vol. 279, pp. E799–E805, 2000.

[11] A. Inui, H. Kitaoka, M. Majima et al., "Effect of the Kobe earthquake on stress and glycemic control in patients with diabetes mellitus," *Archives of Internal Medicine*, vol. 158, no. 3, pp. 274–278, 1998.

[12] E. Pfeiffer, "A short portable mental status questionnaire for the assessment of organic brain deficit in elderly patients," *Journal of the American Geriatrics Society*, vol. 23, no. 10, pp. 433–441, 1975.

[13] L. S. Radloff, "The CES-D scale: a self-report depression scale for research in the general population," *Applied Psychological Measurement*, vol. 1, pp. 385–401, 1977.

[14] S. Cohen and G. M. Williamson, "Perceived stress in a probability sample of the United States," in *The Social Psychology of Health*, S. Spacapan and S. Oskamp, Eds., pp. 31–67, Sage, Newbury Park, Calif, USA, 1988.

[15] T. Rankinen, S.-Y. Kim, L. Pérusse, J. P. Després, and C. Bouchard, "The prediction of abdominal visceral fat level from body composition and anthropometry: ROC analysis," *International Journal of Obesity*, vol. 23, no. 8, pp. 801–809, 1999.

[16] A. S. McKnight and A. J. McKnight, "The automated psychophysical test (APT) for assessing age-diminished capabilities," *Behavior Research Methods, Instruments, & Computers*, vol. 26, pp. 187–191, 1994.

[17] A. S. McKnight and A. J. McKnight, "Multivariate analysis of age-related driver ability and performance deficits," *Accident Analysis and Prevention*, vol. 31, no. 5, pp. 445–454, 1999.

[18] National Diabetes Study Group, "Report of the expert committee on the diagnosis and classification of diabetes mellitus," *Diabetes Care*, vol. 20, no. 7, pp. 1183–1197, 1997.

[19] J. J. Mastrototaro, "The MiniMed continuous glucose monitoring system (CGMS)," *Journal of Pediatric Endocrinology and Metabolism*, vol. 12, no. 3, pp. 751–758, 1999.

[20] J. J. Mastrototaro and T. M. Gross, "Reproducibility of the continuous glucose monitoring system matches previous reports and the intended use of the product," *Diabetes Care*, vol. 26, no. 1, pp. 256–257, 2003.

[21] T. E. Seeman, L. F. Berkman, B. I. Gulanski et al., "Self-esteem and neuroendocrine response to challenge: MacArthur studies of successful aging," *Journal of Psychosomatic Research*, vol. 39, no. 1, pp. 69–84, 1995a.

[22] T. E. Seeman, B. Singer, and P. Charpentier, "Gender differences in patterns of HPA axis response to challenge: MacArthur studies of successful aging," *Psychoneuroendocrinology*, vol. 20, no. 7, pp. 711–725, 1995b.

[23] T. E. Seeman and R. J. Robbins, "Aging and hypothalamic-pituitary-adrenal response to challenge in humans," *Endocrine Reviews*, vol. 15, no. 2, pp. 233–260, 1994.

[24] R. R. Wing, L. H. Epstein, E. Blair, and M. P. Nowalk, "Psychologic stress and blood glucose levels in nondiabetic subjects," *Psychosomatic Medicine*, vol. 47, no. 6, pp. 558–564, 1985.

[25] P. Z. Zimmet, J. R. Wall, R. Rome, L. Stimmler, and R. J. Jarrett, "Diurnal variation in glucose tolerance: associated changes in plasma insulin, growth hormone, and non-esterified fatty acids," *British Medical Journal*, vol. 1, no. 906, pp. 485–488, 1974.

[26] K. S. Polonsky, B. D. Given, L. J. Hirsch et al., "Abnormal patterns of insulin secretion in non-insulin-dependent diabetes mellitus," *New England Journal of Medicine*, vol. 318, no. 19, pp. 1231–1239, 1988.

[27] J. R. Kramer, J. Ledolter, G. N. Manos, and M. L. Bayless, "Stress and metabolic control in diabetes mellitus: methodological issues and an illustrative analysis," *Annals of Behavioral Medicine*, vol. 22, no. 1, pp. 17–28, 2000.

10

The Role of Lifestyle Behaviors on 20-Year Cognitive Decline

D. Cadar,[1,2] H. Pikhart,[2] G. Mishra,[3] A. Stephen,[4] D. Kuh,[1] and M. Richards[1]

[1] *MRC Unit for Lifelong Health and Ageing, London WC1B 5JU, UK*
[2] *Faculty of Population Health Sciences, University College London, London WC1E 6BT, UK*
[3] *School of Population Health, University of Queensland, Herston, QLD 4006, Australia*
[4] *MRC Human Nutrition Research, Elsie Widdowson Laboratory, 120 Fulbourn Road, Cambridge CB1 9NL, UK*

Correspondence should be addressed to D. Cadar, dorina.cadar.09@ucl.ac.uk and M. Richards, m.richards@nshd.mrc.ac.uk

Academic Editor: Allison A. M. Bielak

This study examined the association between smoking, physical activity and dietary choice at 36 and 43 years, and change in these lifestyle behaviors between these ages, and decline in verbal memory and visual search speed between 43 and 60–64 years in 1018 participants from MRC National Survey of Health and Development (NSHD, the British 1946 birth cohort). ANCOVA models were adjusted for sex, social class of origin, childhood cognition, educational attainment, adult social class, and depression; then the lifestyle behaviors were additionally mutually adjusted. Results showed that healthy dietary choice and physical activity were associated, respectively, with slower memory and visual search speed decline over 20 years, with evidence that increasing physical activity was important. Adopting positive health behaviors from early midlife may be beneficial in reducing the rate of cognitive decline and ultimately reducing the risk of dementia.

1. Introduction

With an increase in the ageing population, the number of older people affected by cognitive decline and dementia is continually rising, causing a major public health impact on individuals and governments around the world [1]. Despite major progress in understanding the neurobiology of cognitive impairment and dementia, there are still no clear determinants and complete causal models available for explaining risks for this condition [2]. Substantial evidence suggests that certain lifestyle behaviors (particularly smoking, sedentary lifestyle, and poor dietary choices) predict faster cognitive decline [3–5], and higher risk of dementia [6, 7], while physical, mental and social leisure activities are found to be protective [8, 9]. A study of London civil servants [10] highlights that the number and duration of unhealthy behaviors are associated with subsequent cognitive function in later life. Similar findings from the Suwon Longitudinal Aging Study (SLAS) showed that a combination of multiple positive lifestyle behaviors (such as nonsmoking, vegetable consumption, and social activity) was associated with higher cognitive ability [11]. However, since these behaviors tend to cluster [12, 13], the extent to which apparent effects of one behavior are attributable to (i.e., confounded by) another is uncertain.

In addition, relatively little is known about the longitudinal effects of these behaviors on cognitive decline; yet associations among multiple health behaviors place the emphasis on longitudinal studies, since patterns of behaviors tend to develop over decades, with implications for targeted interventions to change the aggregate public health risk [14]. The life course approach to age-related diseases [15, 16] provides an important opportunity to identify the nature and timing of different environmental contributions to neuronal damage and the risk of dementia across life [17]. The present study therefore focuses on behavioral risk in early midlife, at a stage of the life course when people are still more likely to have control over modifiable risk and protective factors for cognitive decline than in later life.

Although clinically significant cognitive decline and the onset of dementia occur in older age (65+ years), it is important to take in consideration early signs of cognitive decline that appear in midlife. This is because conditions such as dementia develop slowly and silently over the preceding decades [18–20]. Neuroimaging also show pathological changes in midlife before the clinical signs of the disease appear [21, 22]. Consistent with this, subtle cognitive decline begins as least as early as the 5th decade [23, 24].

Risk and protective factors for health can exert their most critical influences at different ages [25]. This is acknowledged by the life course approach and the hypothesis that positive lifestyle behaviors such as nonsmoking, being physically active, and choosing healthier diets may protect cognitive functioning and slow cognitive decline in later life. Fratiglioni et al. identified key periods for potential risk and protective factors [25]. Early life seems to be most critical for the development of cognitive reserve (learning and education) [26], when distal adverse influences (such as poor childhood social circumstances) contribute to the risk of adult disease or later life risk of dementia. Lifestyle behaviors, including those that influence cardiovascular and metabolic risk, become more influential in midlife, although some, such as diet and physical activity, track back into childhood [27, 28], whereas mental and physical activity patterns may continue to moderate these risks into later life [29, 30].

The fact that the lifestyle behaviors are modifiable implies that encouraging a healthy lifestyle may prevent or ameliorate cognitive decline and underlying cerebrovascular and cardiovascular risk factors [31]. Such interventions should take into account the relative beneficial effect of each independent behavior as well as their combined and cumulative effect.

1.1. Present Study. The aim of the current study was to examine the role of individual and combined lifestyle behaviors (smoking, physical activity, and dietary choice) on a 20-year interval of cognitive decline. We used measures of memory and psychomotor speed over this interval, which are sensitive to decline associated with ageing and neurodegeneration. The repeated measures of lifestyle behaviors at 36 and 43 years were used as predictors of cognitive change from 43 to 60–64 years. In addition to the independent and combined effects of these behaviors, we also examined the cumulative effects of these behaviors across early midlife and the changes in these behaviors from one age to another.

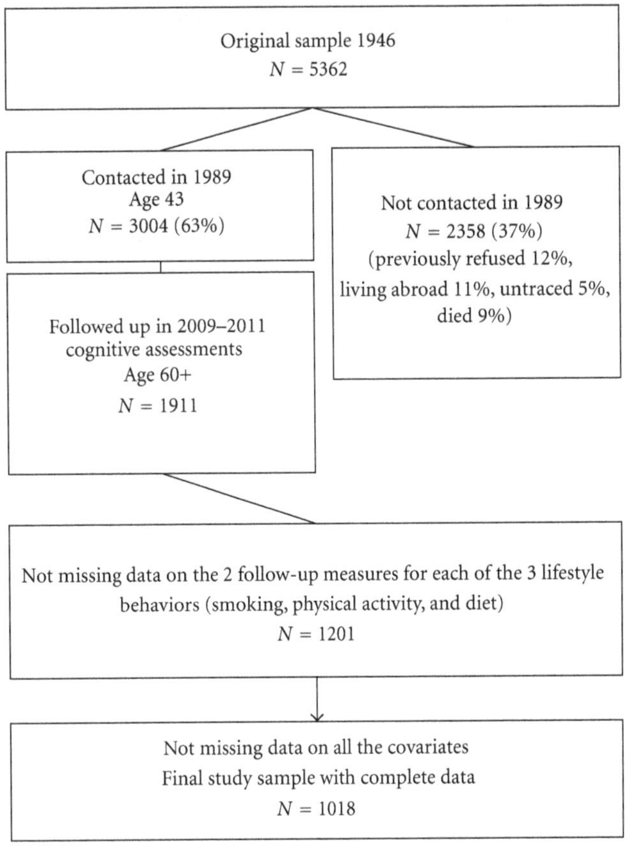

FIGURE 1: Flow chart of lifestyle behaviors, cognitive functioning and covariates data follow up (considered since baseline cognition-at age 43) in the Medical Research Council National Survey of Health and Development.

2. Methods

2.1. Study Members. The Medical Research Council National Survey of Health and Development (NSHD) originally consisted of a socially stratified sample of 5362 children born within marriage in one week in March 1946 in England, Scotland, and Wales [32, 33]. This cohort has been followed up prospectively 23 times, from birth onwards. In 1989, when study members were aged 43 years, 3262 were successfully contacted, of whom 3004 have completed both cognitive tests. Of these, 1911 had successfully completed the most recent cognitive assessment, conducted between 2006 and 2011 when survey members were aged 60 to 64 years (henceforth 60+ years). This data collection began with a postal questionnaire sent to the target 3163 sample [33]. This was followed by an invitation to an assessment by trained nurses at one of six clinical research facilities (based in Cardiff, Birmingham, Edinburgh, London (at UCL and St Thomas' hospitals), and Manchester), or, if preferred, at a home visit. This was supplemented by a further questionnaire sent to those who agreed to a clinic or home visit. These questionnaires, along with additional questions asked by the nurses, updated information on general health, household composition, family structure, socioeconomic status, daily function, life events, and lifestyle. Contact was not attempted for 2198 (718 deaths, 567 living abroad, 594 prior refusals, and 320 permanently lost). From the current respondents, a total of 1,018 study members had nonmissing data for all variables incorporated in these analyses (see Figure 1).

2.2. Ethical Approval. The study protocol received ethical approval from the Greater Manchester Local Research Ethics Committee for the five English sites; from Scotland Research Ethics Committee for the data collection taking place in Edinburgh. Written informed consent was obtained from the study member at each stage of data collection.

2.3. Cognitive Function. Cognitive functioning was measured at 43 and 60+ years using two tests: verbal memory and speed and concentration. The verbal memory test consisted of a 15-item word learning task devised by the NSHD research team. Each word was shown for two seconds. When all 15 words were shown, the study member was asked to write down as many of these as possible, in any order. The total number of words correctly recalled over three identical trials was summed to provide an overall score for short-term verbal memory (maximum score = 45). This was followed by a letter search test (see below), after which an uncued delayed free recall trial was administered.

Speed and concentration were assessed with a letter search task in which participants were required to cross out the letters P and W, randomly embedded within a page of other letters, as quickly as possible within 1 minute. At age 43 years the total number of letters to be searched was 450, and at age 60+ years it was 600. Scores were computed as total number of letters searched.

2.4. Lifestyle Behaviors. Data on lifestyle behaviors were extracted from questionnaires, interview-based prospective information, and diet diaries completed in early midlife (36 and 43 years).

2.5. Smoking. Interview-based prospective information on cigarette smoking frequency was obtained at age 36 and 43 years. Smoking frequency was categorized at each age as 0 (nonsmoker), 1 to 20 (light smoker), or more than 20 cigarettes per day (heavy smokers).

A midlife smoking score was derived by assigning those classified as nonsmokers a value of 0, those as light smokers a value of 1, and those as heavy smokers a value of 2 at each age (36 and 43 years) and then summing the values for the 2 ages whereby an individual with a midlife smoking score of 0 was categorized as nonsmoker, an individual with a midlife smoking score of 1 to 3 was categorized as moderate smoker, and the remaining individuals were categorized as heavy smokers (sum equal 4).

A score for change in smoking behavior was also derived by assigning those classified as nonsmokers at each age a value of 0; those reporting an increase in smoking a score of 1; those who reported a decrease in smoking a score of 2; those who were constantly moderate or heavy smokers across early midlife a score of 3.

2.6. Physical Activity. Physical activity levels were ascertained at ages 36 and 43 years during interviews at the study participants' home. Questions about physical activity at age 36 years were based on the Minnesota leisure time physical activity questionnaire [27, 34]. The questions addressed engagement in sports and recreational activities in the previous month, utilizing a checklist of 27 different leisure time activities. At age 43 years, participation in any sports, vigorous leisure activities, or exercise was reported, although this was based on answers to an open-ended question, rather than the above checklist. However, the monthly frequency of these activities was also reported, enabling a similar categorization to the 36 year measure. At each age, participants were categorized as inactive (reported no participation); moderately active (participated in relevant activities 1–4 times in the previous month at age 36 years, and per month at age 43 years); or most active (participated in relevant activities five or more times in the previous month at age 36 years and per month at age 43 years) [35].

A total physical activity score was derived by assigning those classified as inactive a value of 0, those as moderately active a value of 1, and those as most active a value of 2 at each age (36 and 43 years) and then summing the values for the two ages. This was categorized as inactive (score 0), moderately active (score 1 to 3), and most active (score 4).

A score for change in physical activity behavior, was derived in a similar fashion as for smoking, by assigning those classified as inactive at each age a value of 0; those reporting an increase in activity a score of 1; those who reported a decrease in their physical activity levels a score of 2; those whose physical activity levels were moderate or most active at both ages a score of 3.

2.7. Dietary Choice. Dietary intake was assessed by a five-day diary [36] at both 36 and 43 years. All food and drinks consumed both at and away from home were recorded in the diaries, including brand names of food products, food preparation methods, and recipes used. Participants were asked to record the amount eaten in household measures, with guidance notes and photography provided in the diary to assist in estimating portion size [37]. From this information, an overall score representing level of healthy food choice was derived, by summing scores for four separate criteria: (1) consumption of breakfast (a score of 0 representing no consumption to 1 some days and 2 all days); (2) type of milk (from 0 whole only to 3 skim milk only); (3) type of bread (from 0 white only to 4 wholemeal only); (4) number of daily portions of fruit and vegetables (from 0 to maximum 5 portions per day); a dietary reference score representing the percentage of energy from fat, carbohydrates, and protein (scores from 1-highest to 5-lowest percentages less than 30% energy). The total score was subject to a median split (median = 10 at age 36 years and median = 11 at age 43 years; minimum score 0 and maximum 19) to represent low versus high (energy dense/nutrient poor versus healthier) dietary choice. The range of dietary scores varied from a minimum of 5 to a maximum of 19; $M = 10.22$, SD = 1.84 at age 36; $M = 11.42$, SD = 2.27 at age 43).

A midlife dietary choice score was also derived by assigning those classified as making poorer choices for their diet a value of 0 and those making healthier choices a value of 1 at each age (36 and 43 years) and then summing up the values for the 2 ages. Midlife dietary choice was categorized as making poorer (low) choices at both ages (score 0) and making healthier dietary choices (high) at least at one age (score 1 or 2).

A score for change in diet was also derived. Those classified as choosing a low-quality diet at each age were assigned a value of 0; those reporting an increase from a low-quality to a high-quality diet a score of 1; those who changed to a lower-quality diet a score of 2; those who constantly maintain a high-quality diet were assigned a score of 3.

2.8. Covariates. Based on previous findings, the following variables were treated as potential confounders: sex; father social class; childhood cognitive ability; educational attainment; midlife household occupational social class and depression [14, 38–40].

2.9. Occupational Social Class of Origin. *Occupational social class of origin* was represented by father's social class when participants were aged 11 years, or if this was unknown, at age 4 or 15 years. This was classified as professional managerial intermediate, skilled nonmanual, skilled manual, semi-skilled manual, or unskilled, according to the UK Registrar General's Classification of Occupations [41].

2.10. Prior Cognitive Ability. Childhood cognitive ability at age eight years was represented as the sum of four tests of verbal and nonverbal ability devised by the National Foundation for Educational Research [42]. These tests were (1) reading comprehension (selecting appropriate words to complete 35 sentences); (2) word reading (ability to read and pronounce 50 words); (3) vocabulary (ability to explain the meaning of 50 words); (4) picture intelligence, consisting of a 60-item nonverbal reasoning test.

2.11. Educational Attainment. The highest educational qualification achieved by age 26 years was dichotomized into those with advanced ("A level", taken during the final year of secondary/high school) or higher (university or equivalent) qualifications, versus those below this level.

2.12. Occupational Social Class. Household midlife occupational social class was used at each time of the health behavior (36 or 43 years), or the latest age for longitudinal behavioral measures (see below). This was coded according to the Registrar General (as for social class of origin).

2.13. Depression and Anxiety Symptoms. Frequency and severity of common symptoms of depression and anxiety were assessed by the Psychiatric Symptom Frequency scale (PSF) [43] at age 43 years, and with the 28-item General Health Questionnaire (GHQ) [44] at age 60+.

2.14. Statistical Analyses. Multivariable ANCOVA models were used to test associations between smoking, physical activity, and diet at each age, entered as categorical variables and cognitive decline, used as continuous variables. First, we tested the association between each lifestyle behavior at 36 and 43 years and change in both cognitive outcomes (verbal memory and letter search speed); then we used the cumulative behavior scores for both these ages; finally we tested associations between change in behaviors between these ages and change in the cognitive outcomes between ages 43 and 60+ years. In order to reduce the effect of regression to the mean and because of the difference in size of the letter search matrix at ages 43 and 60+ years, we used conditional models of change by adjusting cognitive scores at age 60+ years for their corresponding score at 43 years [23]. Positive coefficients represent a slower rate of decline, and negative coefficients represented a faster rate of decline. Model 1 adjusted raw associations for sex (since there was no evidence of sex x lifestyle behavior interactions on the outcomes), social class of origin, prior cognitive ability at age 8 years, educational attainment, occupational class, and symptoms of anxiety and depression. Model 2 included these covariates but additionally tested the specificity of lifestyle behaviors by mutually adjusting each for the other behaviors. For cumulative effects, model 2 was further adjusted for the cumulative scores of the additional behaviour; for change in behaviour from 36 to 43, model 2 was mutually adjusted for the change in other lifestyle behaviours. All analyses were based on the sample with complete data on cognitive tests at the 2 time points, lifestyle behaviors at the 2 time points, and all the selected covariates.

3. Results

3.1. Sample Description and Missing Data. Participants with missing scores on memory and visual search at age 43 were more likely to be men, to have less than advanced educational attainment, to be in a manual occupation in midlife, and to have lower cognitive capability scores at age 8 years (all $P < 0.001$). A similar pattern was observed for those without cognitive scores at age 60+. Those with missing scores on memory at age 43 had a marginally higher total anxiety and depression score at the same age than those who underwent memory testing ($P = 0.058$). Those who did not complete data on lifestyle behaviors at both 36 and 43 years had lower cognitive scores for both verbal memory ($P < 0.001$) and visual search ($P = 0.076$; $P = 0.010$) at age 43 and 60+, were more likely to belong to a manual occupation of social class of origin ($P < 0.001$), and had less than advanced levels of educational attainment by age 26 years ($P < 0.001$).

Participants included in the current analysis were mostly nonsmokers at either 36 (76.6%) or 43 years (80.1%) and at least moderately active at ages 36 (68.1%), although less so at 43 years (53.2%), but had a similar quality of diet at both 36 and 43 years (55.4% and 51.1%, respectively, were in the lower median split).

Table 1 shows means for the total verbal memory and visual search speed scores at age 60+, by the three lifestyle behaviors (at 36 and 43 years, and the cumulative and change scores for these ages), by sex, father's social class, educational attainment, and midlife social class and depression of the 1018 participants. All three lifestyle behaviors (smoking, physical activity, and diet) at age 36, 43 years, as cumulative scores or change in behavior were strongly associated with verbal memory at age 60+. The effect was monotonic, with those who did not smoke or decreased their level of smoking; those who were most physically active or increased their level of activity or had a healthier or improved diet, having better memory scores at age 60+. For visual search speed at age 60+ the general trend was for slower function with heavy and increased smoking across early midlife; a positive association for high and increased physical activity; a positive association for consistently high and increased diet quality.

3.2. Association between Lifestyle Behaviors and Memory Decline. Table 2 shows results for the ANCOVAs for each health behavior (at 36 and 43 years, the cumulative and change scores for these ages) and memory decline from 43 to 60+ years. Trends can be observed for associations

TABLE 1: Characteristics and mean scores for memory and search speed at age 60+ years, by lifestyle behaviour profiles and dichotomous covariates.

Variable	N	Memory at age 60+ years	P	Search speed at age 60+ years	P
Smoking at age:					
36 years					
Non-smoker	780	25.00 (5.88)		273.47 (73.13)	
1–20 c/day	200	24.18 (6.37)	<0.001	266.7 (69.88)	0.002
20+ cig/day	38	21.23 (7.33)		233.26 (59.33)	
43 years					
Non-smoker	816	25.05 (5.95)		274.45 (72.55)	
1–20 c/day	159	23.99 (6.05)	<0.001	258.60 (68.67)	0.001
20+ cig/day	43	20.72 (7.05)		242.83 (73.49)	
Midlife score					
Non-smoker	744	25.05 (5.90)		274.51 (73.69)	
Moderate smoker	252	24.07 (6.30)	<0.001	263.48 (67.50)	<0.001
Heavy smoker	22	20.18 (7.25)		221.81 (59.74)	
Change in smoking					
Non-smoker	744	25.05 (5.90)		274.51 (73.69)	
Increase	55	22.89 (5.91)	0.005	254.63 (65.05)	0.011
Decrease	79	24.77 (6.51)		272.29 (60.10)	
Constant med/heavy	140	23.52 (6.60)		255.44 (72.33)	
Physical activity at age:					
36 years					
Inactive	324	23.82 (5.83)		264.87 (72.81)	
Moderate active	275	24.61 (5.98)	<0.001	270.04 (68.14)	0.138
Most active	419	25.44 (6.24)		275.49 (74.58)	
43 years					
Inactive	475	23.85 (6.13)		263.83 (69.38)	
Moderate active	251	25.15 (6.05)	<0.001	267.10 (69.13)	<0.001
Most active	292	25.69 (5.84)		284.76 (78.01)	
Midlife score					
Inactive	221	23.37 (6.01)		259.08 (74.61)	
Moderate active	608	24.81 (5.98)	<0.001	270.87 (68.78)	0.003
Most active	189	25.90 (6.20)		283.43 (79.00)	
Change in physical activity:					
Inactive	221	23.37 (6.01)		259.08 (74.61)	
Increase	164	25.03 (5.35)	<0.001	282.39 (74.40)	0.003
Decrease	354	24.61 (6.30)		266.84 (66.91)	
Constant active	279	25.68 (6.08)		277.72 (74.71)	
Diet at age:					
36 years					
Low quality	564	24.01 (6.19)	<0.001	267.26 (69.12)	0.096
High quality	454	25.55 (5.84)		274.85 (76.14)	
43 years					
Low quality	521	23.72 (6.13)	<0.001	267.24 (69.30)	0.124
High quality	497	25.72 (5.86)		274.21 (75.41)	
Midlife score					
Low quality	234	22.51 (5.90)	<0.001	260.02 (67.96)	0.010
High quality	784	25.34 (5.99)		273.81 (73.41)	
Change in diet:					
Constant low quality	234	22.55 (5.90)		260.02 (67.96)	
Increase	330	25.06 (6.18)	<0.001	272.39 (69.57)	0.022
Decrease	94	23.98 (5.44)		263.80 (71.44)	
Constant high	360	25.96 (5.88)		277.73 (77.16)	

Table 1: Continued.

Variable	N	Memory at age 60+ years	P	Search speed at age 60+ years	P
Sex:					
Male	490	23.72 (5.94)	<0.001	265.36 (71.84)	0.024
Female	528	25.61 (6.07)		275.54 (72.63)	
Father social class					
Non-manual	507	26.28 (5.90)	<0.001	278.69 (75.64)	<0.001
Manual	511	23.12 (5.84)		262.66 (68.16)	
Education:					
<advanced	567	22.77 (5.66)	<0.001	263.03 (70.09)	<0.001
≥advanced	451	27.12 (5.71)		280.21 (74.17)	
Midlife social class at age:					
36 years					
Non-manual	617	26.24 (5.79)	<0.001	280.36 (71.29)	<0.001
Manual	401	22.33 (5.75)		255.69 (71.62)	
43 years					
Non-manual	696	26.08 (5.79)	<0.001	276.31 (71.73)	<0.001
Manual	322	21.72 (5.60)		258.38 (72.42)	
Depression at age:					
43 years					
No symptoms	966	24.80 (6.05)	0.036	271.08 (72.92)	0.403
Depressive symptoms	52	22.98 (6.47)		262.46 (61.78)	
60+ years					
No symptoms	805	24.85 (6.09)	0.194	270.03 (73.61)	0.531
Depressive symptoms	171	24.19 (5.74)		273.87 (69.23)	

between heavy smoking at age 43 and for increase in smoking consumption and faster memory decline at all stages of model adjustment, but these trends were not significant at the $\alpha = 0.05$ level. Directions of associations between physical activity and memory decline were inconsistent across the various categories of this behavior, but none were significant. On the other hand a consistently healthy dietary choice at 36 and 43 years was associated with slower memory decline, although none of the dietary change categories were associated with this outcome.

3.3. Association between Lifestyle Behaviors and Visual Search Speed Decline. Table 3 shows results for the ANCOVAs for each health behavior (at 36 and 43 years, and the cumulative and change scores for these ages) and decline in visual search speed from 43 to 60+ years. Heavy smoking at 43 years was associated with faster decline in search speed compared to nonsmokers after adjustment for the covariates in Model 1, but not at 36 years or at both these ages (the latter an effect of reduced statistic power) and not at 43 years after mutual adjustment for the other health behaviors. Nor were there associations between change in smoking and this outcome. On the other hand high physical activity at 43 years was associated with slower search speed decline, after full adjustment. This was also the case for those most active at both 36 and 43 years and for those who increased their level of activity between these ages. There were no associations at the $\alpha = 0.05$ level between any measure of dietary choice and rate of search speed decline.

4. Discussion

The principal aim of this study was to test associations between lifestyle behaviors in early midlife and cognitive decline over 20 years. Key findings were that a consistently healthy dietary choice was associated with slower memory decline, and that consistently high or increasing physical activity from early midlife to midlife was associated with slower visual search speed decline, independently of each other lifestyle behavior and of social class of origin, childhood cognition, educational attainment, adult social class, and symptoms of anxiety and depression. Smoking was not associated with either cognitive outcome. It should be noted that the current findings for dietary choice and physical activity were not always consistent at different ages across midlife, compared to effects of the cumulative scores and change in behavior between the 2 time points. It will be important to seek replication elsewhere before these findings can be treated as authoritative.

4.1. Strengths and Limitations. Strengths of this study include use of a nationally representative sample; availability of a wide range of prospectively-obtained potential confounders, including childhood cognition to rule out selection by prior ability; a detailed assessment of lifestyle behaviors in midlife, including 5-day diet diaries; estimation of cumulative and change effects with two measures of health behaviors; availability of cognitive outcomes that are age and morbidity sensitive [45, 46]; a 20-year interval for capturing decline in

TABLE 2: Regression coefficients (95% confidence intervals) representing rate of decline in verbal memory from 43 to 60+ years per level increase in each health behavior at 36 and 43 years and per cumulative and change in health behavior scores.

	N (%)	Verbal memory decline 43 to 60+ (95% CI) Model 1	Model 2
Smoking at age:			
36 y			
Non-smoking	780 (76.6)	0.00	0.00
1–20 c/day	200 (19.6)	−0.16 (−0.85, 0.53)	−0.12 (−0.81, 0.57)
20+ cig/day	38 (3.7)	−0.22 (−1.67, 1.22)	−0.17 (−1.62, 1.28)
P value		0.610	0.701
43 y			
Non-smoking	816 (80.1)	0.00	0.00
1–20 c/day	159 (15.6)	−0.08 (−0.83, 0.67)	−0.07 (−0.83, 0.69)
20+ cig/day	43 (4.2)	−1.38 (−2.75, −0.01)	−1.24 (−2.61, 0.11)
P value		0.124	0.165
Midlife score:			
Non-smoker	744 (73.0)	0.00	0.00
Moderate smoker	252 (24.7)	−0.20 (−0.83, 0.43)	−0.12 (−0.76, 0.51)
Heavy smokers	22 (2.1)	−0.22 (−2.10, 1.66)	−0.01 (−1.90, 1.87)
P value		0.535	0.750
Change in smoking:			
Non-smoker	744 (73.0)	0.00	0.00
Increase	55 (5.4)	−1.11 (−2.32, 0.09)	−1.00 (−2.21, 0.21)
Decrease	79 (7.7)	0.10 (−0.91, 1.12)	0.09 (−0.92, 1.11)
Constant med/heavy	140 (13.7)	−0.03 (−0.83, 0.77)	0.04 (−0.78, 0.86)
P value		0.363	0.473
Physical activity at age:			
36 y			
Inactive	324 (31.8)	0.00	0.00
Moderately active	275 (27.0)	−0.06 (−0.76, 0.64)	−0.07 (−0.78, 0.63)
Most active	419 (41.1)	0.21 (−0.42, 0.86)	0.17 (−0.47, 0.82)
P value		0.484	0.571
43 y			
Inactive	475 (46.6)	0.00	0.00
Moderately active	251 (24.6)	0.06 (−0.61, 0.75)	0.02 (−0.65, 0.71)
Most active	292 (28.6)	−0.06 (−0.72, 0.59)	−0.12 (−0.79, 0.54)
P value		0.878	0.731
Midlife score:			
Inactive	221 (21.7)	0.00	0.00
Moderate	608 (59.7)	−0.13 (−0.82, 0.54)	−0.23 (−0.91, 0.45)
Most active	189 (18.5)	−0.16 (−1.05, 0.71)	−0.31 (−1.20, 0.56)
P value		0.697	0.472
Change in activity:			
Inactive	221 (21.7)	0.00	0.00
Increase	164 (16.1)	−0.35 (−1.25, 0.54)	−0.47 (−1.37, 0.43)
Decrease	354 (34.7)	−0.10 (−0.84, 0.63)	−0.18 (−0.92, 0.55)
Constant mod/active	279 (27.4)	−0.06 (−0.87, 0.73)	−0.17 (−0.98, 0.63)
P value		0.871	0.768
Diet at age:			
36 y			
Low-quality diet	564 (55.4)	0.00	0.00
High-quality diet	454 (44.6)	0.38 (−0.17, 0.93)	0.35 (−0.20, 0.91)
P value		0.176	0.212
43 y			
Low-quality diet	521 (51.1)	0.00	0.00
High-quality diet	497 (48.8)	0.20 (−0.34, 0.75)	0.17 (−0.38, 0.73)
P value		0.468	0.549

Table 2: Continued.

	N (%)	Verbal memory decline 43 to 60+ (95% CI) Model 1	Model 2
Midlife score:			
Low-quality diet	234 (22.9)	0.00	0.00
High-quality diet	784 (77.0)	0.71 (0.04, 1.38)	0.70 (0.02, 1.38)
P value		0.037	0.043
Change in diet:			
Low-quality	234 (22.9)	0.00	0.00
Increase in quality	330 (32.4)	0.65 (−0.08, 1.40)	0.65 (−0.10, 1.41)
Decrease in quality	94 (9.2)	0.95 (−0.09, 2.00)	0.91 (−0.14, 1.97)
Constant high-quality	360 (35.3)	0.78 (0.02, 1.53)	0.76 (0.00, 1.54)
P value		0.146	0.180

Model 1: model adjusted for sex, childhood social class, childhood cognition at age 8, SEP (own occupation and education), and depression.
Model 2: model 1 plus other lifestyle behaviors.

these measures upto an age when decline may begin to have functional consequences. In addition, while there are many reports examining associations with single lifestyle behaviors [47–49], very little work has focused on the combined influence of these behaviors on cognitive functioning [10, 11] and none at all to our knowledge on cognitive decline. Furthermore, we believe that the long interval between repeat administrations of the cognitive tests would have minimized potential practice effects.

We should also highlight a number of limitations. First, there was a disproportional loss of those who were less advantaged, in terms of lower childhood cognitive ability, education, and SES, although we have no reason to suspect that this affected the pattern of results observed. Second, all information on lifestyle behaviors was dependent on self-report and was not validated by independent measures, for example, cotinine in the case of smoking. Third, there is the possibility of regression to the mean effect when analyzing cognitive ability data over a long period of time, for example, one may assume that some of those who had high cognitive ability score at age 43 may have lower scores at age 63 years and vice versa. We have tried to reduce this effect by using the conditional model of change [50].

In regard to previous findings in NSHD, the inverse association between physical activity and memory decline from 43 to 53 years reported by Richards et al. [51] was not seen here for 20-year decline. This may be because the previous study had additional specificity through adjusting for non-physical spare-time activities, which would have been too cumbersome in the context of multiple lifestyle behaviors in the present study, or because of the longer period of cognitive change. The associations between physical activity and slower decline in visual search speed and between healthy dietary choice and memory are new findings and were not previously tested in this cohort; in the former case physical activity was not investigated in relation to search speed in the previous study; in the latter case midlife cognition has not previously been studied in relation to diet in this cohort. On the other hand the associations between heavy smoking at age 43 and faster memory decline previously reported between ages 43 and 53 years [40] were not replicated here with the 20-year period of cognitive change from 43 to 60+. The loss of the cumulative midlife heavy smoking-memory decline association may be due low statistical power resulting from the relatively high odds of morbidity and premature mortality in this subgroup (135 study members smoking more than 20 cigarettes per day at age 43 were represented in the previous study, compared to 22 in the present study).

In relation to other cohorts, Sabia et al. found an effect of sex on the association between smoking and cognitive decline in a study of London civil servants. Their results showed that men who smoked showed faster decline than nonsmoking men over a 10-year period, after adjusting for the effects of heart disease, stroke, and lung function on mental abilities, while for women there were no differences in cognitive scores over the same time period. This could be related to a lower number of female participants in contrast to males in the Whitehall II study [52]. In relation to physical activity, leisure-time physical activity at least twice a week in midlife was associated with reduced risk of memory decline in the Cardiovascular Risk Factors, Aging and Incidence of Dementia (CAIDE) study after adjustment for age, sex, education, follow-up time, locomotor disorders, APOE genotype, vascular disorders, smoking, and alcohol consumption [53]. Similarly, in The Mayo Clinic Study of Aging, moderate exercise in midlife or late life was associated with reduced odds of Mild Cognitive Impairment (MCI) [54]. In contrast, results from the Chicago Health and Aging Project reported that physical activity conducted within 2 weeks of the date of baseline cognitive assessment was not associated with risk of cognitive decline in an older population [55].

Our finding that maintained healthy dietary choice was associated with a slower rate of memory decline is consistent with the results of a recent systematic review, which highlighted that a diet high in saturated fat represents an increased risk of cognitive decline and subsequent dementia [6]. The emphasis on identifying specific nutrients associated with cognitive ability in later life, such as antioxidants (vitamin C, E, carotenoids, and polyphenols), minerals, and dietary lipids (total, trans, and saturated mono-and

Table 3: Regression coefficients (95% confidence intervals) representing rate of decline in visual search from 43 to 60+ years per level increase in each health behavior at 36 and 43 years and per cumulative and change in health behavior scores.

	N (%)	Visual search decline 43 to 60+ (95% CI) Model 1	Model 2
Smoking at age:			
36 y			
Non-smoking	780 (76.6)	0.00	0.00
1–20 c/day	200 (19.6)	−1.90 (−11.77, 7.96)	−1.79 (−11.68, 8.09)
20+ cig/day	38 (3.7)	−18.70 (−39.27, 1.86)	−19.44 (−40.05, 1.17)
P value		0.156	0.148
43 y			
Non-smoking	816 (80.1)	0.00	0.00
1–20 c/day	159 (15.6)	−4.19 (−14.92, 6.53)	−2.73 (−13.55, 8.08)
20+ cig/day	43 (4.2)	−19.54 (−38.97, −0.12)	−18.52 (−38.00, 0.94)
P value		0.060	0.103
Midlife score:			
Non-smoker	744 (73.0)	0.00	0.00
Moderate smoker	252 (24.7)	−4.85 (−13.93, 4.21)	−4.82 (−13.93, 4.28)
Heavy smokers	22 (2.1)	−24.80 (−51.61, 2.00)	−25.46 (−52.34, 1.42)
P value		0.078	0.077
Change in smoking:			
Non-smoker	744 (73.0)	0.00	0.00
Increase	55 (5.4)	−13.08 (−30.17, 4.00)	−12.78 (−30.02, 4.45)
Decrease	79 (7.7)	−2.70 (−17.06, 11.64)	−2.65 (−17.09, 11.78)
Constant med/heavy	140 (13.7)	−6.71 (−18.09, 4.67)	−5.82 (−17.44, 5.79)
P value		0.374	0.455
Physical activity at age:			
36 y			
Inactive	324 (31.8)	0.00	0.00
Moderately active	275 (27.0)	2.69 (−7.29, 12.68)	3.20 (−6.80, 13.20)
Most active	419 (41.1)	8.00 (−1.12, 17.13)	8.47 (−0.70, 17.65)
P value		0.081	0.067
43 y			
Inactive	475 (46.6)	0.00	0.00
Moderately active	251 (24.6)	−3.93 (−13.57, 5.69)	−4.37 (−14.03, 5.28)
Most active	292 (28.6)	11.84 (2.55, 21.12)	11.18 (1.78, 20.58)
P value		0.022	0.034
Midlife score:			
Inactive	221 (21.7)	0.00	0.00
Moderate	608 (59.7)	8.32 (−1.33, 17.97)	8.76 (−0.95, 18.47)
Most active	189 (18.5)	16.71 (4.32, 29.10)	17.00 (4.50, 29.51)
P value		0.008	0.008
Change in activity:			
Inactive	221 (21.7)	0.00	0.00
Increase	164 (16.1)	14.45 (1.83, 27.07)	13.78 (1.05, 26.50)
Decrease	354 (34.7)	7.58 (−2.87, 18.03)	7.80 (−2.72, 18.34)
Constant mod/active	279 (27.4)	10.51 (−0.74, 21.77)	10.46 (−0.92, 21.84)
P value		0.127	0.157
Diet at age:			
36 y			
Low-quality diet	564 (55.4)	0.00	0.00
High-quality diet	454 (44.6)	−0.52 (−8.39, 7.34)	−1.74 (−9.67, 6.19)
P value		0.896	0.667
43 y			
Low-quality diet	521 (51.1)	0.00	0.00
High-quality diet	497 (48.8)	0.59 (−7.23, 8.42)	−1.03 (−8.91, 6.84)
P value		0.881	0.797

Table 3: Continued.

	N (%)	Visual search decline 43 to 60+ (95% CI) Model 1	Model 2
Midlife score:			
Low-quality diet	234 (22.9)	0.00	0.00
High-quality diet	784 (77.0)	1.59 (−7.89, 11.09)	−0.64 (−10.28, 9.00)
P value		0.741	0.896
Change in diet:			
Low-quality	234 (22.9)	0.00	0.00
Increase in quality	330 (32.4)	1.53 (−9.04, 12.12)	−0.69 (−11.45, 10.06)
Decrease in quality	94 (9.2)	−1.23 (−16.11, 13.64)	−3.22 (−18.18, 11.74)
Constant high-quality	360 (35.3)	1.63 (−9.09, 12.36)	−1.39 (−12.31, 9.57)
P value		0.972	0.978

Model 1: model adjusted for sex, childhood social class, childhood cognition at age 8, SEP (own occupation and education), and depression.
Model 2: model 1 plus other lifestyle behaviors.

polyunsaturated fats) [56], is now giving way to studies of global diet quality indices, for guidance in modeling dietary risk in relation to cognitive performance [57, 58]. In this context general recommendations are made for high fruit and vegetable consumption and moderation of high-glycemic index foods as cardioprotective, with secondary benefits to cognitive ageing [59]. The reason for the specificity of the diet memory association is unclear. Healthy dietary choice is protective of dementia [60], and evidence shows that dementia is predicted by memory impairment in particular [61, 62]. However, physical exercise, which was specifically associated with search speed, is also protective of dementia [63]. As already noted, however, the apparent loss of the exercise memory association reported by Richards et al. (2003) may be a consequence of not adjusting for non physical leisure activities here [51].

Our results for diet differ to those of The Nutrition et Cognition (NutCog) study, where diet quality was not independently associated with cognitive change over 3-year period. However, cognitive decline in this study was measured over a much shorter interval, although this study did report an association between diet quality and risk factors for nutrition-related chronic diseases, which are also considered to be risk factors for cognitive decline [56].

There are several plausible biological mechanisms underlying associations between physical activity and cognitive decline. Physical activity reduces cardiovascular risk [64], increases cerebral perfusion, and facilitates neurogenesis [65–67]. In contrast, impaired blood flow in the midbrain [68, 69] is a risk factor for subsequent cognitive impairment and dementia. Of interest, physical activity was specifically associated with a slower decline in psychomotor speed, which is consistent with evidence that highly fit individuals respond faster to stimuli [70].

4.2. Conclusions and Implications. In conclusion, our results support evidence that physical activity and healthy dietary choice are protective of aspects of cognitive ageing. These mutually adjusted associations were observed over a 20-year period, in analyses additionally controlling for socioeconomic status, sex, educational attainment, prior cognitive ability, and symptoms of anxiety and depression. Further work on interactions between lifestyle behaviors is recommended. For example, evidence suggests that smokers have poorer dietary choices than nonsmokers [71]; the Mediterranean diet only appears to be an effective protective factor for Alzheimer's disease in those who also exercise [72]. Overall, however, and in view of the enormous financial and societal burden of neurodegenerative diseases, public health interventions based on modifiable lifestyle behaviors across the life course represent high level priorities around the world.

Acknowledgments

D. Cadar, A. Stephen, D. Kuh, and M. Richards are supported by the UK Medical Research Council. H. Pikhart is supported by the Higher Education Funding Council for England (HEFCE). G.Mishra receives support from the Australian National Health and Medical Research Council (APP1000986). No financial disclosures were reported by the authors of this paper. Financial support for this study was provided by the UK Medical Research Council. The authors are grateful to NSHD study members who took part in this latest data collection for their continuing support. They thank members of the NSHD scientific and data collection team at the following centers: MRC Unit for LHA; Medical Research Council (MRC); Clinical Research Facility (CRF) Manchester; WTCRF at the Western General Hospital in Edinburgh; WTCRF at University Hospital Birmingham; WTCRF at University College London Hospital; CRF at the University Hospital of Wales; CRF and Twin Research Unit at St Thomas' Hospital London.

References

[1] A. Wimo and M. Prince, "Alzheimer's disease international world Alzheimer report 2010: the global economic impact of dementia," in *Alzheimer' Disease International*, London, UK, 2010.

[2] L. J. Whalley, F. D. Dick, and G. McNeill, "A life-course approach to the aetiology of late-onset dementias," *The Lancet Neurology*, vol. 5, no. 1, pp. 87–96, 2006.

[3] L. J. Whalley, H. C. Fox, I. J. Deary, and J. M. Starr, "Childhood IQ, smoking, and cognitive change from age 11 to 64 years," *Addictive Behaviors*, vol. 30, no. 1, pp. 77–88, 2005.
[4] B. M. Van Gelder, M. A. R. Tijhuis, S. Kalmijn, S. Giampaoli, A. Nissinen, and D. Kromhout, "Physical activity in relation to cognitive decline in elderly men: the FINE study," *Neurology*, vol. 63, no. 12, pp. 2316–2321, 2004.
[5] I. J. Deary, J. Corley, A. J. Gow et al., "Age-associated cognitive decline," *British Medical Bulletin*, vol. 92, no. 1, pp. 135–152, 2009.
[6] Y. Lee, J. H. Back, J. Kim et al., "Systematic review of health behavioral risks and cognitive health in older adults," *International Psychogeriatrics*, vol. 22, no. 2, pp. 174–187, 2010.
[7] T. K. T. Phung, K. Andersen, L. V. Kessing, and G. Waldemar, "Lifestyle-related risk factors for dementia," *Ugeskrift for Laeger*, vol. 168, no. 40, pp. 3401–3405, 2006.
[8] L. Fratiglioni and H. X. Wang, "Brain reserve hypothesis in dementia," *Journal of Alzheimer's Disease*, vol. 12, no. 1, pp. 11–22, 2007.
[9] L. Fratiglioni, B. Winblad, and E. von Strauss, "Prevention of Alzheimer's disease and dementia. Major findings from the Kungsholmen Project," *Physiology and Behavior*, vol. 92, no. 1-2, pp. 98–104, 2007.
[10] S. Sabia, H. Nabi, M. Kivimaki, M. J. Shipley, M. G. Marmot, and A. Singh-Manoux, "Health behaviors from early to late midlife as predictors of cognitive function," *American Journal of Epidemiology*, vol. 170, no. 4, pp. 428–437, 2009.
[11] Y. Lee, J. Kim, and J. H. Back, "The influence of multiple lifestyle behaviors on cognitive function in older persons living in the community," *Preventive Medicine*, vol. 48, no. 1, pp. 86–90, 2009.
[12] N. P. Pronk, L. H. Anderson, A. L. Crain et al., "Meeting recommendations for multiple healthy lifestyle factors: prevalence, clustering, and predictors among adolescent, adult, and senior health plan members," *American Journal of Preventive Medicine*, vol. 27, pp. 25–33, 2004.
[13] W. Poortinga, "The prevalence and clustering of four major lifestyle risk factors in an English adult population," *Preventive Medicine*, vol. 44, no. 2, pp. 124–128, 2007.
[14] G. Mishra, K. Ball, J. Arbuckle, and D. Crawford, "Dietary patterns of Australian adults and their association with socioeconomic status: results from the 1995 National Nutrition Survey," *European Journal of Clinical Nutrition*, vol. 56, no. 7, pp. 687–693, 2002.
[15] Y. Ben-Shlomo and D. Kuh, "A life course approach to chronic disease epidemiology: conceptual models, empirical challenges and interdisciplinary perspectives," *International Journal of Epidemiology*, vol. 31, no. 2, pp. 285–293, 2002.
[16] D. Kuh, Y. Ben-Shlomo, J. Lynch, J. Hallqvist, and C. Power, "Life course epidemiology," *Journal of Epidemiology and Community Health*, vol. 57, no. 10, pp. 778–783, 2003.
[17] L. J. Launer, "The epidemiologic study of dementia: a life-long quest?" *Neurobiology of Aging*, vol. 26, no. 3, pp. 335–340, 2005.
[18] R. C. Petersen, J. E. Parisi, D. W. Dickson et al., "Neuropathologic features of amnestic mild cognitive impairment," *Archives of Neurology*, vol. 63, no. 5, pp. 665–672, 2006.
[19] M. Lamar, S. M. Resnick, and A. B. Zonderman, "Longitudinal changes in verbal memory in older adults: distinguishing the effects of age from repeat testing," *Neurology*, vol. 60, no. 1, pp. 82–86, 2003.
[20] S. A. Small, Y. Stern, M. Tang, and R. Mayeux, "Selective decline in memory function among healthy elderly," *Neurology*, vol. 52, no. 7, pp. 1392–1396, 1999.
[21] J. T. Becker, S. W. Davis, K. M. Hayashi et al., "Three-dimensional patterns of hippocampal atrophy in mild cognitive impairment," *Archives of Neurology*, vol. 63, no. 1, pp. 97–101, 2006.
[22] N. C. Fox, W. R. Crum, R. I. Scahill, J. M. Stevens, J. C. Janssen, and M. N. Rossor, "Imaging of onset and progression of Alzheimer's disease with voxel-compression mapping of serial magnetic resonance images," *The Lancet*, vol. 358, no. 9277, pp. 201–205, 2001.
[23] M. Richards, B. Shipley, R. Fuhrer, and M. E. J. Wadsworth, "Cognitive ability in childhood and cognitive decline in mid-life: longitudinal birth cohort study," *British Medical Journal*, vol. 328, no. 7439, pp. 552–554, 2004.
[24] A. Singh-Manoux, M. Kivimaki, M. M. Glymour et al., "Timing of onset of cognitive decline: results from Whitehall II prospective cohort study," *British Medical Journal*, vol. 344, no. 7840, 2012.
[25] L. Fratiglioni, S. Paillard-Borg, and B. Winblad, "An active and socially integrated lifestyle in late life might protect against dementia," *The Lancet Neurology*, vol. 3, no. 6, pp. 343–353, 2004.
[26] Y. Stern, "Cognitive reserve," *Neuropsychologia*, vol. 47, no. 10, pp. 2015–2028, 2009.
[27] D. J. L. Kuh and C. Cooper, "Physical activity at 36 years: patterns and childhood predictors in a longitudinal study," *Journal of Epidemiology and Community Health*, vol. 46, no. 2, pp. 114–119, 1992.
[28] V. Mikkilä, L. Räsänen, O. T. Raitakari, P. Pietinen, and J. Viikari, "Longitudinal changes in diet from childhood into adulthood with respect to risk of cardiovascular diseases: the Cardiovascular Risk in Young Finns study," *European Journal of Clinical Nutrition*, vol. 58, no. 7, pp. 1038–1045, 2004.
[29] V. H. Menec, "The relation between everyday activities and successful aging: a 6-year longitudinal study," *Journals of Gerontology B*, vol. 58, no. 2, pp. S74–S82, 2003.
[30] H. Iwasa, Y. Yoshida, I. Kai, T. Suzuki, H. Kim, and H. Yoshida, "Leisure activities and cognitive function in elderly community-dwelling individuals in Japan: a 5-year prospective cohort study," *Journal of Psychosomatic Research*, vol. 72, no. 2, pp. 159–164, 2012.
[31] M. M. Esiri, Z. Nagy, M. Z. Smith, L. Barnetson, A. D. Smith, and C. Joachim, "Cerebrovascular disease and threshold for dementia in the early stages of Alzheimer's disease," *The Lancet*, vol. 354, no. 9182, pp. 919–920, 1999.
[32] M. Wadsworth, D. Kuh, M. Richards, and R. Hardy, "Cohort profile: the 1946 National Birth Cohort (MRC National Survey of Health and Development)," *International Journal of Epidemiology*, vol. 35, no. 1, pp. 49–54, 2006.
[33] D. Kuh, M. Pierce, J. Adams et al., "Cohort Profile: updating the cohort profile for the MRC National Survey of Health and Development: a new clinic-based data collection for ageing research," *International Journal of Epidemiology*, vol. 40, no. 1, Article ID dyq231, pp. e1–e9, 2011.
[34] H. L. Taylor, D. R. Jacobs, and B. Schucker, "A questionnaire for the assessment of leisure time physical activities," *Journal of Chronic Diseases*, vol. 31, no. 12, pp. 741–755, 1978.
[35] R. Cooper, G. D. Mishra, and D. Kuh, "Physical activity across adulthood and physical performance in midlife: findings from a British birth cohort," *American Journal of Preventive Medicine*, vol. 41, no. 4, pp. 376–384, 2011.
[36] G. M. Price, A. A. Paul, F. B. Key et al., "Measurement of diet in a large national survey: comparison of computerized and manual coding of records in household measures," *Journal of

Human Nutrition and Dietetics, vol. 8, no. 6, pp. 417–428, 1995.

[37] C. J. Prynne, A. A. Paul, G. D. Mishra, D. C. Greenberg, and M. E. J. Wadsworth, "Changes in intake of key nutrients over 17 years during adult life of a British birth cohort," *British Journal of Nutrition*, vol. 94, no. 3, pp. 368–376, 2005.

[38] S. Köhler, M. P. J. Van Boxtel, J. Van Os et al., "Depressive symptoms and cognitive decline in community-dwelling older adults," *Journal of the American Geriatrics Society*, vol. 58, no. 5, pp. 873–879, 2010.

[39] J. M. Starr, I. J. Deary, H. C. Fox, and L. J. Whalley, "Smoking and cognitive change from age 11 to 66 years: a confirmatory investigation," *Addictive Behaviors*, vol. 32, no. 1, pp. 63–68, 2007.

[40] M. Richards, M. J. Jarvis, N. Thompson, and M. E. J. Wadsworth, "Cigarette smoking and cognitive decline in midlife: evidence from a Prospective Birth Cohort study," *American Journal of Public Health*, vol. 93, no. 6, pp. 994–998, 2003.

[41] Office of Population Censuses and Surveys, *Classification of Occupations*, HMSO, London, UK, 1970.

[42] D. A. Pigeon, "Tests used in the 1954 and 1957 surveys," in *The Home and the School (appendix 1)*, M. Wadsworth, Ed., Macgibbon & Kee, London, UK, 1964.

[43] M. Lindelow, R. Hardy, and B. Rodgers, "Development of a scale to measure symptoms of anxiety and depression in the general UK population: the psychiatric symptom frequency scale," *Journal of Epidemiology and Community Health*, vol. 51, no. 5, pp. 549–557, 1997.

[44] D. P. Goldberg and V. F. Hillier, "A scaled version of the General Health Questionnaire," *Psychological Medicine*, vol. 9, no. 1, pp. 139–145, 1979.

[45] T. A. Salthouse, "The processing-speed theory of adult age differences in cognition," *Psychological Review*, vol. 103, no. 3, pp. 403–428, 1996.

[46] S. Belleville, N. Rouleau, and N. Caza, "Effect of normal aging on the manipulation of information in working memory," *Memory and Cognition*, vol. 26, no. 3, pp. 572–583, 1998.

[47] K. J. Anstey, C. Von Sanden, A. Salim, and R. O'Kearney, "Smoking as a risk factor for dementia and cognitive decline: a meta-analysis of prospective studies," *American Journal of Epidemiology*, vol. 166, no. 4, pp. 367–378, 2007.

[48] D. T. Nash, "Nutritional and exercise aspects of cognitive impairment," *Journal of Clinical Lipidology*, vol. 1, no. 4, pp. 242–247, 2007.

[49] K. Yaffe, D. Barnes, M. Nevitt, L. Y. Lui, and K. Covinsky, "A prospective study of physical activity and cognitive decline in elderly women women who walk," *Archives of Internal Medicine*, vol. 161, no. 14, pp. 1703–1708, 2001.

[50] M. Aickin, "Dealing with change: using the conditional change model for clinical research," *The Permanente Journal*, vol. 13, no. 2, pp. 80–84, 2009.

[51] M. Richards, R. Hardy, and M. E. J. Wadsworth, "Does active leisure protect cognition? Evidence from a national birth cohort," *Social Science and Medicine*, vol. 56, no. 4, pp. 785–792, 2003.

[52] S. Sabia, A. Elbaz, A. Dugravot et al., "Impact of smoking on cognitive decline in early old age: the Whitehall II cohort study," *Archives of General Psychiatry*, vol. 69, no. 6, pp. 627–635, 2012.

[53] S. Rovio, I. Kåreholt, E. L. Helkala et al., "Leisure-time physical activity at midlife and the risk of dementia and Alzheimer's disease," *The Lancet Neurology*, vol. 4, no. 11, pp. 705–711, 2005.

[54] Y. E. Geda, R. O. Roberts, D. S. Knopman et al., "Physical exercise, aging, and mild cognitive impairment a population-based study," *Archives of Neurology*, vol. 67, no. 1, pp. 80–86, 2010.

[55] M. T. Sturman, M. C. Morris, C. F. Mendes De Leon, J. L. Bienias, R. S. Wilson, and D. A. Evans, "Physical activity, cognitive activity, and cognitive decline in a biracial community population," *Archives of Neurology*, vol. 62, no. 11, pp. 1750–1754, 2005.

[56] B. Shatenstein, G. Ferland, S. Belleville et al., "Diet quality and cognition among older adults from the NuAge study," *Experimental Gerontology*, vol. 47, no. 5, pp. 353–360, 2012.

[57] E. Kesse-Guyot, H. Amieva, K. Castetbon et al., "Adherence to nutritional recommendations and subsequent cognitive performance: findings from the prospective Supplementation with Antioxidant Vitamins and Minerals 2 (SU.VI.MAX 2) study," *American Journal of Clinical Nutrition*, vol. 93, no. 1, pp. 200–210, 2011.

[58] N. Scarmeas, Y. Stern, M. X. Tang, R. Mayeux, and J. A. Luchsinger, "Mediterranean diet (MeDi) and risk of Alzheimer's disease (AD)," *Neurology*, vol. 66, no. 5, p. 309, 2006.

[59] V. Solfrizzi, V. Frisardi, D. Seripa et al., "Mediterranean diet in predementia and dementia syndromes," *Current Alzheimer Research*, vol. 8, no. 5, pp. 520–542, 2011.

[60] Y. Gu, J. W. Nieves, Y. Stern, J. A. Luchsinger, and N. Scarmeas, "Food combination and alzheimer disease risk: a protective diet," *Archives of Neurology*, vol. 67, no. 6, pp. 699–706, 2010.

[61] B. Hanseeuw and A. Ivanoiu, "Performance on the RI-48 cued recall test best predicts conversion to dementia at the 5- and 10-year follow-ups," *Dementia and Geriatric Cognitive Disorders Extra*, vol. 1, no. 1, pp. 258–266, 2011.

[62] E. Aretouli, O. C. Okonkwo, J. Samek, and J. Brandt, "The fate of the 0.5s: predictors of 2-year outcome in mild cognitive impairment," *Journal of the International Neuropsychological Society*, vol. 17, no. 2, pp. 277–288, 2011.

[63] M. Hamer and Y. Chida, "Physical activity and risk of neurodegenerative disease: a systematic review of prospective evidence," *Psychological Medicine*, vol. 39, no. 1, pp. 3–11, 2009.

[64] S. J. Colcombe, K. I. Erickson, N. Raz et al., "Aerobic fitness reduces brain tissue loss in aging humans," *Journals of Gerontology A*, vol. 58, no. 2, pp. 176–180, 2003.

[65] J. Prickaerts, G. Koopmans, A. Blokland, and A. Scheepens, "Learning and adult neurogenesis: survival with or without proliferation?" *Neurobiology of Learning and Memory*, vol. 81, no. 1, pp. 1–11, 2004.

[66] C. W. Cotman and C. Engesser-Cesar, "Exercise enhances and protects brain function," *Exercise and Sport Sciences Reviews*, vol. 30, no. 2, pp. 75–79, 2002.

[67] S. A. Neeper, F. Gómez-Pinilla, J. Choi, and C. W. Cotman, "Physical activity increases mRNA for brain-derived neurotrophic factor and nerve growth factor in rat brain," *Brain Research*, vol. 726, no. 1-2, pp. 49–56, 1996.

[68] A. Edman, L. Edenbrandt, J. Freden-Lindqvist, M. Nilsson, and A. Wallin, "Asymmetric cerebral blood flow in patients with mild cognitive impairment: possible relationship to further cognitive deterioration," *Dementia and Geriatric Cognitive Disorders Extra*, vol. 1, no. 1, pp. 228–236, 2011.

[69] B. V. Zlokovic, "Neurovascular pathways to neurodegeneration in Alzheimer's disease and other disorders," *Nature Reviews Neuroscience*, vol. 12, no. 12, pp. X723–X738, 2011.

[70] W. W. Spirduso, "Physical fitness, aging, and psychomotor speed: a review," *Journals of Gerontology*, vol. 35, no. 6, pp. 850–865, 1980.

11

Older People and Social Connectedness: How Place and Activities Keep People Engaged

Irene H. Yen,[1] Janet K. Shim,[2] Airin D. Martinez,[3] and Judith C. Barker[4]

[1] *Department of Medicine, University of California, San Francisco, 3333 California Street, Suite 335, San Francisco, CA 94118, USA*
[2] *Department of Social and Behavioral Sciences, University of California, San Francisco, 3333 California Street, Suite 455, San Francisco, CA 94143-0612, USA*
[3] *Community Track Program, Department of Health, Johns Hopkins Bloomberg School of Public Health, Behavior and Society, 624 N. Broadway, HH 753, Baltimore, MD 21205, USA*
[4] *Department of Anthropology, History, and Social Medicine, University of California, San Francisco, 3333 California Street, Suite 485, San Francisco, CA 94143-0850, USA*

Correspondence should be addressed to Irene H. Yen, irene.yen@ucsf.edu

Academic Editor: Frank Oswald

To understand how older adults perceive and navigate their neighborhoods, we examined the implications of activity in their neighborhoods for their health. We interviewed 38 adults (ages 62–85) who lived in San Francisco or Oakland, California. Seven key themes emerged: (1) people express a wide range of expectations for neighborliness, from "we do not bother each other" to "we have keys to each other's houses", (2) social distance between "other" people impede a sense of connection, (3) ethnic differences in living arrangements affect activities and activity locations, (4) people try to stay busy, (5) people able to leave their homes do many activities outside their immediate residential neighborhoods, (6) access to a car is a necessity for most, and (7) it is unusual to plan for the future when mobility might become limited. Multiple locations influence older adults' health, including residential neighborhoods. Older adults value mobility, active lives, and social connections.

1. Introduction

The phenomenon known as "aging in place" refers to the people wanting to stay in their residence as they age [1–3]; indeed, in the US only, about 5% of people age 55 and over move each year, and half of those who do move stay in the same county [4]. Therefore, understanding the dynamic of older adults in their residential neighborhoods is important for social policy and public health programs in an aging US. As people age and their physical mobility decreases, it is assumed that their geographic world shrinks [5]. While it is relatively unclear at what ages, what levels of functional ability, or in what ways or why older adults pare down the territory in which they act, the residential neighborhood is assumed to be at the center of range. Here, neighborhood refers to individuals' perceptions of their residential environment. This could be a historically recognized area with a name (e.g., Chinatown) or an area that is bounded by certain streets generally accepted by those who live within it to be a neighborhood. In this paper, we examine the perceptions and uses older people make of their neighborhood and the implications for health.

A review of the quantitative literature (1997–2007) describing how neighborhoods might be associated with health for older adults identified some key limitations: (1) primarily cross-sectional studies, (2) not taking into consideration specific characteristics of older people (e.g., functional capacity and household composition), and (3) few studies which featured ethnic minority study samples [6]. Most of the quantitative literature focuses on a particular segment of the older population and describes the negative effects of living in areas with higher proportions of low-income people, highlighting crime, isolation, and psychological distress [7]. As a result, there remains a gap in the literature about what resources neighborhoods might provide to a more socioeconomically and ethnically diverse population of older adults, barriers to accessing those resources, key features or qualities of neighborhoods that support or maintain older adult health, and whether these qualities differ by ethnicity of the older adult.

Qualitative research has examined the meanings of place for older adults and how they cope with loss (e.g., changes in the social interactions, their ability to engage with place as their capacity declines) as they age [8]. While the literature still lacks studies of ethnic minorities [9], because of its approach, qualitative methods can be more expansive than quantitative literature. Qualitative researchers conceptualize space with a focus on social relations, the power dynamics of those relations, how space is produced and reproduced, and how space contributes to identity formation [10, 11].

We sought to address the gaps in the quantitative literature by embarking on a qualitative interview study with the ultimate objective to translate these qualitative findings into survey methodology to do larger-scale studies. Two conceptual frameworks guided our investigation: social and physical insidedness [12] and environmental press [13]. We describe these briefly here. The geographer, Rowles, developed concepts of connectedness to neighborhoods and other places, specifically for older people. Rowles' term for these concepts was "place attachment." Place attachment is created through peoples' senses of places' social and physical insidedness. Social insidedness comes from everyday social exchanges over long periods of time resulting in an integration into the social fabric and an overarching identification with a locale. Physical insidedness comes from familiarity and routine within specific settings [12]. Places are redefined in the course of engaging with them. The relative importance of any attribute shifts with varied activities and memories [14]. The concept of place attachment has expanded to include cognitive and emotional bonding as well as behavioral, physical, and social connection to a community [15].

Environmental press is one of the earliest and most comprehensive ecological models of aging [13] and suggests how neighborhood environment influences health. Lawton argued that individuals behave within their environments ("person-environment fit") and respond to environmental demands ("press") depending on their abilities to cope with those demands. As people age, they experience physical and social losses, such as losses in vision, mobility, cognitive capacity, and in social support provided by kin and friends. These losses affect their interactions with their environments. Accessing resources is a means of coping. This involves a person's ability to perceive the demands that are present, interpret them as manageable, and act appropriately in response to the demand by strategically deploying the assets they command. Environmental press can be positive, negative, or neutral [13, 16–20].

More recent developments in environmental gerontology have emerged and expanded the place attachment and environmental frameworks, explicitly contributing concepts of behavior, agency, and emphasizing that these are dynamic processes [21]. The Wahl and Oswald Conceptual Framework on P-E Relationships in Later Life highlights autonomy, identity, and well-being, proposing two parallel pathways: (1) experiences (e.g., familiar routines and relationships with neighbors) leading to belonging (e.g., place attachment) and (2) behavior (e.g., moving to change conditions as an adaptation to aging) leading to agency (e.g., altered person-environment fit). Belonging and agency both contribute to well-being. As people age, their level of agency to cope with environmental press may shift. If they are or become over time more physically frail, they may be more confined and vulnerable to negative characteristics (e.g., fewer stores, poor public transit, and lack of friends) [22]. Accompanying the changing dynamic where environment can bring more presses on the individual, one's affective connection to neighborhood may change (e.g., friends move away and feelings of connection or belonging weaken). So, if a person lives in a neighborhood for two or three decades, place attachment may increase over time and then decline with deteriorating cognitive and physical function.

The epidemiologic literature investigating how neighborhoods affect health could benefit from stronger conceptual underpinnings [23, 24]. In this literature, health is often studied in the negative, such as risk for morbidity or mortality. As such, a conceptual framework that highlights the environmental characteristics that provoke adaptation is consistent with that literature that emphasizes negative effects of poor areas such as high crime and inadequate services. The concept of belonging highlights social exchanges, routines, and attachment that develop within settings over time. Investigating belonging promotes understanding positive aspects of health, as in well-being and quality of life. Wahl and Oswald's conceptual framework (2010) highlights the intersections of the individual's behaviors within an environment together with their social experience (e.g., connections or attachment). This perspective can capture older adults' activity and how it relates to their environment, as well as identify positive environmental factors that enable older adults to use their neighborhoods. This conceptual background guided this project, as it collected qualitative data from a multiethnic sample to identify the types of resources that people use in their residential settings to maintain or improve their overall well-being.

2. Materials and Methods

2.1. Data Collection. Face-to-face interviews took place in participants' homes or a location of the participant's choosing. Interviews were conducted in English or Spanish, lasted between 30 and 180 minutes, were digitally recorded, and transcribed verbatim. After the interview, we asked the respondents to answer a brief demographic survey that included a question on self-rated health. Participants received a $25 gift card as a "thank you." Study procedures were approved by the University of California, San Francisco (UCSF) Institutional Review Board.

To create an interview guide, we reviewed research literature that documented associations between neighborhood environment and health in older adults. We created a list of overarching topics on the basis of reported associations in the research, the two conceptual frameworks (place attachment and environmental press), and the gaps we located (e.g., not taking into consideration specific characteristics of older adults and defining neighborhood as census or administrative boundaries). Examples of these topics are name of the neighborhood, time in neighborhood, positive or negative characteristics of neighborhood, activities undertaken in the neighborhood, changes in the neighborhood over time, typical activities in a week, and other activities. Within each overarching topic, we generated a set of specific questions to elicit people's accounts of their lived experiences, typical activities (e.g., exercise, food shopping and volunteer activities), the person-environment dynamic, how their activities might contribute to place attachment, and whether the environment created press on the person while engaging in typical activities (e.g., if food shopping was difficult because stores were far away).

In order to allow participants to describe their experiences in their own words, questions were open-ended with probes as necessary. New questions were added on the basis of the analysis of earlier interviews. The new interview questions were then applied to subsequent interviews. For example, several participants in early interviews were very active and going to a variety of destinations on a regular basis either by driving or through adept use of public transit. In subsequent interviews, we asked about typical activities and how they got to the locations, rather than focus more narrowly on activities in the residential neighborhood.

2.2. Sampling. We recruited a purposive sample of older adults from diverse ethnic groups with a range of economic circumstances, aiming for a total of 40 participants. We recruited participants through the organizational contacts of the University of California San Francisco's Center for Aging in Diverse Communities and through professional and personal contacts of one of the authors (IHY).

Eligibility criteria included (a) aged 65 or older, (b) self-identified as White, African American or Black, Asian American, or Latino/Hispanic, (c) lived in Oakland or San Francisco, (d) lived in the same residential neighborhood for at least one year at the time of the interview, and (e) spoke either English or Spanish. Recognizing the population trends discussed above, we wanted to include participants from four ethnic groups in our interview sample, those that are strongly represented in the San Francisco Bay Area. We aimed to split the sample of 40 as evenly as possible across the four ethnic groups; moreover, recognizing that in all included groups women have a longer life expectancy than men, we aimed to interview six women and four men in each of the four ethnic groups.

Excluded were people who lived in predominantly low-income neighborhoods. Excluded neighborhoods were determined on the basis of the research team's prior experience in these areas, Chambers of Commerce data, and representations in the local media. There were two reasons for this exclusion criterion. First, was the necessity to keep the amount of variation among study participants to a manageable level given the desire to target a widely diverse group, on the basis of age, sex, and ethnicity. Second, the decision was made to concentrate the sample selection in order to maximize the chances of exploring positive features of neighborhoods.

2.3. Analysis. Two of the authors analyzed transcripts by systematically coding text independently, guided by the interview topics as well as themes that emerged from the data [25]. Analysis took place in several stages. All transcripts were coded by the lead author and another coauthor. Transcripts were read separately and assigned codes that related to the topics and questions in the interview guide as well as other codes that they saw emerging from the data. An initial set of codes was developed. On the basis of this initial coding, a preliminary organization of the codes was constructed, loosely grouped together into larger categories or thematic domains. Subsequent transcripts were coded provoking refinement of codes and thematic domains. Coders met to discuss each transcript and the codes. Any differences of view for any of the coding for transcripts were discussed and resolved until consensus was reached. Discussions during the joint coding meetings also identified new and emergent topics and themes. The coders wrote analytic memos to describe the implications and details of these codes and the larger categories that helped organize the codes [25–27]. All codes were assigned to text blocks using QSR NVivo version 2.0 (QSR International 2006). All authors discussed and concurred with the final list of codes that were applied, the subsequent findings and interpretations of data, and linkages to the conceptual framework.

3. Results

Our final sample, diverse in terms of ethnicity and sex, comprised 38 persons ages 62 to 85 (see Table 1). When age data were checked on completion of the interviews, two people were found to be under the age of 65. Their data is included in this report because their health and activity status were very similar to that of participants over 65 years old. They lived in a variety of neighborhoods, ranging from the suburban hills in Oakland to Oakland's Chinatown and, in San Francisco, the well-to-do Pacific Heights area, the Castro (known for its gay community), and the Richmond district (known for Russian and Chinese immigrant communities).

On the basis of the analytic process described above, we identified seven key themes that fit within the Wahl and Oswald person-environment processes and place attachment framework. For experience or place attachment (belonging), there was a cluster of three themes highlighting social relations and living arrangements: (1) people express a wide range of expectations for neighborliness, from "we don't bother each other" to "we have keys to each other's houses", (2) perceptions of "social distance" between older people and "other" people (e.g., different ages or race/ethnicities) impede a sense of connection in neighborhoods, and (3) ethnic differences in living arrangements affect activities and activity locations—living with extended family, taking care of grandchildren being more common for Latinas. A second cluster of themes highlighted how behaviors might contribute to agency: (4) people try to stay busy, (5) people

TABLE 1: Descriptive information of respondents ($n = 38$).

Demographic characteristics	Overall n (%)
Age	Mean = 74 (range: 62–85)
Sex	
Men	14 (37%)
Women	24 (63%)
Race/ethnicity	
White	9 (24%)
African American	9 (24%)
Latino	10 (26%)
Asian	10 (26%)
City	
San Francisco	20 (52%)
Oakland	18 (48%)
Housing tenure—own	25 (66%)
Educational attainment	
Did not graduate from high school	6 (16%)
High school graduate	4 (11%)
Some college	10 (26%)
College degree	8 (21%)
Graduate degree	6 (16%)
Missing	4 (11%)
Living arrangements	
Lives alone	18 (47%)
Lives with spouse or significant other	14 (37%)
Lives with adult child	6 (16%)
Car ownership—yes	21 (55%)
Years living in neighborhood	
<10	10 (26%)
11–20	7 (18%)
21–40	13 (34%)
41+	7 (18%)
Self-rated health	
Excellent	4 (11%)
Very good	15 (13%)
Good	9 (24%)
Fair	5 (13%)
Poor	2 (5%)
Missing	3 (8%)

able to leave their homes do many activities outside their immediate residential neighborhoods, and (6) access to a car is a necessity for most people. A final theme emerged that indicated that many participants (those who were quite socially and physically active) did not anticipate transitioning into another phase of life should their activity levels decline and their relationship with their home and neighborhood environments shift: (7) it is unusual to plan for the future when mobility might become limited.

People Express a Range of Expectations for Neighborliness, from "We Don't Bother Each Other" to "We Have Keys to Each Other's Houses." Participants described a range of experiences with their neighbors, from detachment to friendships. Having detached or limited social relations with neighbors was common. In general, they expressed satisfaction with the way things were. At times, people noted that over several years, the turnover in neighbors had created a situation where they were not familiar with their neighbors. In these instances, they also pointed out that the newer neighbors were working age and busy during the day. The differing schedules between the older adults and the working adults meant lower likelihood of running into each other coming and going. One woman (82, Caucasian) did not know many of her neighbors, saying:

> *I don't know anybody who lives up here. We did know somebody who lived up here, but they moved away, so I guess we don't know anybody else. I know [name], who lives right behind us. . . . The other people I just wouldn't recognize if I bumped into them on a street.*

An 83-year-old, African American woman had a conflict with her neighbors regarding parked cars. The neighbors eventually stopped parking their cars in a way that blocked other people from walking on the sidewalk and then the relationship stabilized: "Yeah, and so I enjoy them, because it's like I said, they don't bother me and I don't bother them. . ." From this woman's perspective, a good relationship with neighbors was a relatively distant one, defined by not being a bother to one another.

In a couple of instances, people seemed to indicate that this detachment was not completely consensual. A 62-year-old African American woman who lived in a subsidized senior housing apartment building talked about relations with some of her neighbors in a similar fashion:

> Participant: *Another lady down the hall, she passed away, she was very nice lady. . . . but some of these Black people here, they look at you like you're crazy or somethin'. They don't bother with you.*
>
> Interviewer: *Why do you suppose that is?*
>
> Participant: *They don't want to get involved with you.*

Some participants desired detached relations, because they preferred not knowing so much about their neighbors or being fodder for neighborhood gossip. One woman (69, African American) avoided extended conversations with her neighbor across the street so that he would not talk about her to others or attribute comments to her. In another instance, a participant was resigned not to know her neighbors well. An Asian woman (age 74), when asked about changes in the neighborhood, responded that she did not know of many: "Not really, but maybe some." She added, "You know, here in America you don't, not too much socializing in this neighborhood," attributing her lack of knowledge of what was happening in her neighborhood to the lack of socializing within it.

Participants also described relationships with neighbors at the other end of the spectrum where they looked out for each other's homes, had keys to each others' houses, and called regularly to check on each other. One man (78, African American) talked about keeping an eye out on a neighbor's home when she leaves for a few days:

> *Well, like the lady across the street, she's a widow, she's about eighty-three. Whenever she goes to see one of her daughters she'd let me know, "I'm going to be gone three days, four days." I watch the house to see if anybody's coming around or what have you.*

This participant indicated that he watched her house even when she was not out of town and made a point to talk to her at least once a week to make sure she was okay. Another participant (84, Caucasian woman) explained that a group of her neighbors have each others' house keys:

> Interviewer: *When any of your neighbors go away for trips or anything, do they ever ask you to look in on their place?*
>
> Participant: *Well, yeah. We do that for each other. The corner house, myself and the other house, we all have keys to each others' homes. They have my key, I have their keys. Which makes it nice. Helps.*

African American participants were more likely to mention keeping to themselves or not bothering or being bothered by their neighbors than did other participants. One African American woman (age 69) mentioned that she preferred that there were no sidewalks where she lived, because it deterred people from walking around her neighborhood. Latino participants were more likely to highlight social ties to people they knew through church, rather than those in the neighborhood.

"Social Distances" with People from "Other Groups". Twenty of the 38 participants had lived in their neighborhoods for over twenty years. These people often observed that there had been a lot of change in the composition of the neighborhood population and that they used to know more of their neighbors. A common experience was that the participant would recall that when their children were young, they knew neighbors who also had school-aged children. Over time, households would relocate as children moved out. The newer neighbors might be working aged, away during the day, busy with their own young children, and less available for intermittent neighborhood socializing. Sometimes, the lack of familiarity caused uncertainty or insecurity. People's discomfort was frequently a result of perceived social distance from the neighbors, being far apart in age or of a different ethnicity. A man (70, Latino) commented on young people hanging around in the neighborhood, giving him a feeling of insecurity:

> *In the outskirts of our neighborhood there's been more kind of young kids congregating on corners. On the business district there's more young Black and Latino kids, maybe sometimes a White kid, too, but Black and Latino kids, kind of acting rowdy, loud.*

Later, in response to a question of whether there was anything he did not like about his neighborhood, he added:

> *What I don't like is the sense that it's become a little more dangerous, you know, in terms of reading about assaults, and seeing kids acting out, you know, on the street. You know, fifteen year olds, acting crazy.*

An older woman (84, Caucasian) who lived near a high school mentioned staying clear of the shopping area near her home when it was lunchtime. She commented:

> *We used to have some kids walking around and not going to school and stuff like that. But I think that goes on all over. But the only time you're really kind of bothered with it is if you go up here at lunchtime when they're all out having lunch. But you learn to stay home and avoid it so, that's about it.*

Groups of young people were seen as a threat or a nuisance. There was a sense that older adults and young people belonged to separate groups while occupying the same space. People mentioned a sense of vulnerability in part due to being older with less capacity to defend oneself.

Another sort of social distance described by some was with regard to relations with people from ethnic groups different from the participant's. Latinos and African Americans mentioned tensions with Asians. A woman (62, African American) who lived in a subsidized senior housing complex mentioned that her Chinese neighbors greeted her, which she found surprising:

> *"Cause you know Chinese people don't... Some of them don't talk to Black people. And that was unusual for them when I was walkin' the hall she spoke to me and talked to me and asked me how I was doin". And I was just surprised that she would talk to me.*

Another woman (85, Latina) described her Chinese neighbors as not particularly friendly:

> *The Europeans and the Latinos are more friendly; the Chinese are ... they're not so. Well, there's one nearby to me. The only thing [she/he] says is "hello", that's all. [She/he] doesn't come by to talk, just a hello, that's all.* [Translated from Spanish]

Language may have been a factor in this dynamic around social distance. Another Latina (age 65) was concerned that storeowners in her neighborhood were taking advantage of the residents by overcharging their merchandise:

> *The only problem we have with the stores, is that almost all are run by Arabs. They are, how can*

> *I say this, abusive, because they have checkout machines. The items have very small labels and the prices are always faded so it's not possible to see how much something costs. After you pay, they give you a receipt, but there's no ink, so you can't see what the price was. This is a problem for us.* [Translated from Spanish]

Asian respondents were less forthcoming about the topic of social distance though they commented about ethnic composition of their neighborhoods. An 80-year-old Asian man described that the proportions of Chinese neighbors changed over the 50 years he lived in the neighborhood. During some periods, there were more and during other periods, there were less. He mentioned this fluctuation two or three times during the interview. When asked what this fluctuation meant for his experience living in the neighborhood, he would not or could not say. A 74-year-old Asian man said it made no difference to him if his neighbors were Asian or not. Yet, he was clear that some of his closer neighbors were Chinese, while he himself was Filipino. He did say that he liked to go places to engage with Filipinos, "I will always try to go to the place where there are so many Filipinos. To me, it's enough. But when I see Filipinos, I talk to them."

Ethnic Differences in Living Arrangements Affect Activities and Activity Locations. Latina participants tended to live with other family members, in particular adult children, more than did the White, African American, or Asian participants. Four of the Latinas lived with adult children. In two of these instances, their primary activity was to look after grandchildren during the work week. In contrast, one White woman (age 71) lived with her adult daughter. However, it was not until the end of the interview, when asked whether neighbors looked after her home when she went out of town that she mentioned her daughter lived with her. The woman did very little with her daughter regularly, including sharing meals. One African American man (age 66) lived with two of his grandsons who would drive him to places, because he had chronic health problems and some difficulty walking. An Asian couple (both aged 74-years) had retired from work in the Philippines and were living with an adult son. Apart from these four people, all the other African American, White, and Asian participants lived alone ($n = 14$) or with spouses ($n = 12$). Similar to the Latina women, one of the Asian women (age 81) had been living with one of her sons looking after her grandchildren (e.g., taking them to school in the morning, picking them up in the afternoon, and cooking dinner for the family). As the grandchildren grew up and became involved in more activities, she then moved into an apartment in a nearby city that had been purchased for her by her children.

Living arrangements somewhat affected use of services, in combination with an individual's gender and type of neighborhood (i.e., whether there were retail services close by and/or easy access to public transport). Living in close proximity to family was important for all participants. Those who had children living close by could easily get assistance when necessary. For example, an 85-year-old Latina woman was an avid gardener; her son would help her carry large bags of soil or mulch. People who lived alone did all their own food shopping, with the exception of one person who had significant mobility issues. If people lived in a suburban area with no retail close by, they would drive, often selecting the destination on the basis of prices or if they had other errands to do on the way. If people lived with a spouse, usually the woman did more of the food shopping. For one couple who lived close to shopping, the man did all the shopping because the woman had difficulty walking. They had a fixed income. He used the shopping list as his reason for walking in the morning to look at price differences at the various stores close to their home. A Latina woman (age 66) who lived with her daughter and the daughter's family might accompany her daughter to the store; however, most of her activity day during the week was at the senior center near her daughter's work and her granddaughter's school.

People Try to Stay Busy. Many of the participants were very active with social activities, work, volunteering, classes, and leisure travel. Several people talked about being "on the go," wanting to get out every day. In some cases, people intentionally went out to keep mentally and physically active. One woman (69, African American), who was in poor health by her own assessment, commented on how she likes to be on the go:

> Interviewer: *Would you say that you spend more time inside at home than out and about? Or is it half and half?*
>
> Participant: *I would say maybe half and half because I'm a goer. Yeah, and if I feel okay, I be out.*

Another woman (68, Latina) talked about being involved in many different activities:

> *Well, I don't have family, I don't have anyone. I am not going to sit around. I am involved in many things with the church and other things I do during the day. I don't stay here.* [Translated from Spanish]

Ten of these 38 respondents participated in regular and varied volunteer activities. These included helping drive people who attend the same church to doctor's appointments, holding premature babies in a hospital clinic, visiting patients in hospitals, and helping at a meal program for the homeless. Even people who did not drive but who were interested and had the time did volunteer activities at home. For example, an 80-year-old Asian woman knitted hats and blankets for premature babies in the hospital: "I don't have to go anywhere; I just stay home and do it. And what I do is I knit hats and doilies for the hospital, and make baby afghans." Activity levels seemed to be a result of personality (being more or less outgoing), physical functioning (ability to get out), and the desire to maintain a similar level of activity as when the person was younger (possibly to retain a younger outlook). One woman (82, Caucasian), when talking about not knowing many of her neighbors, mentioned that she's more introverted and likes to stay at home:

> *My husband is just the opposite, he likes people. He thinks I should be more active than I am, but I'm not. I remember that in my family, my mother was the extrovert. She was the one who knew everybody and their business. But I just don't. I'd rather stay home and read.*

A 78-year-old African American widower mentioned forcing himself to get out to socialize and do things:

> *Well, if you go to a senior place you're around somebody all of the time, and they have activities going on. So that's the key to me to going someplace else where they have activities going on. ... Activities for your body and for your mind.*

A 64-year-old African American man, who was in relatively frail health (with gout and arthritis), regularly took a bus to his former neighborhood in order to spend time with friends. He was living in subsidized housing for seniors, located in a thriving, vibrant neighborhood in San Francisco. His friends live in an area, known for crime and disadvantage, where there is a larger concentration of African American residents. This man may not have had place attachment in his residential neighborhood, but he did have it in another neighborhood, which he regularly visited.

Perhaps in part because people are generally busy in mainstream US culture, older adults express a value in staying busy. There did not seem to be a difference amongst respondents by gender or race/ethnicity about the level of busyness [28, 29].

People Able to Leave Their Homes Do Many Activities Outside Their Immediate Residential Neighborhoods. Half of the participants went out of their neighborhoods at least once a week for a variety of reasons. In addition to the activities listed above, weekly activities included going to the movies, participating in hobby or social groups (e.g., bowling league and hiking group), food shopping, caregiving for a friend or relative, window shopping at the mall, or visiting family. Other regularly occurring (monthly or quarterly) events included going to doctor's appointments and picking up prescriptions. The neighborhood was not a key location for the majority of these activities. The most common activity done close to home, mentioned by 13 of the participants, was walking in their neighborhoods. Half of the participants lived close to retail areas with a large array of businesses or were within easy walking distance to smaller commercial districts where there might be a café, a few stores, and a couple of restaurants.

Combined with the emphasis of striving to be busy and on the go described above, this theme highlights the sometimes extensive geographic distance covered by many older adults on a regular basis. While each person's sense of neighborhood physical boundaries differed, activities outside perceived residential boundaries were very common. For example, an 82-year-old man went to the movies twice a week, generally travelling on foot and by bus to go to his favorite theatre about three miles away from his home. A 69-year-old woman drove about seven miles from her home in Oakland to Oakland's Chinatown, two to three times per week, to volunteer activities and buy food. A 78-year-old man travelled by bus Monday through Friday morning five miles to a senior center in the Mission District of San Francisco to visit with friends.

Two people did not leave their neighborhoods. One woman (age 63, African American) had severe arthritis and needed someone to do her grocery shopping for her. Her busyness came in the form of watching television and speaking to siblings on the telephone frequently. The other (an 84-year-old Asian woman) lived in a retail-rich area of San Francisco and did some errands in her neighborhood. When she left the neighborhood, it was for doctors appointments.

Access to a Car Is a Necessity for Most. Related to the theme above, having easy access to a car was a perceived to be a necessity. Twenty-one people either drove themselves or had access to a car when, for example, a child or grandchild would drive the person where they needed to go. A woman living in Oakland (72, Caucasian) said, "Well, we wouldn't be able to stay here without being able to drive. I suppose we could use taxis, but that would be the only alternative." A 69-year-old, African American man in Oakland said, "I would say that there are no stores. And that's one of the major difficulties of living here is that if you don't have an automobile you're up the creek."

It Is Unusual to Plan for a Future When Mobility Might Be Limited. As noted above, we spoke to many people who were socially and physically active, commonly driving outside of their neighborhoods for their activities. We asked people if they had made plans for a time when they might not be so mobile or able to get out so easily (e.g., if they could no longer drive). Five participants were living with an adult child. One couple who had retired in the US from another country, assumed that at a certain point when they were frailer, they would move back to their home country for access to affordable support services. A Latina woman, widowed, originally from Nicaragua, mentioned a similar plan. The others assumed they would continue to live with their adult child and would be able to rely on them. Three participants mentioned that if a time came when they could not get around easily, they would likely move in with an adult child living close by. Some people indicated that they would move to an institution. Others mentioned that they have thought about having a paid caregiver move in to their home. More commonly, people had not given too much thought about it:

> *I think I'm just going to rely on my daughters, or my granddaughter by that time. ... I have a couple of girlfriends who live up here in the same situation I am, and, you know, we have talked about that, how maybe we can help each other*

drive or something. But, no, I have to admit I have not given it a lot of serious thought. (69, African American woman)

Most of the participants adhered to the aspiration to age in place and stay in their current living situations for as long as possible. Given the high level of activity that these older adults maintained and their reliance on the car to be so active, we anticipate that it will become increasingly important to understand how to support older people and their desired activities and lifestyles as they become frailer.

4. Discussion

The US population is aging and is increasingly non-white. Current population projections for the US predict that by 2050, the proportion of non-Whites over age 65 will double (from 19% to 39% of the population of age 65 and older people), the proportion of Latinos will triple (from 6% to 18%), the proportion of African Americans will increase by one-third (from 9% to 12%), and the proportion of Asians will nearly triple (from 3% to 8%) [30]. Understanding how neighborhoods and other places affect older adults from different ethnic backgrounds could contribute to policies to address ethnic health disparities.

Through qualitative interviews, we learned about urban older adults' activities both in their residential environments and elsewhere. Participants spent time in their neighborhoods walking and had varying levels of engagement with their neighbors. For participants who were physically able to move about, other than walking or socializing, if the neighborhood did not include retail locations (as was more common in Oakland than San Francisco), then it was not the setting for regular activities. Participants drove their cars to many other destinations to volunteer, exercise, shop, and socialize.

When applied to these data, the Wahl and Oswald conceptual framework (2010) uncovers some new perspectives on the neighborhood-health dynamic for older adults. Since many of these older adult participants maintain a high level of "busyness" and travel to nonneighborhood locations for a variety of activities, this suggests that it is common to live on a geographic scale greater than the residential neighborhood and that social and material needs are fulfilled by doing activities in a broader space. This has implications for social policy addressing "aging in place," suggesting the need to provide access to spaces beyond the residential setting. The neighborhood does provide opportunities for social interactions and at times social connections, a basis for the experience-to-belonging piece of the Wahl and Oswald framework (2010). But for the most part, participants in our study largely described detached and distant relations with their neighbors and furthermore expressed satisfaction with this state of affairs. Indeed, the social distance theme reflects a trajectory from that of a form of place attachment (knowing ones neighbors well and having lots in common because children are going to the same schools) to a position of feeling a poorer fit with the neighbors, a form of environmental press, with the change in composition to households that are different in age and/or ethnicity. At the time of the interview, for a relative few, the social ties within neighborhoods were positive characteristics, but in most other cases, the social interactions were sources of tensions or negative environmental press, using the language of Lawton's person-environment framework. Lawton's conceptualization of environment encompassed the personal environment (e.g., spouses and coworkers) and the group environment which referred to the influences of an aggregation of individuals (e.g., neighbors) [31, 32]. The age, race/ethnicity, and language composition of others in the neighborhood contributed to whether these factors were perceived to be part of the press that the environment imposed, and that limited engagement in the neighborhood or, conversely, as a resource residents could used to be meet environmental demands.

We found that people prefer to stay busy and their ability to do so is heavily dependent on having access to a car. Indeed, while all but three people very much wanted to continue living where they were, their primary social and shopping activities occurred outside of their immediate neighborhoods. When asked to think about a time when they might not be able to drive or get around on their own, most people had not given serious consideration as to what they would do under those circumstances. Therefore, for those without access to a car or for those who have no relatives close by and who would likely experience constrained mobility in the future, the features and resources within the neighborhood are and would be important.

As concepts in environmental gerontology have been refined in the last twenty years, the dynamic process of aging has been more explicitly incorporated [22, 33, 34]. With our participants, chronological age did not clearly correspond to physical function or limitations. The youngest three participants, all African American, were in the poorest health. This is consistent with the trend that African Americans develop chronic conditions at younger ages than their White counterparts [35–37]. On the other hand, one of the oldest participants, also African American, had no chronic conditions, and was extremely active, visiting people in the hospital, attending community meetings, and active in her church. Chronological age is not necessarily the most optimal categorization for these participants. These complexities further corroborate the Wahl-Oswald conceptual framework (2010), especially the pathway from agency to identity. Moreover, the arrows along this pathway could potentially also be bidirectional, with the possibility that identity affects behavior, and in turn agency. For our participants, "identity" is tied to group identity, which is informed by social definitions and positions, often less tied to geography, and which motivate behaviors through which individuals seek to affirm and reinforce those identities.

Our longer-term objective in conducting these interviews is to translate the findings to conduct larger-scale survey research. The quantitative research literature on neighborhood-health associations for older adults sometimes uses age (as measured by the proportion of people age 65 and older in the census tract) or ethnic composition (quantified by measures of segregation) among the important demographic characteristics to describe the neighborhood. Our qualitative study supports the significance and continued inclusion of these variables. Our participants confirm what past research, in particular on intentional communities for older adults or age-segregated residential facilities [38, 39], has found, namely, that older people felt more comfortable if there were other older persons living nearby. There was a sense among our participants that younger neighbors were busy with their lives, coming and going, with not much time or interest in older people or any of the other neighbors.

For ethnic composition, existing evidence and our study findings are more equivocal. Studies have reported that African Americans who live in areas with higher proportions of African Americans have poorer health compared to African Americans who live in areas with lower proportions of African Americans [40, 41]. Other studies have reported that older Latinos who lived in areas with higher proportions of Latinos have better health than Latinos who live in areas with lower proportions of Latinos [42, 43]. The participants in this study did report tensions or uncomfortable interactions with people from other countries or who spoke other languages. Feeling different than, being taken advantage of, or overlooked by racially and ethnically dissimilar neighbors appeared to constitute sources of environmental press with negative effects on neighborhood engagement. Ethnic diversity can be experienced as dissimilarity, as not belonging, as the opposite of place attachment, when residents perceive it to stand in the way of forming social ties to neighbors. The literature also clearly shows that racial/ethnic concentration, when it is a product of segregation, marginalization, and disinvestment in particular communities, is not conducive to health. Our qualitative data support the notion that rather than neighborhood racial/ethnic composition, in and of itself, being important to health, it is a combination of a neighborhood's composition and attendant social, economic, and political resources—or a lack thereof—that are meaningful for residents' health.

Epidemiologists seek to conduct large-scale, longitudinal studies in multiple locations to produce generalizable population-based findings. The findings from this qualitative research project can be used to inform the contents of a survey for a larger-scale study. On the basis of the key themes reported here, future studies should ask questions about older adults' perceptions of their neighborhood boundaries, where else they regularly spend time, the extent to which they are influenced by the social and physical environment of other neighborhoods in which they spend a significant amount of their time, and their use and reliance on a car or public transit. Future research could extend the Wahl-Oswald framework to these other locations, sometimes referred to as activity spaces [44] and consider the possibility that older adults find and experience place attachment in these more geographically distant places as well as close to home. To date, modest associations have been reported for the neighborhood influence on health status for older adults. Investigating other activity spaces for their resources, demands, and attachments could suggest other mechanisms through which place influences health for older adults.

Acknowledgments

This study was supported by a grant from the National Institute on Aging (K01 AG 027273). The authors thank the participants for their interviews, Anita Stewart for advice and mentoring, Jochebed Catungal for data support, and an anonymous reviewer for critical comments.

References

[1] AARP, *A National Study on Housing and Home Modification Issues: Executive Summary*, American Association of Retired Persons, Washington, DC, USA, 2000.

[2] J. D. Fisher, D. S. Johnson, J. T. Marchand, T. M. Smeeding, and B. B. Torrey, "No place like home: older adults and their housing," *The Journals of Gerontology: Series B*, vol. 62, no. 2, pp. S120–S128, 2007.

[3] S. M. Golant, "Deciding where to live: the emerging residential settlement patterns of retired Americans: new forms of retirement enclaves," *Generations*, vol. 26, no. 2, pp. 66–73, 2002.

[4] A. Kochera, A. Straight, and T. Guterbock, *Beyond 50.05 A Report to the Nation on Livable Communities: Creating Environments for Successful Aging*, AARP Public Policy Institute, Washington, DC, USA, 2005.

[5] J. L. Wiles, R. E. S. Allen, A. J. Palmer, K. J. Hayman, S. Keeling, and N. Kerse, "Older people and their social spaces: a study of well-being and attachment to place in Aotearoa New Zealand," *Social Science and Medicine*, vol. 68, no. 4, pp. 664–671, 2009.

[6] I. H. Yen, Y. L. Michael, and L. Perdue, "Neighborhood environment in studies of health of older adults: a systematic review," *American Journal of Preventive Medicine*, vol. 37, no. 5, pp. 455–463, 2009.

[7] N. Krause, "Neighborhood deterioration, religious coping, and changes in health during late life," *Gerontologist*, vol. 38, no. 6, pp. 653–664, 1998.

[8] C.C. Cook, P. Martin, M. Yearns, and M. L. Damhorst, "Attachment to "place" and coping with losses in changed communities: a paradox for aging adults," *Family and Consumer Sciences Research Journal*, vol. 35, no. 3, pp. 201–214, 2007.

[9] G. Becker, "Meanings of place and displacement in three groups of older immigrants," *Journal of Aging Studies*, vol. 17, no. 2, pp. 129–149, 2003.

[10] W. Benjamin, *One Way Street*, New Left Books, London, UK, 1979.

[11] A. E. Smith, *Ageing in Urban Neighbourhoods: Place Attachment and Social Exclusion. Ageing and the Lifecourse*, The Policy Press, Bristol, UK, 2009.

[12] G. D. Rowles, "Geographicl dimensions of social support in rural Appalachia," in *Aging and Milieu: Environmental Perspectives on Growing Old*, G. D. Rowles and R. J. Ohta, Eds., pp. 111–130, Academic Press, New York, NY, USA, 1983.

[13] M. P. Lawton and L. Nahemow, "Ecology and the aging process," in *The Psychology of Adult Development and Aging*, C. Eisdorfer and M. P. Lawton, Eds., pp. 464–488, American Psychological Association, Washington, DC, USA, 1973.

[14] S. C. Howell, "The meaning of place in old age," in *Aging and Milieu*, G. D. Rowles and R. J. Ohta, Eds., pp. 97–110, Academic Press, New York, NY, USA, 1983.

[15] F. Oswald, A. Hieber, H. W. Wahl, and H. Mollenkopf, "Ageing and person-environment fit in different urban neighbourhoods," *European Journal of Ageing*, vol. 2, no. 2, pp. 88–97, 2005.

[16] M. P. Lawton and B. Simon, "The ecology of social relationships in housing for the elderly," *Gerontologist*, vol. 8, no. 2, pp. 108–115, 1968.

[17] M. P. Lawton, "Social ecology and the health of older people," *American Journal of Public Health*, vol. 64, no. 3, pp. 257–260, 1974.

[18] M. P. Lawton, "Housing the elderly. Residential quality and residential satisfaction," *Research on Aging*, vol. 2, no. 3, pp. 309–328, 1980.

[19] M. P. Lawton, "Environment and other determinants of well-being in older people," *Gerontologist*, vol. 23, no. 4, pp. 349–357, 1983.

[20] M. P. Lawton, "Competence, environmental press, and the adaptation of older people," in *Aging and the Environment: Theoretical Approaches*, M. P. Lawton and P. G. Windley, Eds., pp. 33–59, Springer, New York, NY, USA, 1982.

[21] H.-W. Wahl and F. Oswald, "Environmental perspectives on ageing," in *The SAGE Handbook of Social Gerontology*, D. Dannefer and C. Phillipson, Eds., pp. 111–124, Sage, London, Uk, 2010.

[22] F. Oswald, D. Jopp, C. Rott, and H.-W. Wahl, "Is aging in place a resource for or risk to life satisfaction?" *Gerontologist*, vol. 51, no. 2, pp. 238–250, 2011.

[23] P. O'Campo, "Invited commentary: advancing theory and methods for multilevel models of residential neighborhoods and health," *American Journal of Epidemiology*, vol. 157, no. 1, pp. 9–13, 2003.

[24] A. V. Diez Roux, "Neighborhoods and health: where are we and were do we go from here?" *Revue d'Epidemiologie et de Sante Publique*, vol. 55, no. 1, pp. 13–21, 2007.

[25] A. Strauss and J. Corbin, "Grounded theory methodology: an overview," in *Handbook of Qualitative Research*, N. K. Denzin and Y. S. Lincoln, Eds., Sage, Thousand Oaks, Calif, USA, 1994.

[26] M. B. Miles and A. M. Huberman, *Qualitative Data Analysis: A Sourcebook of New Methods*, Sage, Newbury Park, Calif, USA, 2nd edition, 1993.

[27] K. Charmaz, "Grounded theory," in *Rethinking Methods in Psychology*, J. Smith, R. Harre, and L. Van Langenhove, Eds., Sage, London, Uk, 1995.

[28] D. J. Ekerdt, "The busy ethic: moral continuity between work and retirement," *The Gerontologist*, vol. 26, no. 3, pp. 239–244, 1986.

[29] S. Katz, "Busy Bodies: activity, aging, and the management of everyday life," *Journal of Aging Studies*, vol. 14, no. 2, pp. 135–152, 2000.

[30] Federal Interagency Forum on Aging-Related Statistics, *Older Americans: Key Indicators of Well-Being*, US Government Printing Office, Washington, DC, USA, 2008.

[31] K. D. Moore, K. VanHaitsma, K. Curyto, and A. Saperstein, "A pragmatic environmental psychology: a metatheoretical inquiry into the work of M. Powell Lawton," *Journal of Environmental Psychology*, vol. 23, no. 4, pp. 471–482, 2003.

[32] M. P. Lawton, *Environment and Aging*, Center for the Study of Aging, Albany, NY, USA, 1986.

[33] P. B. Baltes and J. Smith, "Multilevel and systemic analyses of olde age: theoretical and empirical evidence for a fourth age," in *Handbook of Theories of Aging*, V. L. Bengston and K. W. Schai, Eds., pp. 153–173, Springer, New York, NY, USA, 1999.

[34] P. B. Baltes and J. Smith, "New frontiers in the future of aging: from successful aging of the young old to the dilemmas of the fourth age," *Gerontology*, vol. 49, no. 2, pp. 123–135, 2003.

[35] M. J. Brown, "Hypertension and ethnic group," *British Medical Journal*, vol. 332, no. 7545, pp. 835–836, 2006.

[36] A. P. Carson, G. Howard, G. L. Burke, S. Shea, E. B. Levitan, and P. Muntner, "Ethnic differences in hypertension incidence among middle-aged and older adults: the multi-ethnic study of atherosclerosis," *Hypertension*, vol. 57, no. 6, pp. 1101–1107, 2011.

[37] Centers for Disease Control. Diabetes and Women's Health Across the Life Stages: A Public Health Perspective, 2011, http://www.cdc.gov/diabetes/pubs/women/index.htm.

[38] F. M. Carp, "Some components of disengagement," *The Journals of Gerontology*, vol. 23, no. 3, pp. 382–386, 1968.

[39] S. R. Sherman, "Patterns of contacts for residents of age segregated and age integrated housing," *The Journals of Gerontology*, vol. 30, no. 1, pp. 103–107, 1975.

[40] T. A. LaVeist, "Racial segregation and longevity among African Americans: an individual-level analysis," *Health Services Research*, vol. 38, no. 6, part 2, pp. 1719–1733, 2003.

[41] S. V. Subramanian, D. Acevedo-Garcia, and T. L. Osypuk, "Racial residential segregation and geographic heterogeneity in black/white disparity in poor self-rated health in the US: a multilevel statistical analysis," *Social Science and Medicine*, vol. 60, no. 8, pp. 1667–1679, 2005.

[42] G. V. Ostir, K. Eschbach, K. S. Markides, and J. S. Goodwin, "Neighbourhood composition and depressive symptoms among older Mexican Americans," *Journal of Epidemiology and Community Health*, vol. 57, no. 12, pp. 987–992, 2003.

[43] K. Eschbach, G. V. Ostir, K. V. Patel, K. S. Markides, and J. S. Goodwin, "Neighborhood context and mortality among older Mexican Americans: is there a barrio advantage?" *American Journal of Public Health*, vol. 94, no. 10, pp. 1807–1812, 2004.

[44] S. A. Matthews, "The salience of neighborhood. Some lessons from sociology," *American Journal of Preventive Medicine*, vol. 34, no. 3, pp. 257–259, 2008.

12

Perceived Effectiveness of Elder Abuse Interventions in Psychological Distress and the Design of Culturally Adapted Interventions: A Qualitative Study in the Chinese Community in Chicago

XinQi Dong,[1] E-Shien Chang,[1] Esther Wong,[2] and Melissa Simon[3]

[1] *Chinese Health, Aging, and Policy Program, Rush Institute for Healthy Aging, Rush University Medical Center, 1645 West Jackson Blvd, Suite 675, Chicago, IL 60612, USA*
[2] *Chinese American Service League, Chicago, IL, USA*
[3] *Northwestern University, Feinberg School of Medicine, Chicago, IL, USA*

Correspondence should be addressed to XinQi Dong; xinqi dong@rush.edu

Academic Editor: F. Richard Ferraro

This qualitative study examines US Chinese older adults' views on the perceived effectiveness, challenges, and cultural adaptations of elder abuse interventions to psychological distress in the Chinese community in Chicago. A community-based participatory research approach was implemented to partner with the Chinese community. A total of 37 community-dwelling Chinese older adults (age 60+) participated in focus group discussions. Data analysis was based on grounded theory framework. Our findings suggest that older adults perceived social support, empowerment, and community-based interventions design as most effective to promote psychological well-being of victims. The perceived preferences were similar between elder abuse victims and non-victims. Strategies to culturally adapt evidence-based interventions were proposed with respect to nurturing filial piety values, familial integrations, and increased independence. Research and educational outreach initiatives were also discussed. This study has wide policy and practice implications for designing and deploying interventions to reduce psychological distress with respect to elder abuse outcome. Cultural relevancy of health interventions is important in the context of the Chinese communities. Collective federal, state, and community efforts are needed to support the culturally appropriate design and implementation of interventions suitable for the needs of the Chinese older adults.

1. Introduction

Elder abuse, sometimes referred to as elder mistreatment or elder maltreatment, is an important global health issue. Elder abuse manifests in various forms including physical abuse, sexual abuse, psychological abuse, caregiver neglect, and financial exploitation [1]. Available data suggest that 10% of US older adults aged 60 or older experience one or multiple forms of abuse [2, 3]. Despite the accessibility of Adult Protective Services in all fifty states, an overwhelming number of abused older adults may pass through healthcare system undiagnosed and overlooked. Associated with increased risk of morbidity and mortality, elder abuse continues to affect the quality of lives among vulnerable older adults [4–7]. Of particular importance is the adverse health outcome of elder abuse on victims' psychological well-being. Abused older adults exhibit symptoms of depression, anxiety, fear, and unworthiness, amongst other forms of psychological distress [8].

The associations between elder abuse and psychological distress highlight the urgent need for developing intervention programs addressing both elder abuse and psychopathology. Even though elder abuse has great public health relevance to health care professionals, social services providers, and the community gatekeepers and leaders, we have incomplete understanding of evidence-based prevention and intervention strategies to assist victims of elder abuse [9, 10]. A number of studies have started to examine the effectiveness of different intervention programs to reduce psychological distress, including increased social support for both victims and perpetrators [11–13], victim empowerment [14], advocacy interventions [14–16], and cognitive behavior activation [17]. However, research on interventions to reduce psychological distress with respect to elder abuse outcome remains scarce [18]. A recent systematic review further reported that existing interventions had limited effects on improving the social and psychological well-being of victims [10].

In addition, there exist structural, cultural, and social barriers in help seeking among the victims. For elder abuse victims, barriers to obtaining services may include physical frailty, cognitive impairment, and dependence on the abusers [19]. At the same time, victims may also serve in a caregiving or support capacity to their dependents or abusive family members, which in turn create different but equally challenging barriers to the victims' willingness and acceptance of needed services for themselves [20]. The issue of cultural diversity surrounding elder abuse further exemplifies a major complexity in advancing the field of elder abuse intervention. There exist knowledge gaps in understanding the cultural complexities of effective psychological well-being care supporting victims of elder abuse, particularly for minority older adults including African, Hispanic, and Asian populations [21].

Chinese population is one of the fastest growing minority groups in the U.S. Population estimates suggest that there are 4.0 million Chinese Americans in the United States, comprising 23% of the Asian American. Much of the health concern of Chinese older adults is deeply related to family caregiving guided by filial piety virtues. In Confucius teachings, filial piety dictates children's obligatory roles and responsibilities of caregiving to aging parents [22, 23]. Whereas respect for seniors is a deep-rooted cultural tradition, recent research suggests that elder abuse is an existing and pervasive health issue facing U.S. Chinese older adults [5, 24]. However, we are unaware of any studies that have examined the perceptions and preferred programs to reduce psychological distress from the perspectives of community-dwelling Chinese American older adults. Improved understanding of important factors shaping effective care for older adults' psychological well-being brings significant implications for health care professionals, social services providers, and health policy makers.

In order to expand our knowledge base on elder abuse interventions in a community-dwelling population of Chinese older adults, the goals of this qualitative study were to (1) elicit the perceived effectiveness of elder abuse interventions in reducing psychological distress, (2) explore similarities and differences in intervention preferences between the victim group and nonvictim group, and (3) identify strategies to culturally adapt evidence-based intervention programs to reduce psychological distress in the Chinese aging population.

2. Methods

2.1. Conceptual Framework and Definition. This study followed the conceptual framework of sociocultural context of elder abuse suggested by the National Research Council [1]. In this framework, elder abuse is defined as "intentional actions that cause harm or create a serious risk of harm (whether or not harm is intended) to a vulnerable elder by a caregiver or other person who stands in a trust relationship to the elder; or failure by a caregiver to satisfy the elder's basic needs or to protect the elder from harm." The Socio-Cultural Context model focuses on the comprehensive assessment of vulnerability factors while considering the socio-cultural context and social embeddedness, which refers to the set of people in the social network between older adult and trusted others. It is the interactions among these components in which elder abuse may take place, while at the same time guiding the proposed analysis in this report.

2.2. Community-Based Participatory Research Approach. Community-based participatory research (CBPR) design has been reported as an important model for exploring the issues of elder abuse in minority communities [25, 26]. Described as "a systematic inquiry with the participation of those affected by the issue being studied, for the purpose of education and taking action or affecting social change" [27], CBPR allows researchers, community leaders, stakeholders, and members alike to form a synergistic collaboration for community changes. In order to fully engage Chinese community through the preparation, conduct, and findings dissemination of research processes, a community-academic collaboration was formed between Rush University Medical Center and Chinese American Service League (CASL), the oldest and largest social service agency dedicated to serving Chinese immigrants in the Midwest. In order to maximize cultural and linguistic sensitivity of our research efforts, we formed a community advisory board to provide overall guidance ranging from research conceptualization and preparation to the conduct and findings review [6]. Board members were stakeholders and leaders enlisted through civic, health, social and advocacy groups, community centers, and clinics. Residents and opinion leaders were also invited to join the bimonthly meetings.

Since the inception of this synergistic community-academic collaboration, elder abuse has been identified as a pervasive health issue facing the Chinese community. A number of initiatives were undertaken to improve our understandings in this complex public health concern. We investigated cultural perception of elder abuse in the Chinese community through focus group discussions and in-depth interviews [5–7]. A recent advocacy effort also included the commemoration of the World Elder Abuse Awareness Day (WEAAD). Proclaimed by President Obama, WEAAD is now observed every year on June 15 in the U.S. as the opportunity to learn the signs of elder abuse and to empower older adults with tools and information necessary to overcome abusive situations [28]. The Chicago community commemorated WEAAD for the first time in CASL. Residents were invited to join focus group discussions regarding their views on elder abuse interventions. All study procedures were approved by the Rush University Medical Center Institutional Review Board.

2.3. Study Design and Procedure. This study utilizes both survey questionnaires and semistructured focus group methods to investigate the experience of elder abuse among U.S. Chinese older adults. We invited seniors who experienced elder abuse as well as those who did not experience elder abuse to participate. Our sample size was 37. In order to ensure diverse opinions, we planned to recruit one-third of elder abuse victims and two-thirds of nonvictims in the study sample.

Elder abuse was measured using a self-reported instrument derived from the Hwalek-Sengstok Elder Abuse Screening Test (H-S/EAST) and the Vulnerability to Abuse Screening Scale (VASS) (Hwalek and Sengstock, 1986; Schofield and Mishra, 2003). Sample questions included if participants felt uncomfortable with someone in the family, have been called names or put down, or been forced by someone to do things their belongings without have been taken permission. In addition, basic sociodemographic information was collected, including age, sex, education, marital status, household, country of origin, years of residing in the U.S. and preferred language.

Participants were then invited to participate in semistructured focus group discussions. Health behavior and interventions are highly culturally mediated issues. Focus group technique is an important qualitative research technique. It is particularly well suited for an exploratory study for which previous health literature is limited and for generating hypotheses and models of human behavior [29]. Focus group participants were recruited in accordance with the following eligibility criteria: (1) aged sixty years or older, (2) self-identified as Chinese, and (3) reside in Chicago. Prior to survey questionnaires and focus group discussions, study participants gave written consents. All materials were prepared in simplified Chinese, traditional Chinese, and English. In order to ensure cultural sensitivity of the study, participants were then divided into four focus groups according to their preferred dialect, including Cantonese or Mandarin [30]. Focus group interviews were guided by trained facilitators affiliated with CASL. Participants' perception of elder abuse interventions, perceived barriers, and facilitators of intervention programs were explored by the following questions.

(1) In general, what components in elder abuse interventions will be most effective to reduce psychological distress of abused seniors in our community?

(2) What components or approach in elder abuse interventions will probably not work in reducing psychological distress of abused seniors in our community?

(3) What are the creative ways or measures you can think of to improve the interventions components?

(4) How do we overcome these challenges to promote intervention programs in accordance with Chinese cultural and linguistic contexts?

The length of discussions was determined by the levels of interaction among participants. The facilitators proceeded with topics when responses were exhausted.

2.4. Data Analysis. For analysis purpose, we performed descriptive statistical analysis based on survey results. In accord with the standard diagnosis of a positive screen, the screening was considered positive for elder abuse or neglect if a patient answered yes to any of the screening questions.

With respect to qualitative data, grounded theory provided a general framework to analyze and develop themes and theories [31–33]. A bilingual research assistant first transcribed audio recordings into Chinese transcripts (different dialects used the same Chinese characters). The original Chinese transcripts were then imported into NVivo software (NVivo, version 9) for analysis. Two bicultural and bilingual researchers analyzed data in Chinese iteratively. Following grounded theory, they first labeled the texts with key words and phrases. The key words were coded and analyzed for emerging categories. Two coders then compared and discussed their sets of categories collectively to evolve dominant themes. The categorization of each response was not finalized until consensus was reached. Each category was reviewed and a short summary was written for each category. Quotes from the Chinese transcripts that captured participants' opinions and sentiments were then translated into English and incorporated to support each theme. The essence of discussions could be truly captured by working with the original language in which the focus groups took place.

3. Results

3.1. Characteristics of the Study Population by the Presence of Abuse. A total of 37 participants enrolled in the project (Table 1). Among these, 11 participants (29.7%) reported at least one item in the abuse screening tool in the domain of psychological, physical, financial abuse and exploitation. There were more men than women who screened positive for abuse. In the victim group, the majority (72.7%) were married and received 0–8 years of education (36.4%) or 13 or more years of education (36.4%). All of the participants who screened positive to abuse emigrated from Mainland China.

3.2. Perceived Effectiveness of Elder Abuse Interventions. We explored the perceived effectiveness of elder abuse interventions in reducing psychological distress using open-ended questions. Intervention programs identified as most effective to least effective included social support, empowerment, community-based interventions, advocacy, and psychological interventions (Table 2).

Of all the dimensions identified, the majority of responses fell into the category of social support. Specifically, increased peer group support, family support, and community support were viewed as beneficial elements to reduce distress of abused victims. For instance, support group that reduces social isolation and further informs seniors of their rights may be helpful to victims. As one participant described,

TABLE 1: Characteristics of the study population by the presence of elder abuse.

Any abuse	Yes (N = 11)	No (N = 26)
Age group, number (%)		
60–69	5 (45.5)	8 (30.8)
70–79	6 (54.5)	12 (46.2)
80+	0 (0.0)	6 (23.1)
Sex, number (%)		
Men	7 (63.6)	9 (34.6)
Women	4 (36.4)	17 (65.4)
Education levels, years (%)		
0–8 years	4 (36.4)	12 (46.2)
9–12 years	3 (27.3)	9 (34.6)
13 or more	4 (36.4)	5 (19.2)
Marital status, number (%)		
Married	8 (72.7)	19 (73.1)
Single	1 (9.1)	0
Widowed	2 (18.2)	7 (26.9)
Number of people in the household, number (%)		
1	3 (27.3)	6 (23.1)
2-3	7 (63.6)	14 (53.8)
4 or more	1 (9.1)	5 (19.2)
Origin, number (%)		
Mainland	11 (100)	25 (96.2)
Hong Kong	0	0
Taiwan	0	1 (3.8)
Others	0	0
Number of years in the U.S., number (%)		
1–10	3 (27.3)	6 (23.1)
11–20	2 (18.2)	7 (26.9)
21–30	5 (45.5)	10 (38.5)
31 or more	1 (9.1)	3 (11.5)
Language ability, number (%)		
Cantonese	8 (72.2)	17 (65.4)
Mandarin	2 (18.2)	2 (7.7)
English	1 (9.1)	0 (0.0)
Toishanese	0 (0.0)	7 (26.9)

"If you have a speaker that experienced elder abuse to come in and actually talk to the elders, then elders can connect with someone who understands what they are going through".

Empowerment was identified as an effective process to help individuals maximize their confidence, skills, and abilities in order to regain control of their lives. Many participants perceived education as the first step to inform victims of their rights. In addition, participants also pointed to increased financial independence of victims as an initial step. Many participants held favorable views toward interventions delivered by community-based social services organizations. Community-based organizations that offer bilingual and bicultural services have been viewed as a safe haven by immigrant older adults and perceived as the only available help resource for immigrants [5–7]. Participants perceived the easy access, prompt response, and flexibility to integrate interventions into existing programs as a plus to community-based intervention module. Advocacy and psychological intervention garnered least favorable views from our data analysis.

3.3. Similarities and Differences on Perceptions of Intervention Component between Victims and Nonvictims Groups. In addition, this study investigated the similarities and differences regarding preferences on the intervention components between the victims and nonvictims (Table 3). The majority of responses on preferred intervention programs from victims fell into community-based interventions and empowerment, whereas for nonvictim respondents, empowerment, and social support components received the most favorable views. Psychological interventions, including behavioral interventions and behavioral activations, remained least favorable by both groups.

3.4. Perceived Challenges to Each Intervention Component. This study also captured the potential challenges in the design of interventions from the perspectives of older adults (Table 4). A most commonly perceived challenge to advocacy pertains to the fear of limited actions. Participants expressed that advocacy programs would not be effective if the design and implementation only set out to enhance victim self-care without actionable goals. Advocacy could easily be interpreted as "knowledge" or "a type of explanation to abusive situations" and thus may be rendered less effective. Furthermore, participants were aware of the potential implementation barriers to other programs, such as empowerment and psychological interventions. Participants commented that empowerment programs would only be helpful if linking with other elements, such as counseling or peer group support element, that is, "empowerment does not work; if victims are not provided with direct counseling help (and support), then nothing can be resolved".

The benefits of psychological interventions to reduce psychological distress of victims remained least evident throughout the discussion. We suspect that the concept of behavioral activation or cognitive behavioral therapy may be foreign to community-dwelling older adults; hence there exists limited understanding on its benefits. Participants expressed the major challenge pertaining to negative perceptions on psychological interventions and behavior interventions. There may be a high level of reluctance and shame in joining such interventions.

Last, many seniors perceive intervention as a way to advocate for victims and their family members that "the community has to do something about it to provide them (victims) the protection and care that they deserve".

Table 2: Perceived effectiveness of elder abuse intervention.

Themes	Subthemes	Representative statements
Social support	Peer group support	"I think you can have increased support from victims themselves, like support group type of things. If you have a speaker that experienced elder abuse to come in and actually talk to the elders, then elders can connect with someone who understands what they are going through. The speaker can share his help-seeking experiences and provide guidance to other peers too."
	Family support	"As family friends and relatives, we need to be patient and listen to their problems." "They need family and relatives to lend ears to hear their problems."
	Community support	"(...) we need to get a support group together in the community centers. Before older adults realize any potential abusive situations, they can go to the support groups and let professionals intervene at the earliest possibility. Then perhaps we can prevent abuse from happening." "I was thinking that maybe there should be a place for those elders to enjoy the time or to talk about their problems with people there to help."
	Phone calls and hotlines	"I hope there is a bilingual hotline number to call, if anything comes up."
Empowerment	Education	"Education is the first step. They (victims) need to have a clear understanding of what elder abuse is so that they know what is going on." "If everyone conforms to Chinese traditional values to respect seniors, there would be no abuse at all. Therefore, education is important. If we educate everyone, then we can stop abuse."
	Counseling	"Counseling is important too, so that victims can talk freely about their distress and frustrations." "I think if a senior is abused, he/she will be very sad and painful. If we don't provide counseling help, we will not be able to relate to that type of turmoil and provide solutions. So I think counseling will be really critical."
	Enhance financial independence	"We need to improve the financial situations of abused seniors. If they can stand on their own feet financially, it may help them overcome abusive situations and decrease their risks to be victimized."
Community-based intervention	Interventions delivered through community agencies	"I think the options we have may all be effective. But if I must pick one, I would think community-based intervention would work best in our community, since seniors always turn to community social services agencies for help." "I think the community-based intervention model would work. If seniors have problems, community organizations can always step in and help."
	Integrate services to existing social service agencies	"I think we should educate homemakers about elder abuse. On the one hand, they can help us communicate and outreach to seniors. On the other hand, if they encounter any clients who may be victimized by abuse, they can help report the cases. Homemakers should be more aware of these types of issues and advocate for seniors."
Advocacy	Understand current situation and identify potential solutions	"We need to provide seniors with viable solutions. This could be one of the most important methods. Make sure the seniors are willing to listen. Newspapers and advertisement may be important as ways to advocate for their rights. And provide them with potential solutions and ways out of the abusive relationships."
Psychological intervention	Behavior activation	"It is important do something positive to alleviate their distress. For instance, I like painting. If I am distressed or frustrated, I would paint. It helps express my feelings and frustrations. These types of changes may help victims as well."

3.5. Strategies to Culturally Adapt Elder Abuse Interventions in Chinese Communities. In light of the perceived challenges in the design of interventions, we also solicited ways to adapt existing elder abuse interventions for Chinese seniors in accordance with Chinese cultural and linguistic characteristics (Table 5). Most of the responses fell in the category of improving filial piety practice as a way to improve social support. As one participant claimed, "Parents will feel much better if their children are filial. This is the best measure to help seniors". The importance of educating and nurturing filial piety values was echoed throughout the discussions.

In addition, our analysis showed that improved peer support by organizing community social events and activities may be a viable option to increase cultural sensitivity of intervention programs. One participant proposed that support group discussions may be integrated with existing cultural programs offered by community centers. Participants also called for more research and educational outreach efforts

Table 3: Similarities and differences on perceived preferences of intervention components between victims and nonvictims groups.

Among victims	Proportion of responses	Among nonvictims	Proportion of responses
Community-based intervention	31.5%	Empowerment	32.3%
Empowerment	31.5%	Social support	27.9%
Social support	22.2%	Community based intervention	22%
Advocacy	9.3%	Advocacy	8.8%
Psychological	5.5%	Psychological	8.8%

Table 4: Perceived challenges in the design of intervention.

Themes	Subthemes	Representative statements
Advocacy	Advocacy will be helpful if linking to actual actions to stop abuse	"I think advocacy is not going to be useful unless you help seniors to take real actions. You need actual changes to stop abuse, not only advocating for the rights of seniors." "Among all the components, I think advocacy is least useful. Advocacy is only knowledge, a type of explanation to tell people what to do. It is too far reached and actual impact is unclear."
	The root of the issue is to stop abusers	"We should think about the abuser. Why are they abusing the elderly? Maybe the abusers have some problems or stress management issues; we should also talk to them and see how they feel."
Empowerment	Empowerment will be helpful if linked with counseling	"Empowering seniors is an added value to the intervention. It does not help solve the real problem." "Empowerment does not work. If victims were not provided with counseling . . .(and support), nothing can be resolved. Victims will still feel lonely and frustrated."
Psychological intervention	The concept may be foreign to community seniors and hence decrease the chance of using this intervention	"Some people don't even want your help, they would be like, go away, I don't need it, it's going to make my life worse for me. . .that's what older people might think...Are they going to accept that? If they go to therapy, they may say that they don't think they have any problems. Older people have that attitude. So how are you going to persuade them to go to therapy and change any types of behaviors?"

Health surveys were perceived as a helpful way to equip older adults with necessary health sciences knowledge. In addition, rigorous research contributes to the identification of seniors at high risks of abuse as well as those "who need the most help from us". Last, increasing religious involvement was recognized as a helpful strategy. Participants linked religious attendance with increased social support, and thus it may be an effective intervention for victims.

4. Discussion

In this first exploratory study of perceived effectiveness, challenges, and cultural adaptations of elder abuse interventions among community-dwelling Chinese older adults, our findings suggest that older adults viewed social support, empowerment, and community-based interventions design as most effective to vulnerable victims. The preferences were similar between victim and nonvictims. Strategies to tailor interventions toward Chinese cultural beliefs were also proposed with respect to nurturing filial piety values, familial integration, and improving independence of victims.

This qualitative investigation provides new insights on how minority older adults viewed different abuse intervention components and strategies to overcome intervention barriers. First, our findings provide direction for violence-related intervention services. A multidisciplinary approach that includes strengthening the informal support system including family members, friends, and community gatekeepers as well as facilitating access to formal services building on the health care system warrants exploration in this context.

It has been argued that older adults with fewer psychosocial resources or more psychosocial deficits seem to be more vulnerable to elder abuse, and elder abuse seems particularly

TABLE 5: Strategies to culturally adapt elder abuse interventions in the chinese communities.

Themes	Subthemes	Representative statements
Improve social support	Improve and nurture filial piety	"Parents will feel much better if their children are filial. This is the best way to help seniors. Much better than improving other types of social support. So we need to educate our children and grandchildren and try to avoid family conflicts." "Abusive situations can be much improved upon if children are filial. If they respect seniors, they will feel much better. Wouldn't you say that this is the best way to improve the mental health of victims?"
	Improve peer support	"We can organize more social events and activities for older adults. I think Chinese seniors are often lonely. Especially those who may encounter problems and conflicts at home. If we can get them to go to those support groups, it will help ease their minds." "Seniors need to make more friends, especially with those who are currently undergoing similar issues. We need to get Chinese victims all together, like having them go to the same group discussion in community centers after some sort of painting classes or tai-chi classes."
Provide financial independence	Enhance victims' financial independence	"The U.S. government should be attentive of the social welfare needs of immigrant older adults. I think if abused seniors have more financial means, or financially more stable, they may not need to depend on the abusers at all, which will help improve their independence."
Research	Provide education through research and workshops	"We need to organize more educational workshops and group activities. It will be helpful if seniors are educated and informed of the benefits to interventions." "We need more research and health surveys that gather comprehensive health information of seniors. We will be able to document the health and well-being of seniors this way and reach out to those who need the most help from us."
Religion	Provide victims with religious support	"I believe we can try to help them by increasing their religion involvement. If they have higher religious attendance, they may be able to get more social support as well."

detrimental to psychological well-being for victims [34]. Our data suggest that the increased social support from family, friends, and supports is viewed as amongst the most effective interventions in increasing psychosocial resources of victims. This finding resonates with respect to important Chinese traditional values of filial obligations of respect and care from older adults. Despite acculturation challenges brought about by immigration, many traditional values and practices are still entrenched in this community. The utilization of family power in intervention designs warrants further attention.

It is also worth noting that advocacy and psychological interventions received limited appraisal among participants. Advocacy programs aim to enhance abused victims' self-care by helping them to make sense of the situation, identify potential solutions, and achieve the goals they have set [24]. From the limited empirical evidence, the effect of advocacy intervention designed to improve quality of life and mental health of Chinese abused women remained to be seen [14–16]. Similarly, whereas cognitive behavior model remained less favorable, some researches suggest that it can be a viable model in Chinese American population, with a few modifications [35, 36]. Systematic research is needed to explore the effectiveness of the different components of the advocacy and psychological intervention for the various forms of elder abuse.

In addition, given that community-based intervention module is appraised by Chinese older adults in this study, future research is needed to move forward to designing multicomponent elements of interventions suitable for the needs of minority older adults. For instance, studies in tribal communities found that interventions that offer combinations of individual or family counseling, case management, skills training, and behavior management strategies may be more effective than interventions that only provide a peer support group [37]. Measures that provide the opportunity for older adults, caregivers, families, and health professionals to come together to prevent and mitigate elder abuse in a community setting may be a novel option for Chinese older adults.

Furthermore, the results highlight the need to alleviate older adults' fears and shame in disclosing abuse. Our findings reveal that there exist more similarities than differences in the preferences of intervention programs between susceptible victims and nonvictims. Although the finding may be due to a small sample size effect, the violence and mental health stigma may indeed affect older adults' willingness to enroll in intervention programs. Health care providers should consider outreach programs particularly designed to reduce the stigma of violence and caregiver stress among Chinese immigrant families.

Last, conducting participatory research approach allows us to prioritize sensitive cultural context and increase the relevance of our research findings to actionable intervention goals [38, 39]. When culture is continually evolving, the ability to identify factors that are amendable to adaptation to the Chinese population would help ensure that the health intervention is sensitive to the needs and concerns of victims. Our synergetic academic-community collaboration helps raise awareness and understanding of the complexities in elder abuse situations and further empower older adults and their family members.

There are several limitations to this study. First, the data used in this investigation were from a small sample of Chinese older adults. Future studies should consider working with diverse Chinese immigrants in a population-based study design. Second, the sample used was purposively selected from the Chinese community in Chicago, and hence, our results may not be generalizable to other Chinese populations, including suburban groups, Chinese ethnic minority groups, or rural Chinese populations, as they may be subjected to varying degrees of social and economic influence [40]. Systematic examinations of the longitudinal risk and protective factors and of effect size are needed to devise targeted intervention studies. In addition, given the extent of the different types of elder abuse and variation in risk and protective factors and perpetrator characteristics, we did not investigate evidence-based interventions for the specific dyads that may be at particularly high risk for elder abuse. Rigorously designed intervention studies and measures of relevant outcomes of elder abuse are particularly needed.

Nonetheless, this study provides insights on the policy and practice implications for designing and deploying intervention to reduce psychological distress with respect to elder abuse outcome in Chinese aging communities. Cultural relevancy of health interventions is critical in this vulnerable population. Cultural sensitivity in health intervention programs entails more than matching languages or locations preferred by the local community members. Rather, incorporating the cultural, social, and structural contexts in the targeted community contributes to the salience of policy impact [41, 42]. In addition, health care professionals should consider outreach programs particularly designed to increase familial, social, and community support for vulnerable older adults. Collective federal, state, and community efforts are needed to support the culturally appropriate training and education on elder abuse interventions.

5. Conclusion

We conclude that, from the perspectives of community-dwelling Chinese older adults, elder abuse interventions hold promise for improving the psychological well-being of victims. Our results further underscore the urgent need of designing culturally and linguistically sensitive evidence-based interventions tailored toward the needs of diverse aging populations.

References

[1] National Research Council, *Elder Mistreatment: Abuse, Neglect And Exploitation in an Aging America*, The National Academies Press, Washington, DC, USA, 2003.

[2] S. R. Beach, R. Schulz, N. G. Castle, and J. Rosen, "Financial exploitation and psychological mistreatment among older adults: differences between African Americans and non-African Americans in a population-based survey," *The Gerontologist*, vol. 50, no. 6, pp. 744–757, 2010.

[3] R. Acierno, M. A. Hernandez, A. B. Amstadter et al., "Prevalence and correlates of emotional, physical, sexual, and financial abuse and potential neglect in the United States: The National Elder Mistreatment study," *American Journal of Public Health*, vol. 100, no. 2, pp. 292–297, 2010.

[4] X. Dong, M. Simon, C. Mendes De Leon et al., "Elder self-neglect and abuse and mortality risk in a community-dwelling population," *Journal of the American Medical Association*, vol. 302, no. 5, pp. 517–526, 2009.

[5] X. Q. Dong, E.-S. Chang, E. Wong, B. Wong, and M. A. Simon, "How do U.S. Chinese older adults view elder mistreatment? Findings from a community-based participatory research study," *Journal of Aging and Health*, vol. 23, no. 2, pp. 289–312, 2011.

[6] X. Dong, E.-S. Chang, E. Wong, and M. Simon, "Working with culture: lessons learned from a community-engaged project in a Chinese aging population," *Aging Health*, vol. 7, no. 4, pp. 529–537, 2011.

[7] X. Q. Dong, M. A. Simon, T. T. Beck et al., "Elder abuse and mortality: the role of psychological and social wellbeing," *Gerontology*, vol. 57, no. 6, pp. 549–558, 2011.

[8] X. Dong, R. Chen, E. Chang, and M. Simon, "Elder abuse and psychological well-being: a systematic review and implications for research and policy—a mini review," *Gerontology*, vol. 59, pp. 132–142, 2013.

[9] X. Dong, "Advancing the field of elder abuse: future directions and policy implications," *Journal of American Geriatric Society*, vol. 60, pp. 2151–2156, 2012.

[10] J. Ploeg, J. Fear, B. Hutchison, H. MacMillan, and G. Bolan, "A systematic review of interventions for elder abuse," *Journal of Elder Abuse and Neglect*, vol. 21, no. 3, pp. 187–210, 2009.

[11] A. J. Sowden, S. Tilford, F. Delaney, M. Vogels, S. Gilbody, and T. A. Sheldon, "Mental health promotion in high risk groups," *Quality and Safety in Health Care*, vol. 6, no. 4, pp. 219–225, 1997.

[12] B. G. Knight, S. M. Lutzky, and F. Macofsky-Urban, "A meta-analytic review of interventions for caregiver distress: recommendations for future research," *The Gerontologist*, vol. 33, no. 2, pp. 240–248, 1993.

[13] H.-F. Hsieh, J.-J. Wang, M. Yen, and T.-T. Liu, "Educational support group in changing caregivers' psychological elder abuse behavior toward caring for institutionalized elders," *Advances in Health Sciences Education*, vol. 14, no. 3, pp. 377–386, 2009.

[14] A. F. Tiwari, F. Salili, R. Y. Chan, E. K. Chan, and D. Tang, "Effectiveness of an empowerment intervention in abused Chinese women," *Hong Kong Medical Journal*, vol. 16, pp. 25–28, 2010.

[15] A. Tiwari, D. Y. T. Fong, K. H. Yuen et al., "Effect of an advocacy intervention on mental health in Chinese women survivors of intimate partner violence: a randomized controlled trial," *Journal of the American Medical Association*, vol. 304, no. 5, pp. 536–543, 2010.

[16] J. Ramsay, Y. Carter, L. Davidson et al., "Advocacy interventions to reduce or eliminate violence and promote the physical and psychosocial well-being of women who experience intimate partner abuse," *Cochrane Database of Systematic Reviews*, vol. 8, no. 3, Article ID CD005043, 2009.

[17] Y. Dai, S. Zhang, J. Yamamoto et al., "Cognitive behavioral therapy of minor depressive symptoms in elderly Chinese Americans: a pilot study," *Community Mental Health Journal*, vol. 35, no. 6, pp. 537–542, 1999.

[18] A. Papadopoulos and J. La Fontaine, *Elder Abuse Therapeutic Perspectives in Practice*, Winslow, Bicester, UK, 2000.

[19] P. Brownell and D. Heiser, "Psycho-educational support groups for older women victims of family mistreatment: a pilot study," *Journal of Gerontological Social Work*, vol. 46, no. 3-4, pp. 145–160, 2006.

[20] P. Brownell, "Mental health and criminal justice issues among perpetrators of elder abuse," *Journal of Elder Abuse and Neglect*, vol. 11, no. 4, pp. 81–94, 1999.

[21] J. Miranda, G. Bernal, A. Lau, L. Kohn, W.-C. Hwang, and T. LaFromboise, "State of the science on psychosocial interventions for ethnic minorities," *Annual Review of Clinical Psychology*, vol. 1, pp. 113–142, 2005.

[22] P.-C. Lan, "Subcontracting filial piety: elder care in ethnic Chinese immigrant families in California," *Journal of Family Issues*, vol. 23, no. 7, pp. 812–835, 2002.

[23] Mencius and D. C. Lau, *Mencius (Penguin Classics)*, Penguin Classics, London, UK, 2005.

[24] E. Chang, M. A. Simon, E. Wong et al., "Elder mistreatment in a community-dwelling population: findings from a large cohort of U.S. Chinese older adults," *The Gerontologist*, vol. 52, no. S1, p. 37, 2012.

[25] P. A. Holkup, T. Tripp-Reimer, E. M. Salois, and C. Weinert, "Community-based participatory research: an approach to intervention research with a native american community," *Advances in Nursing Science*, vol. 27, no. 3, pp. 162–175, 2004.

[26] X. Dong, "Cultural diversity and elder abuse: implication for research, education, and policy," *Generations: Journal of the American Society on Aging*, vol. 36, pp. 40–42, 2012.

[27] L. W. Green and S. L. Mercer, "Can public health researchers and agencies reconcile the push from funding bodies and the pull from communities?" *American Journal of Public Health*, vol. 91, no. 12, pp. 1926–1929, 2001.

[28] The White House, *Presidential Proclamation—World Elder Abuse Awareness Day, 2012*, Office of the Press Secretaty, The White House, 2012.

[29] R. Krueger, *Focus Groups: A Practical Guide for Applied Research*, Sage, Thousand Oaks, Calif, USA, 1994.

[30] E. E. Suh, S. Kagan, and N. Strumpf, "Cultural competence in qualitative interview methods with asian immigrants," *Journal of Transcultural Nursing*, vol. 20, no. 2, pp. 194–201, 2009.

[31] L. A. Curry, I. M. Nembhard, and E. H. Bradley, "Qualitative and mixed methods provide unique contributions to outcomes research," *Circulation*, vol. 119, no. 10, pp. 1442–1452, 2009.

[32] B. G. Glaser and A. C. Strauss, *The Discovery of Grounded Theory*, Aldine, Chicago, Ill, USA, 1967.

[33] A. C. Strauss and J. Corbin, *Basics of Qualitative Research: Grounded Theory Procedures and Techniques*, Sage, Newbury Park, Calif, USA, 1990.

[34] Y. Luo and L. J. Waite, "Mistreatment and psychological well-being among older adults: exploring the role of psychosocial resources and deficits," *Journals of Gerontology B*, vol. 66, no. 2, pp. 217–229, 2011.

[35] E. K. Shen, L. E. Alden, I. Söchting, and P. Tsang, "Clinical observations of a Cantonese cognitive-behavioral treatment program for Chinese immigrants. Special issue: culture, race, and ethnicity in psychotherapy," *Psychotherapy*, vol. 43, no. 4, pp. 518–530, 2006.

[36] S. W.-H. Chen and D. S. Davenport, "Cognitive-behavioral therapy with Chinese American clients: cautions and modifications," *Psychotherapy*, vol. 42, no. 1, pp. 101–110, 2005.

[37] P. A. Holkup, E. M. Salois, T. Tripp-Reimer, and C. Weinert, "Drawing on wisdom from the past: an elder abuse intervention with tribal communities," *The Gerontologist*, vol. 47, no. 2, pp. 248–254, 2007.

[38] L. C. Tillman, "Culturally senstive research approaches: an African-American perspective," *Educational Researcher*, vol. 31, pp. 3–12, 2002.

[39] L. H. Rogler, "The meaning of culturally sensitive research in mental health," *American Journal of Psychiatry*, vol. 146, no. 3, pp. 296–303, 1989.

[40] W. Li, "Changing Chinese settlement," in *Ethnoburb: The New Ethnic Community in Urban America*, W. Li, Ed., pp. 53–78, University of Hawaii Press, Honolulu, Hawaii, USA, 2009.

[41] M. W. Kreuter, N. A. Lezin, and L. A. Young, "Evaluation community-based collaborative mechanisms: implications for practioners," *Health Promotion Practice*, vol. 1, no. 1, pp. 49–63, 2000.

[42] B. Resnick, P. Inguito, D. Orwig et al., "Treatment fidelity in behavior change research: a case example," *Nursing Research*, vol. 54, no. 2, pp. 139–143, 2005.

13

Apathy as Marker of Frail Status

Roberta Semprini,[1] Adele Lubrano,[1] Giulia Misaggi,[1] and Alessandro Martorana[1,2]

[1] Clinica Neurologica, Dipartimento di Neuroscienze, Università di Roma "Tor Vergata", Via Montpellier, 00133 Rome, Italy
[2] IRCCS Santa Lucia, Via Ardeatina, 00179 Rome, Italy

Correspondence should be addressed to Alessandro Martorana, martorana@med.uniroma2.it

Academic Editor: John Knight

Frailty is a complex and dynamic condition associated with aging. This condition is characterised by the difficult adaptation of an old subject to new challenges occurring during life. Frailty is supposed to be due to the progressive decrease of physiological reserves and multiorgan and multisystem change. It coincides with a reduced or absent resilience. In general comorbidities like hypertension, heart disease, inflammation and infectious diseases are potential risk factors for and psychophysical decline. The aim of this work is to highlight the importance of impaired cognition as factor predisposing to frailty. The authors are convinced and suggest that the presence of neurobehavioral disturbance like apathy associated to impaired executive function could be the major predisposing factor for frailty and unsuccessful aging. Unfortunately available literature largely underestimates the presence of these factors. Thus to better identify markers of frailty, a good neuropsychological assessment and the evaluation of behavioural disturbances are suggested.

1. Introduction

Aging is a complex phenomenon which features have recently gained interest. In general aging is characterised by the progressive accumulation of deficits taking place in different individuals and in different pathways (molecular, cellular, psychological, and psychosocial, etc.), and with a variety of rates proper of each individual, that may depend on the interplay between intrinsic and extrinsic factors [1, 2].

Associated to aging we recognise a nonspecific condition defined "frail-old" or "frailty syndrome". This is a condition that has long been considered synonymous of disability and comorbidity since it is prevalent in old age. Frailty is a condition that expose an old subject to be vulnerable to many non threatening-illness conditions, although they are not recognised as precipitating factors [3, 4].

A good definition of normal aging, even in general terms [5], may be useful to better understand the concept of frailty and its features.

Normal aging is widely considered a physiological condition during which natural reserves progressively decrease, while still supporting an acceptable functioning of essential organs, in a steady state. Thus aging is considered a dynamic event in which a progressive dysregulation of homeostatic conditions makes the organs and systems less or nonresilient [6, 7].

Many variables (biologic, metabolic, psychosocial, etc.) may play a significant role in the evolution of aging process. The association of these variables, which are different among individuals, with comorbidities (hypertension, heart disease, diabetes, bone fractures, infectious diseases) are considered responsible for the quality and rate of aging. Thus, the absence of disabilities and unimpaired cognition might be considered the features of successful aging [8]. Conversely, unsuccessful aging could be the result of the association between disabilities and cognitive decline. Considerable evidence points to impairment of executive function as a key contributor to age-related declines in a range of cognitive tasks [9].

Therefore, frailty could be considered a dynamic condition set between successful and unsuccessful aging.

Following the "Frailty Task Force" of the American Geriatric Society frailty has been considered a clinical syndrome defined by the presence of 3 or more of the following symptoms: unintentional weight loss, self-reported exhaustion, weakness, slow walking speed, and low physical activity.

Clinical signs are represented by undernutrition, sarcopenia, balance and gait disorders, and osteopenia. These features are expected to hesitate in increased risk of falls, worsening mobility or reducing it.

Several conditions have been identified as possibly related to a frail status and thus responsible almost in part for decline of old person.

Aging itself is generally accepted to be accompanied by altered metabolic processes like increased free radicals production, telomere shortening, and mitochondrial dysfunction; changes associated to extrinsic conditions like inflammatory status (IL-6, TNF; CRP) and common comorbidities (chronic illness like diabetes, hypertension, coronary heart disease, obesity, malignancies) may be responsible for frailty and life-shortening [10–14]. In this view, frailty may be considered as a condition which precedes in a subclinical manner, such that when resilience is overwhelmed it becomes manifest concomitantly with the appearance of chronic illness. At the same time altered resilience could be the result of altered volition and motor planning, thus the result of impaired executive functions. This in turn could be responsible for hypomobility and reduced autonomy and as a consequence might render someone frail that successfully aged. In this view impaired cognition may be a precipitating factor that shifts a subject from the prefrail to the frail status [15].

The aim of this work is to discuss the role of altered cognitive conditions of aged person and in particular we will focus on executive functions and apathy in aging.

2. Executive Functions

Cognitive impairment is the primary determinant of disability in late life, and at all ages, cognitive function is the foundation of individual capacity to meet the challenges of any disabling condition [16].

Executive functions refer to a variety of higher cognitive processes that are related to the function of frontal lobes. In general this area of the brain is able to integrate the formation flow arising from many sensory systems set in both anterior and posterior brain, necessary for goal-directed action and also for the control of attentional resources which are considered basic for daily living activities [17]. In general anterior parts of frontal lobes are involved in aspects of self-regulation (inhibition or self-awareness) while posterior parts are involved in reasoning process [18].

PFC and striatum are the main regions of the frontal lobe involved in the control of executive functions [19, 20]. In both regions dopaminergic system plays an essential role as a modulator of cortico-striatal functions, acting through its receptors, namely, D1-like and D2-like [21–23]. Changes of the dorsolateral prefrontal-caudate circuits are considered responsible for disexecutive function, which lead mainly to a subcortical dysfunction. Frontal lobes are involved in the pathophysiology of many neurological and psychiatric disorders and are also highly susceptible to changes of aging [15, 24, 25].

During normal aging synaptic changes of frontal cortex and associated to changes of the striatum (like altered dendritic pruning, decrease of neurotransmitters efficiency, in particular of dopaminergic system, and also the presence of diffuse white matter lesions) [26] are considered responsible for poor performance on executive tasks in healthy old subjects, as demonstrated in neuropsychological studies. Moreover executive functions contribute also to motor planning and therefore to maintain gait stability. As a consequence an impairment of pre-frontal-striatal circuit could be also responsible of gait instability and slow walking speed observed in healthy old subjects.

Gait instability and slow speed during walking are considered risk factors for falls and disability.

Thus it is conceivable to suggest that, as depicted previously about the features of frail patient, impairment of executive functions during normal aging could represent the marker to distinguish a successful aging from a prefrail status, however not sufficient to determine frailty of a subject.

Our suggestion is that, more importantly, the presence of apathetic behavior could represent reasonably a precipitating factor for frailty.

3. Apathy and Aging

Apathy is a behavioural syndrome common in normal physiological aging and is also part of the psychiatric spectrum of mental illness, and of many neurodegenerative disorders like Alzheimer's disease Apathy is an observable behavioural syndrome consisting in a quantitative reduction of voluntary (or goal-directed) behaviours [27]. Therefore, apathy occurs when the systems that generate and control voluntary actions are altered. In this view apathy can be defined as the quantitative reduction of self-generated voluntary and purposeful behaviour and necessarily has not to be considered a clinical aspect of depression (see [28, 29]).

In general the basal ganglia and their connection with the prefrontal cortex are deputed to decision making. Hence, any dysfunction of this frontostriatal circuit may be responsible for apathetic behaviour.

Anatomical circuits of apathy are represented by cortical areas like the prefrontal cortex (neo-, paleo-, and archeocortex, amygdala, and hippocampus) and the ventral basal ganglia (limbic striatum or better the nucleus accumbens, midbrain ventral tegmental area, medial tip of subthalamic nucleus, centromedian, and parafascicular nuclei of the thalamus) [19, 30–32]. The roles played by prefrontal cortex (PFC) and by nucleus accumbens (NAcc) render these structures as the most involved in the appearance of apathy [33, 34].

PFC has an essential role in cognitive and executive processes that involve motivation, emotion learning, and memory. PFC integrates sensory and limbic information and promotes goal-directed behavior through efferent projections to the NAcc. In addition, PFC sends outputs to other limbic areas such as the hippocampus and amygdale, which in turn modulate the activity of the NAcc through excitatory-glutamatergic projections.

NAcc receives inputs from cortical areas (neocortex, hippocampus, amygdala) and envy inputs to the ventral pallidum, which represents the output nuclei of the ventral basal

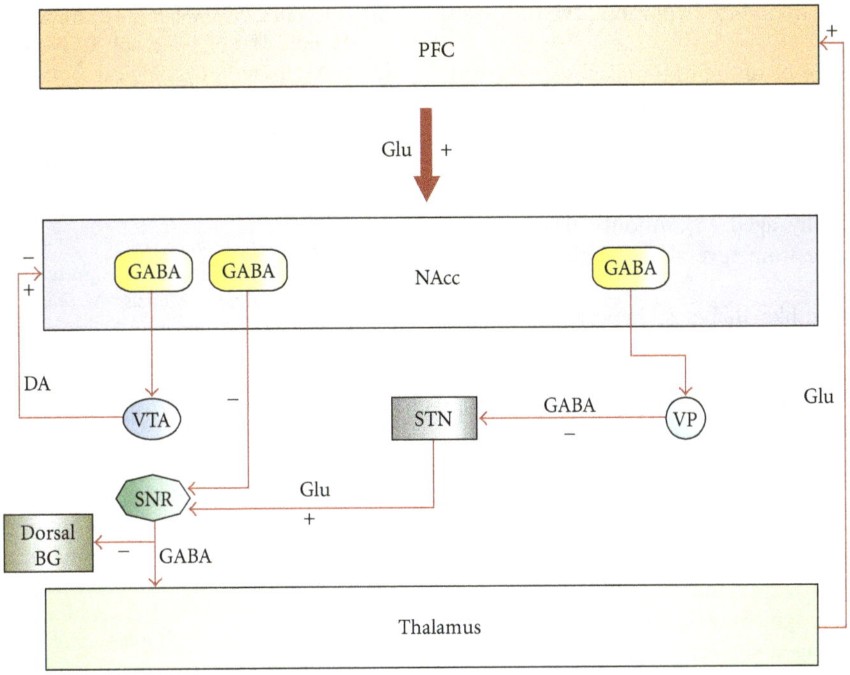

FIGURE 1: Schematic representation of basal ganglia circuit. In this scheme the nucleus accumbens (NAcc) is an interface through which limbic (glutamatergic) structures influence motor activity, in a way that limbic structures can influence behavior, under control of meso-limbic (dopaminergic structures) system (Ventral Tegmental Area neurons).

ganglia system. This is a region that through its connection with the thalamic nuclei transfers information back to the cortex. This arrangement is made to select relevant signals from background noise arising from multiple inputs and to transfer it back to the cortex in order to generate output signal to target nuclei. Put in this frame NAcc has been proposed to play a role in emotion, and more generally in limbic-motor integration (see Figure 1). This hypothesis has been based on the anatomical organization of the NAcc which suggests that this nucleus is an interface through which limbic (glutamatergic) structures influence motor activity, and that these limbic influences on behavior could in part be controlled by mesolimbic (dopaminergic structures) system. Ideally any morphologic alteration in these brain regions can potentially induce apathetic symptoms.

Following Levy and Dubois's work [27], apathy has to be considered heterogeneous disorder that may be ascribed at least to three different phenomena, each related to a specific topography in basal ganglia. The first involves the affective-emotional processing, thus the medial PFC connection with amygdala and NAcc, the second involves the cognitive processing, thus the lateral PFC and caudate nucleus connection, and the third involves the so-called "auto-activation" processing, which is observed in the severe cases of apathy. In these cases a link with pallidal dysfunction o extensive cortical lesions was supposed.

During normal aging it is conceivable to suppose that due to morphological and metabolic changes of cortical neurons as well as of subcortical nuclei, disorder of emotional-affective processing may appear. PFC and hippocampus have been demonstrated to show particular vulnerability during normal aging. Subtle regional changes of dendritic branching or altered mechanisms of neural plasticity have been experimentally demonstrated in lab animals and also in humans [35–39]. These changes are also associated with reduced levels of neurotransmitters like acetylcholine, glutamate, GABA, and dopamine decrease with age (Chen et al. [40]). Such alterations may reasonably be responsible for appearance of apathetic behavior in old subject. In this view, several reports showed that dopamine transmission is particularly vulnerable with age, in particular reduction of the accumbal dopamine transporter and of cortical dopamine receptors (both D1-like and D2-like, where D2-like seems to be prevalent) in aged subjects ([41], Volkow et al. [42]; Ishibashi et al. [43]; and Bäckman et al. [44]). These changes were related to PFC cognitive deficits and in particular were related to executive function impairment [45]. Even reward processing which has been demonstrated to be tuned by dopamine is altered in aged subjects [44, 46, 47]. Thus, dopamine appears particularly as vulnerable to aging. Given the particular deficits of dopamine transmission and the role played by this transmitter in the control of PFC-basal ganglia circuit, it is conceivable to suppose that such changes could be responsible for apathetic behavior in old subject. Moreover, apathy increases with age in healthy old population [48], and its presence is considered an early sign of cognitive decline [49].

4. The Apathy as Marker of Frail Status

Prefrail or frailty syndrome is considered dynamic conditions where the reduced resilience of a subject might induce changes responsible for disability, hypomobility, and even death.

Certainly the absence of disabilities and also preserved cognition, as mentioned previously, represent the target for a good aging.

Population-based studies performed in old healthy adults demonstrated that only 30% of population examined can be defined as successfully aged [8]. About 70% of subjects unfortunately suffer from several disabilities that may shorten their life.

Certainly disabilities like diabetes, hypertension, and heart disease of infections are easily identified and often patient's history shows how these were able to interfere with aging compromising the possible recovery. Sarcopenia, undernutrition, and inflammatory status are conditions that may be easily measured [3, 4].

Conversely cognition and neuropsychiatric disturbances in healthy old subjects are infrequently evaluated among old healthy subjects [50–52]. They are considered typical disturbances of patients with frank cognitive decline and thus evaluated among cognitively impaired patients, and rarely among normally aged subjects [53]. Such condition renders the weight of impaired cognition and of apathy on nondemented healthy subjects underestimated.

Recently few studies [25, 54, 55] outlined the necessity for measures of cognitive abilities and of neuropsychiatric inventory among aged subject. Indeed, the presence of apathy during aging might be responsible for hypomobility and reduced volition on one hand; on the other hand it may be the principal cause of carelessness and as a consequence of progressive worsening of comorbidities.

In this view, the presence of apathy, which we are strongly convinced that it is underestimated among aged adults, could represent the marker of a prefrail status predisposing a subject to become frail.

From our consideration emerges the need for further studies to better identify the real impact of apathy and impaired executive functions on frailty syndrome.

Conflict of Interests

The authors have no conflict of interests to disclosure.

References

[1] A. B. Mitnitski, A. J. Mogilner, and K. Rockwood, "Accumulation of deficits as a proxy measure of aging," *The Scientific World Journal*, vol. 1, pp. 323–336, 2001.

[2] T. B. L. Kirkwood, "Time of our lives. What controls the length of life?" *EMBO Reports*, vol. 6, supplement 1, pp. S4–S8, 2005.

[3] T. Fulop, A. Larbi, J. M. Witkowski et al., "Aging, frailty and age-related diseases," *Biogerontology*, vol. 11, no. 5, pp. 547–563, 2010.

[4] P. O. Lang, J. P. Michel, and D. Zekry, "Frailty syndrome: a transitional state in a dynamic process," *Gerontology*, vol. 55, no. 5, pp. 539–549, 2009.

[5] H. Bergman, L. Ferrucci, J. Guralnik et al., "Frailty: an emerging research and clinical paradigm—issues and controversies," *Journals of Gerontology A*, vol. 62, no. 7, pp. 731–737, 2007.

[6] F. E. Yates, "Complexity of a human being: changes with age," *Neurobiology of Aging*, vol. 23, no. 1, pp. 17–19, 2002.

[7] L. A. Lipsitz, "Physiological complexity, aging, and the path to frailty," *Science of Aging Knowledge Environment*, vol. 2004, no. 16, article pe16, 2004.

[8] C. A. Depp and D. V. Jeste, "Definitions and predictors of successful aging: A comprehensive review of larger quantitative studies," *American Journal of Geriatric Psychiatry*, vol. 14, no. 1, pp. 6–20, 2006.

[9] E. L. Glisky, "Changes in cognitive function in human aging," in *Brain Aging: Models, Methods, and Mechanisms*, D. R. Riddle, Ed., Frontiers in Neuroscience, chapter 1, CRC Press, Boca Raton, Fla, USA, 2007.

[10] D. J. Gunnell, M. Okasha, G. D. Smith, S. E. Oliver, J. Sandhu, and J. M. P. Holly, "Gender gap in longevity and disability in older persons," *Epidemiologic Reviews*, vol. 23, no. 2, pp. 343–350, 2001.

[11] L. P. Fried, "Establishing benchmarks for quality care for an aging population: caring for vulnerable older adults," *Annals of Internal Medicine*, vol. 139, no. 9, pp. 784–786, 2003.

[12] R. Klein, B. E. K. Klein, and M. D. Knudtson, "Frailty and age-related macular degeneration: the beaver dam eye study," *American Journal of Ophthalmology*, vol. 140, no. 1, pp. 129–131, 2005.

[13] K. Bandeen-Roche, Q. L. Xue, L. Ferrucci et al., "Phenotype of frailty: characterization in the Women's Health and Aging Studies," *Journals of Gerontology A*, vol. 61, no. 3, pp. 262–266, 2006.

[14] M. D. Rothman, L. Leo-Summers, and T. M. Gill, "Prognostic significance of potential frailty criteria," *Journal of the American Geriatrics Society*, vol. 56, no. 12, pp. 2211–2216, 2008.

[15] J. K. Johnson, L. Y. Lui, and K. Yaffe, "Executive function, more than global cognition, predicts functional decline and mortality in elderly women," *Journals of Gerontology A*, vol. 62, no. 10, pp. 1134–1141, 2007.

[16] F. Malouin, C. L. Richards, and A. Durand, "Normal aging and motor imagery vividness: implications for mental practice training in rehabilitation," *Archives of Physical Medicine and Rehabilitation*, vol. 91, no. 7, pp. 1122–1127, 2010.

[17] J. R. Hollerman, L. Tremblay, and W. Schultz, "Involvement of basal ganglia and orbitofrontal cortex in goal-directed behavior," *Progress in Brain Research*, vol. 126, pp. 193–215, 2000.

[18] V. Elderkin-Thompson, G. Hellemann, D. Pham, and A. Kumar, "Prefrontal brain morphology and executive function in healthy and depressed elderly," *International Journal of Geriatric Psychiatry*, vol. 24, no. 5, pp. 459–468, 2009.

[19] S. N. Haber and J. L. Fudge, "The primate substantia nigra and VTA: integrative circuitry and function," *Critical Reviews in Neurobiology*, vol. 11, no. 4, pp. 323–342, 1997.

[20] S. Tekin and J. L. Cummings, "Frontal-subcortical neuronal circuits and clinical neuropsychiatry: an update," *Journal of Psychosomatic Research*, vol. 53, no. 2, pp. 647–654, 2002.

[21] D. M. Haluk and S. B. Floresco, "Ventral striatal dopamine modulation of different forms of behavioral flexibility," *Neuropsychopharmacology*, vol. 34, no. 8, pp. 2041–2052, 2009.

[22] S. B. Floresco and O. Magyar, "Mesocortical dopamine modulation of executive functions: beyond working memory," *Psychopharmacology*, vol. 188, no. 4, pp. 567–585, 2006.

[23] S. B. Floresco, O. Magyar, S. Ghods-Sharifi, C. Vexelman, and M. T. L. Tse, "Multiple dopamine receptor subtypes in the medial prefrontal cortex of the rat regulate set-shifting," *Neuropsychopharmacology*, vol. 31, no. 2, pp. 297–309, 2006.

[24] Y. Braw, S. Aviram, Y. Bloch, and Y. Levkovitz, "The effect of age on frontal lobe related cognitive functions of unmedicated depressed patients," *Journal of Affective Disorders*, vol. 129, no. 1–3, pp. 342–347, 2011.

[25] G. Allali, F. Assal, R. W. Kressig, V. Dubost, F. R. Herrmann, and O. Beauchet, "Impact of impaired executive function on gait stability," *Dementia and Geriatric Cognitive Disorders*, vol. 26, no. 4, pp. 364–369, 2008.

[26] E. C. Klostermann, M. N. Braskie, S. M. Landau, J. P. O'Neil, and W. J. Jagust, "Dopamine and frontostriatal networks in cognitive aging," *Neurobiology of Aging*. In press.

[27] R. Levy and B. Dubois, "Apathy and the functional anatomy of the prefrontal cortex-basal ganglia circuits," *Cerebral Cortex*, vol. 16, no. 7, pp. 916–928, 2006.

[28] R. S. Marin, S. Firinciogullari, and R. C. Biedrzycki, "The sources of convergence between measures of apathy and depression," *Journal of Affective Disorders*, vol. 28, no. 2, pp. 117–124, 1993.

[29] R. S. Marin, S. Firinciogullari, and R. C. Biedrzycki, "Group differences in the relationship between apathy and depression," *Journal of Nervous and Mental Disease*, vol. 182, no. 4, pp. 235–239, 1994.

[30] M. Amalric and G. F. Koob, "Functionally selective neurochemical afferents and efferents of the mesocorticolimbic and nigrostriatal dopamine system," *Progress in Brain Research*, vol. 99, pp. 209–226, 1993.

[31] S. N. Haber, K. Kunishio, M. Mizobuchi, and E. Lynd-Balta, "The orbital and medial prefrontal circuit through the primate basal ganglia," *Journal of Neuroscience*, vol. 15, no. 7, pp. 4851–4867, 1995.

[32] S. N. Haber and B. Knutson, "The reward circuit: Linking primate anatomy and human imaging," *Neuropsychopharmacology*, vol. 35, no. 1, pp. 4–26, 2010.

[33] J. L. Cummings, "Frontal-subcortical circuits and human behavior," *Archives of Neurology*, vol. 50, no. 8, pp. 873–880, 1993.

[34] R. S. Marin, B. S. Fogel, J. Hawkins, J. Duffy, and B. Krupp, "Apathy: a treatable syndrome," *Journal of Neuropsychiatry and Clinical Neurosciences*, vol. 7, no. 1, pp. 23–30, 1995.

[35] P. R. Hof and J. H. Morrison, "The aging brain: morphomolecular senescence of cortical circuits," *Trends in Neurosciences*, vol. 27, no. 10, pp. 607–613, 2004.

[36] Z. Petanjek, M. Judaš, I. Kostović, and H. B. M. Uylings, "Lifespan alterations of basal dendritic trees of pyramidal neurons in the human prefrontal cortex: a layer-specific pattern," *Cerebral Cortex*, vol. 18, no. 4, pp. 915–929, 2008.

[37] E. B. Bloss, W. G. Janssen, B. S. McEwen, and J. H. Morrison, "Interactive effects of stress and aging on structural plasticity in the prefrontal cortex," *Journal of Neuroscience*, vol. 30, no. 19, pp. 6726–6731, 2010.

[38] J. M. Juraska and N. C. Lowry, "Neuroanatomical changes associated with cognitive aging," *Current Topics in Behavioral Neurosciences*. In press.

[39] G. Kalpouzos, J. Persson, and L. Nyberg, "Local brain atrophy accounts for functional activity differences in normal aging," *Neurobiology of Aging*, vol. 33, no. 3, pp. 623.e1–623.e13, 2012.

[40] K. H. Chen, E. A. Reese, H. W. Kim, S. I. Rapoport, and J. S. Rao, "Disturbed neurotransmitter transporter expression in Alzheimer's disease brain," *Journal of Alzheimer's disease*, vol. 26, no. 4, pp. 755–766, 2011.

[41] T. H. McNeill, L. L. Koek, and J. W. Haycock, "The nigrostriatal system and aging," *Peptides*, vol. 5, no. 1, pp. 263–268, 1984.

[42] N. D. Volkow, J. S. Fowler, G. J. Wang et al., "Decreased dopamine transporters with age in health human subjects," *Annals of Neurology*, vol. 36, no. 2, pp. 237–239, 1994.

[43] K. Ishibashi, K. Ishibashi, K. Ishii et al., "Regional analysis of age-related decline in dopamine transporters and dopamine D2-like receptors in human striatum," *Synapse*, vol. 63, no. 4, pp. 282–290, 2009.

[44] L. Bäckman, U. Lindenberger, S. C. Li, and L. Nyberg, "Linking cognitive aging to alterations in dopamine neurotransmitter functioning: recent data and future avenues," *Neuroscience and Biobehavioral Reviews*, vol. 34, no. 5, pp. 670–677, 2010.

[45] K. Mizoguchi, H. Shoji, Y. Tanaka, W. Maruyama, and T. Tabira, "Age-related spatial working memory impairment is caused by prefrontal cortical dopaminergic dysfunction in rats," *Neuroscience*, vol. 162, no. 4, pp. 1192–1201, 2009.

[46] J. C. Dreher, A. Meyer-Lindenberg, P. Kohn, and K. F. Berman, "Age-related changes in midbrain dopaminergic regulation of the human reward system," *Proceedings of the National Academy of Sciences of the United States of America*, vol. 105, no. 39, pp. 15106–15111, 2008.

[47] T. M. Gill, P. J. Castaneda, and P. H. Janak, "Dissociable roles of the medial prefrontal cortex and nucleus accumbens core in goal-directed actions for differential reward magnitude," *Cerebral Cortex*, vol. 20, no. 12, pp. 2884–2899, 2010.

[48] H. Brodaty, A. Altendorf, A. Withall, and P. Sachdev, "Do people become more apathetic as they grow older? A longitudinal study in healthy individuals," *International Psychogeriatrics*, vol. 22, no. 3, pp. 426–436, 2010.

[49] C. U. Onyike, J. M. E. Sheppard, J. T. Tschanz et al., "Epidemiology of apathy in older adults: the cache county study," *American Journal of Geriatric Psychiatry*, vol. 15, no. 5, pp. 365–375, 2007.

[50] Y. E. Geda, R. O. Roberts, D. S. Knopman et al., "Prevalence of neuropsychiatric symptoms in mild cognitive impairment and normal cognitive aging: population-based study," *Archives of General Psychiatry*, vol. 65, no. 10, pp. 1193–1198, 2008.

[51] D. Seitz, N. Purandare, and D. Conn, "Prevalence of psychiatric disorders among older adults in long-term care homes: a systematic review," *International Psychogeriatrics*, vol. 22, no. 7, pp. 1025–1039, 2010.

[52] T. Okura, B. L. Plassman, D. C. Steffens, D. J. Llewellyn, G. G. Potter, and K. M. Langa, "Prevalence of neuropsychiatric symptoms and their association with functional limitations in older adults in the United States: The aging, demographics, and memory study," *Journal of the American Geriatrics Society*, vol. 58, no. 2, pp. 330–337, 2010.

[53] C. De Jager, A. D. Blackwell, M. M. Budge, and B. J. Sahakian, "Predicting cognitive decline in healthy older adults," *American Journal of Geriatric Psychiatry*, vol. 13, no. 8, pp. 735–740, 2005.

[54] D. A. Cahn-Weiner, P. F. Malloy, P. A. Boyle, M. Marran, and S. Salloway, "Prediction of functional status from neuropsychological tests in community-dwelling elderly individuals," *Clinical Neuropsychologist*, vol. 14, no. 2, pp. 187–195, 2000.

[55] S. Borson, "Cognition, aging, and disabilities: conceptual issues," *Physical Medicine and Rehabilitation Clinics of North America*, vol. 21, no. 2, pp. 375–382, 2010.

14

Prevalence of Frailty Indicators and Association with Socioeconomic Status in Middle-Aged and Older Adults in a Swiss Region with Universal Health Insurance Coverage

Idris Guessous,[1,2,3] Jean-Christophe Luthi,[2] Christopher Barrett Bowling,[4,5] Jean-Marc Theler,[1] Fred Paccaud,[2] Jean-Michel Gaspoz,[1] and William McClellan[3]

[1] *Unit of Population Epidemiology, Division of Primary Care Medicine, Department of Community Medicine, Primary Care, and Emergency Medicine, Geneva University Hospitals, 4 Rue Gabrielle-Perret-Gentil, 1211 Geneva 14, Switzerland*
[2] *Community Prevention Unit, University Institute of Social and Preventive Medicine, 10 Route de la Corniche, 1010 Lausanne, Switzerland*
[3] *Department of Epidemiology, Rollins School of Public Health, Emory University, 1518 Clifton Road, Atlanta, GA 30322, USA*
[4] *Birmingham/Atlanta Geriatric Research Education and Clinical Center, Atlanta Veterans Affairs Medical Center, 1670 Clairmont Road, Atlanta, GA 30322, USA*
[5] *Department of Medicine, Emory University, 1518 Clifton Road, Atlanta, GA 30322, USA*

Correspondence should be addressed to Idris Guessous; idris.guessous@hcuge.ch

Academic Editor: Jack Cannon

Frailty prevalence in older adults has been reported but is largely unknown in middle-aged adults. We determined the prevalence of frailty indicators among middle-aged and older adults from a general Swiss population characterized by universal health insurance coverage and assessed the determinants of frailty with a special focus on socioeconomic status. Participants aged 50 and more from the population-based 2006–2010 Bus Santé study were included ($N = 2{,}930$). Four frailty indicators (weakness, shrinking, exhaustion, and low activity) were measured according to standard definitions. Multivariate logistic regressions were used to determine associations. Overall, 63.5%, 28.7%, and 7.8% participants presented no frailty indicators, one frailty indicator, and two or more frailty indicators, respectively. Among middle-aged participants (50–65 years), 75.1%, 22.2%, and 2.7% presented 0, 1, and 2 or more frailty indicators. The number of frailty indicators was positively associated with age, hypertension, and current smoking and negatively associated with male gender, body mass index, waist-to-hip ratio, and serum total cholesterol level. Lower income level but not education was associated with higher number of frailty indicators. Frailty indicators are frequently encountered in both older and middle-aged adults from the Swiss general population. Despite universal health insurance coverage, household income is independently associated with frailty.

1. Introduction

Frailty is a biological syndrome that results from cumulative declines across multiple physiologic systems and causes vulnerability to adverse outcomes [1]. Frailty predicts adverse outcomes such as hospitalization and death [2, 3] and is considered as a modifiable predictor of disability [4]. Frailty is partly reversible, especially in its initial phase [4], and the identification of frail adults followed by effective interventions could potentially prevent disability and other adverse outcomes. Studies among older adults, generally defined as people aged 65 years and over, suggest that the prevalence of frailty is variable and has been reported to range from 4.0% to 59.1% of studied populations [5]. Comparable information about the prevalence of frailty among populations younger than 65 years is limited [6]. Gathering data among middle-aged subjects is important given that frailty phenotype finds its ideal application in nondisabled subjects [7].

Socioeconomic status (SES) may contribute to the variability in prevalence among older individuals [8–10]. Life (including early life) course social and health conditions linked to frailty among older adults are often present earlier in adulthood [11, 12]. However the association of SES with frailty among middle-aged adults has not been extensively studied. We address these issues in this study by describing the prevalence of frailty and assessing the association between frailty and lower SES in a population-based study of middle-aged and older adults with uniform access to healthcare.

2. Methods

2.1. Study Population. We used data from the Bus Santé study. The Bus Santé study is an annual cross-sectional population-based survey that collects information on cardiovascular risk factors in the Canton of Geneva (Switzerland) [13]. Subjects are randomly selected throughout each survey year to generate a representative sample of the canton's noninstitutionalized residents aged 35 years and older. Eligible subjects are identified using a list of legal residents provided by the local government. Stratified random sampling is used to select participants by gender within each 10-year age stratum, selecting the number of participants that is proportional to the corresponding population distribution. The 2006–2010 participation rates varied between 60% and 68%. The Bus Santé study complied with the Declaration of Helsinki and was approved by the Institutional Ethics Committee of the University of Geneva. All participants gave written informed consent.

2.2. Data Collection. Participants are examined by trained health professionals. Each participant completes several self-administered, standardized questionnaires. Anthropometric measures, including height, weight, and waist circumference, and blood pressure (BP) are obtained following specified protocols. In a temperature-controlled room, body weight was measured with the subject lightly dressed without shoes using a medical scale (precision 0.5 kg), and standing height is measured using a medical gauge (precision 1 cm). Body mass index (BMI) was defined as weight/height^2. Waist and hip circumferences (cm) were measured in duplicate with an anthropometric tape while the subjects were wearing light clothing. Waist circumference was measured at the minimum circumference between the iliac crest and the rib cage. Hip circumference was measured at the maximum protuberance of the buttocks, and the waist-to-hip ratio was calculated. BP was measured three times on the right arm after at least 10 min rest in the seated position, using a clinically validated automated oscillometric device (Omron HEM-907, Matsusaka, Japan) with a standard cuff or a large cuff if arm circumference was ≥33 cm. The average of the three BP readings was used for analyses. Hypertension was defined as mean SBP ≥ 140 mmHg or mean DBP ≥ 90 mmHg or presence of antihypertensive medication.

Smoking was defined as present if a participant reported to be a current smoker at the time of examination. Diabetes was defined as a fasting glucose ≥7 mmol/L and/or the presence of antidiabetic drug treatment (insulin or oral drugs). Other cardiovascular diseases (CVDs) and risk factors were defined by affirmative answers to the following questions: "Have you ever been told that you had high cholesterol/myocardial infarction/arterial thrombosis?"

Glucose, total and HDL plasma cholesterol, and triglycerides were assayed by using commercially available enzymatic kits (Bayer Technicon Diagnostics, CV 1.4%, 1.2%, and 1.5%, for glucose, cholesterol, and triglycerides, resp.).

2.3. Frailty Indicators. Frailty indicators were assessed by using standardized measures in participants aged 50 or more. These indicators approximated four of the five frailty constructs described by Fried et al. [2]. Frailty indicators used are defined below.

2.3.1. Weakness. Weakness was defined as the gender specific and BMI adjusted lowest 20% grip strength. The grip strength test was performed on the right hand, using the mean of the three measurements with a hydraulic hand dynamometer (Baseline Evaluation Instruments, New York).

2.3.2. Low Activity. Low activity was defined as the gender specific lowest 20% energy expenditure. Energy expenditure in kcal/week was measured using a validated physical activity frequency questionnaire (PAFQ) [14].

2.3.3. Shrinking. Shrinking was defined as self-reported unintentional weight loss. Participants were asked whether they had lost unintentionally weight during the past year: "In the last 12-month *[sic]*, have you unintentionally lost weight?"

2.3.4. Exhaustion. Exhaustion was defined as self-reported exhaustion. Participants were asked whether they had a feeling of generalized weakness in the past year: "In the last 12-month *[sic]*, did you have a feeling of generalized weakness or lack of energy?"

2.4. Socioeconomic Status. Self-reported education and income were used to characterize SES. Education level and monthly household income were categorized into 3 groups (education: high (≥13 years), middle (9–12 years), and low (<8 years); monthly household income: <4,999 CHF, 5,000–9499 CHF, and >9,500 CHF (1 CHF ≈ 1 US$ in September 2014)).

2.5. Statistical Analyses. To account for the survey year-specific age and gender structure estimates and associations were weighted using the 2010 Geneva Census population. Weighted means (standard errors, SE) and frequencies of study variables were calculated. Participants were grouped into three groups according to the number of frailty indicators: 0 frailty indicators, 1 frailty indicator, and 2 or more frailty indicators. The latter category was used because the number of participants with 3 or 4 frailty indicators was small. To account for the sampling procedure, survey procedures

TABLE 1: Participants' characteristics overall and by type of frailty indicator present, Bus Santé study, Geneva 2006–2010, $N = 2{,}930$.

Participant characteristic	All $N = 2930$ 100%	Weakness $N = 586$ 13.8%	Exhaustion $N = 197$ 7.0%	Shrinking $N = 188$ 6.3%	Low activity $N = 586$ 18.3%
Age, years, mean (SE)	60.0 (0.1)	72.8 (0.1)	58.5 (0.5)	60.9 (0.6)	63.4 (0.3)
Age 50–65 years (%)	73.6	0.0	7.6	5.7	14.4
Age ≥ 65 years (%)	26.4	52.2	5.4	7.7	29.0
Women (%)	51.0	54.2	66.1	61.5	53.6
Swiss nationality (%)	78.8	79.4	76.9	74.7	79.0
Education level (%)					
Low	15.6	23.9	16.8	25.7	17.8
Middle	45.5	47.4	41.8	44.1	46.0
High	38.9	28.7	41.4	30.3	36.2
Household income (%)					
<4999	22.7	47.6	35.7	35.8	28.5
5000–9499	41.9	38.8	32.4	36.6	38.8
>9500	35.4	13.7	31.9	27.6	32.6
Hypertension (%)	47.5	70.2	53.4	49.9	53.1
Diabetes (%)	6.6	9.1	8.6	8.1	7.3
Myocardial infarction (%)	2.4	4.9	2.0	3.2	2.5
Angina pectoris (%)	2.7	4.9	5.4	4.4	2.9
Arterial obstruction (%)	2.9	5.6	8.1	4.6	2.7
Current smoker (%)	15.9	9.8	19.5	27.9	17.4
Body mass index, kg/m^2, mean (SE)	26.1 (0.2)	26.4 (0.2)	28.0 (1.5)	24.9 (0.4)	24.7 (0.6)
Waist-to-hip ratio, mean (SE)	0.88 (0.00)	0.90 (0.00)	0.87 (0.01)	0.86 (0.01)	0.87 (0.01)
Serum total cholesterol, mmol/L, mean (SE)	5.63 (0.02)	5.58 (0.04)	5.59 (0.07)	5.51 (0.07)	5.60 (0.04)
Serum HDL cholesterol, mmol/L, mean (SE)	1.45 (0.01)	1.47 (0.02)	1.43 (0.03)	1.48 (0.03)	1.50 (0.02)
Serum triglycerides, mmol/L, mean (SE)	1.31 (0.02)	1.24 (0.02)	1.43 (0.08)	1.30 (0.07)	1.27 (0.03)

(SAS surveyfreq, surveymeans, and surveyreg) were used with the weights option added for each procedure using the 2010 Geneva Census population age and gender structures as weights. We compared groups using the Rao-Scott Chi-square test and F test for categorical and continuous variables, respectively.

We used polytomous multivariate logistic regression to determine and test the associations of potential factors, including socioeconomic factors, CVD, and cardiovascular risk factors, with the number of frailty indicators (1 frailty indicator versus 0, 2+ frailty indicators versus 0). Polytomous logistic regression modeling allows for simultaneous estimation of the probability of multiple outcomes. Middle-aged and older categories were defined as age of 50–64.9 years and ≥65 years, respectively. To determine whether the adjusted associations of SES (i.e., household income and education) with frailty indicators were different in middle-age and older participants, statistical interaction of age category with household income and education was tested, respectively. Citizenship was self-reported and categorized as Swiss or non-Swiss. Analyses were limited to participants with all variables of interest available.

All P values were 2-tailed with significance set at <0.05. All analyses were performed using SAS software version 9.2 (SAS Institute, Inc., Cary, North Carolina).

3. Results

3.1. Participants' Characteristics. Out of the 3,117 subjects aged 50 years and more who participated in the Bus Santé study between 2006 and 2010, 2,930 (95.0%) were included in the analyses. The major reason for exclusion was absence of blood sample. Participants' characteristics are presented in Table 1. Overall mean (SE) age was 60.0 (0.1) and 26.4% were aged 65 years or more. Half were women and 78.8% were Swiss. Hypertension and diabetes were present in 47.5% and 6.6%, respectively. Monthly household income of <4,999 CHF, 5,000–9499 CHF, and >9,500 CHF was reported by 23%, 42%, and 35% of the cohort.

3.2. Frailty Indicators. Low activity and weakness were the most frequently observed frailty indicators; 18.3% and 13.8% of the participants presented low activity and weakness, respectively. Exhaustion was reported in 7.0% and shrinking in 6.3% (Table 1). Among middle-aged participants exhaustion, shrinking, and low activity were present in 7.6%, 5.7%, and 14.4%, respectively. No middle-aged participant presented weakness. Among participants aged 65 or more, weakness, exhaustion, shrinking, and low activity were present in 52.2%, 5.4%, 7.7%, and 29.0%, respectively. Among the 2,930 participants, 0, 1, or 2 or more frailty indicators were present

Table 2: Participants' characteristics by the number of frailty indicators present, Bus Santé study, Geneva, 2006–2010, N = 2,930.

Participant characteristic	0 frailty indicator N = 1711 63.5% % or mean (SE)	1 frailty indicator N = 921 28.7% % or mean (SE)	2 or more frailty indicators N = 298 7.8% % or mean (SE)	P value*
Age, years, mean (SE)	57.5 (0.1)	63.0 (0.3)	68.8 (0.5)	<0.0001
Women (%)	47.8	56.1	57.8	<0.0001
Age 50–65 years (%)	87.1	57.2	24.7	<0.0001
Age ≥ 65 years (%)	12.9	42.8	75.3	<0.0001
Swiss nationality (%)	78.5	80.3	75.1	0.183
Education level (%)				
Low	13.4	18.0	24.4	
Middle	44.9	47.6	42.4	<0.0001
High	41.6	34.4	33.2	
Household income (%)				
<4999	16.6	28.8	49.0	
5000–9499	43.5	41.5	31.0	<0.0001
>9500	39.9	29.7	20.1	
Hypertension (%)	42.5	53.6	64.9	<0.0001
Diabetes (%)	5.8	7.5	8.8	0.069
Myocardial infarction (%)	2.1	2.9	3.6	0.170
Angina pectoris (%)	2.1	3.2	5.1	0.009
Cerebral or legs vascular obstruction (%)	2.2	3.7	5.6	0.001
Current smoker (%)	15.4	16.9	16.6	0.569
Body mass index, kg/m^2, mean (SE)	26.3 (0.2)	25.7 (0.2)	26.0 (1.3)	0.076
Waist-to-hip ratio, mean (SE)	0.89 (0.00)	0.88 (0.00)	0.88 (0.01)	0.326
Serum total cholesterol, mmol/L, mean (SE)	5.64 (0.02)	5.65 (0.03)	5.48 (0.06)	0.027
Serum HDL cholesterol, mmol/L, mean (SE)	1.44 (0.01)	1.46 (0.01)	1.50 (0.02)	0.045
Serum triglycerides, mmol/L, mean (SE)	1.31 (0.02)	1.34 (0.03)	1.20 (0.03)	0.009

*Rao-Scott Chi-square test for dichotomous and categorical variables and F tests for continuous variables.

in 63.5%, 28.7%, and 7.8%, respectively (Table 2). Among participants with 2 or more frailty indicators, 75.3% were of the age of 65 and older. Among middle-aged participants (50–64.9 years), 0, 1, and 2 or more frailty indicators were present in 75.1%, 22.2%, and 2.7%, respectively. Among older participants (≥65 years), 31.2%, 46.6%, and 22.3% had 0, 1, and 2 or more frailty indicators (Figure 1).

Characteristics differed across group defined by the number of frailty indicators present (Table 2). The mean age and proportion of women and Swiss increased with the increasing number of frailty indicators. Both education level and monthly household income were associated with the number of frailty indicators.

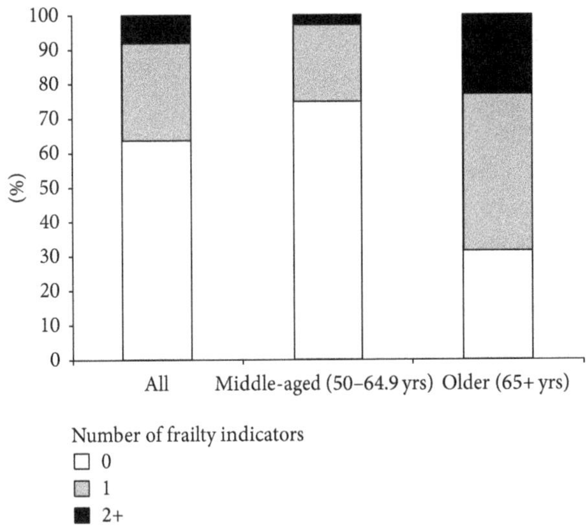

Figure 1: Prevalence of participants with 0, 1, and 2 or more frailty indicators, by age group, Bus Santé study, Geneva, 2006–2010, N = 2,930.

3.3. Determinants of the Number of Frailty Indictors. In the polytomous multivariate logistic regression analyses, the number of frailty indicators was positively associated with age, hypertension, and current smoking status and negatively associated with male gender, BMI, waist-to-hip ratio, and total cholesterol (Table 3). The associations with male gender and BMI were significant only when comparing participants with 1 frailty indicator to participants without frailty indicator. The association with total cholesterol was significant only when comparing participants with 2 or more frailty indicators to participants without frailty indicator.

Monthly household income was negatively and independently associated with having more frailty indicators. Compared to participants with high monthly income level, participants with low monthly income level were 31% more likely to have 1 frailty indicator and two times more likely to have 2 or more frailty indicators. Education level was

TABLE 3: Multivariate associations (odds ratios OR, 95% CI) of characteristics with groups of number of frailty indicators, Bus Santé study, Geneva, 2006–2010, $N = 2,930$.

Participant characteristic	Frailty indicators group (ref = 0)	OR (95% CI)
Age ≥ 65 years versus 50–65 years	2+ versus 0	19.4 (13.5–27.9)*
	1 versus 0	4.9 (4.0–6.0)*
Male	2+ versus 0	1.02 (0.66–1.59)
	1 versus 0	0.72 (0.55–0.94)*
Swiss nationality	2+ versus 0	0.77 (0.54–1.11)
	1 versus 0	1.05 (0.83–1.32)
Education		
Low	2+ versus 0	1.17 (0.75–1.83)
	1 versus 0	1.28 (0.96–1.71)
Middle	2+ versus 0	0.82 (0.58–1.16)
	1 versus 0	1.09 (0.89–1.35)
High	2+ versus 0	Ref
	1 versus 0	Ref
Household income		
<4999 CHF	2+ versus 0	2.16 (1.36–3.44)*†
	1 versus 0	1.31 (1.00–1.72)*
5000–9499 CHF	2+ versus 0	0.83 (0.55–1.27)
	1 versus 0	0.94 (0.75–1.17)
>9500 CHF	2+ versus 0	Ref
	1 versus 0	Ref
Hypertension	2+ versus 0	1.88 (1.32–2.68)*
	1 versus 0	1.40 (1.15–1.70)*
Diabetes	2+ versus 0	1.19 (0.66–2.15)
	1 versus 0	1.20 (0.83–1.72)
Myocardial infarction	2+ versus 0	0.78 (0.37–1.64)
	1 versus 0	0.96 (0.54–1.71)
Angina pectoris	2+ versus 0	1.69 (0.83–3.43)
	1 versus 0	1.24 (0.73–2.10)
Cerebral or legs vascular obstruction	2+ versus 0	1.70 (0.85–3.41)†
	1 versus 0	1.40 (0.81–2.44)
Current smoker	2+ versus 0	1.83 (1.19–2.81)*
	1 versus 0	1.43 (1.03–1.68)*
Body mass index, kg/m^2	2+ versus 0	0.99 (0.89–1.10)
	1 versus 0	0.96 (0.93–0.99)*
Waist-to-hip ratio	2+ versus 0	0.02 (0.01–0.40)*
	1 versus 0	0.73 (0.15–3.68)
Serum total cholesterol, mmol/L	2+ versus 0	0.82 (0.69–0.98)*
	1 versus 0	0.98 (0.89–1.09)
Serum triglycerides, mmol/L	2+ versus 0	0.98 (0.76–1.27)
	1 versus 0	1.12 (0.99–1.26)
Serum HDL cholesterol, mmol/L	2+ versus 0	1.57 (0.95–2.59)
	1 versus 0	1.09 (0.82–1.47)

All models are adjusted for survey year, age, gender, Swiss nationality, education level, monthly household income, hypertension, diabetes, myocardial infarction, angina pectoris, arterial obstruction, current smoking status, BMI, waist-to-hip ratio, serum total cholesterol, serum triglycerides, and serum HDL cholesterol.

*Statistically significant associations (P value < 0.05); †statistically significant interactions (P value < 0.05) with age category (50–64.9 years versus 65 years or more).

(1 CHF ≈ 1 US$.)

not independently associated with the number of frailty indicators.

We found a statistical interaction of age category (50–64.9 versus ≥65 years) with household income but not with education. The positive associations of household income with 2 or more frailty indicators were stronger among middle-aged participants than older participants.

4. Discussion

Using population-based data from a Swiss region with universal health insurance coverage, we found that the prevalence of frailty indicators was high in adults aged 50 or more. Frailty indicators were frequently reported in middle-aged adults (50–64.9 years) too; one-fourth had at least one frailty indicator.

The prevalence of frailty indicators increased with age which is in line with previous observations. Previous population-based studies have however rarely reported the prevalence of frailty among large enough sample of middle-aged participants. The prevalence of frailty in community-dwelling middle-aged and older Europeans participating in a large survey in 2004 has been reported; it ranged from 5.8% to 27.3% [6]. Compared to other countries, Switzerland was characterized by a low prevalence of frailty. Of note, only 882 participants were included in the Swiss part of the 2004 survey and the participation rate was low (37.6%). Out of the 882, only 470 participants were of the age of 50–65 yrs. Among this middle-aged group, the prevalence of exhaustion, weakness, shrinking, and low activity was 25.4%, 2.5%, 5.2%, and 11.2%, respectively [6]. Thirty-six percent and 1.3% were prefrail (1-2 frailty indicators) and frail (3+ frailty indicators), respectively [6]. Using a larger sample in an urban region of Switzerland (Geneva), our results further suggest that frailty is not uncommon in middle-aged adults.

Frail subjects are characterized by rapid decline of functional status even after minor perturbations and effective interventions to prevent disability in frail older persons who have been identified [15]. The identification of frail middle-aged adults followed by effective interventions could potentially prevent disability in older persons. Of note, given the general lack of data on frailty among middle-aged adults, there is currently no robust information on the impact of frailty in middle-aged participants on health in later life. However, given that frailty is a continuous process and that the risk of adverse outcome is sought to increase gradually from nonfrailty to prefrailty and frailty [2], it is likely that—without intervention—frailty before age of 65 years increased the risk of frailty and adverse outcome thereof after age of 65 years. Nevertheless, the natural history of frailty during middle and late life course remains to be described in cohort studies and the efficacy of interventions in middle-aged frail adults determined by experimental studies.

We found a negative association between monthly household income and the number of frailty indicators. Compared to adults with monthly household income <9,500 CHF, adults with monthly household income <5,000 CHF were more likely to have frailty indicators. This relationship persisted after adjustment for major potential confounders including age, gender, nationality, smoking, cardiovascular risk factors, and chronic diseases as well as education level. Of note, interaction of age with household income was statistically significant, suggesting that the association of income with frailty is not modified by age. Our results suggested that the association with frailty is stronger among middle-aged than older adults. We found no independent association with education. Previous results on the associations of education with frailty have been inconsistent [16, 17].

Previous data on SES and frailty have been collected among people aged 65 years and over. Using a dataset from a health survey of 4,000 people aged 65 years and over living in all regions of Hong Kong, Woo et al. reported associations of geographic districts and socioeconomic status with frailty [18]; those of low SES had a higher risk of frailty. In the Cardiovascular Health Study (CHS) Hirsch et al. found that SES was not associated with frailty among African Americans [19]. Yet a previous report of the CHS that included Caucasian and African American participants aged 65 or more found that those who were frail had less education and lower income [2]. Both income and education were independently associated with incident frailty among the Women's Health Initiative study participants aged 65 to 79 [20]. In a cross-sectional analysis of the Women's Health and Aging studies (women aged 65 years or more), low education and low income were associated with frailty [8]. In an old adults (70+ yrs) Mexican population, having a poor self-perceived economic situation was more common in frail participants [21]. In community-dwelling individuals aged 65 and older in England, less wealth and greater neighborhood deprivation were associated with greater frailty [22]. Finally, in a small (n = 640) cross-sectional study of community-dwelling persons aged 75 and older in Lleida, Spain, education was not associated with frailty, while the association of frailty with income approached statistical significance [23]. We found that the association of income with frailty persisted after adjustment for comorbidity. This observation challenges the suggestion that social inequalities in frailty are mediated by comorbidity [10].

The association of SES and income with frailty is of particular importance in a Swiss region with universal healthcare coverage. Theou et al. recently reported that country level of frailty is correlated with national economic indicators. Our results highlight the fact that, even in a high-income country such as Switzerland, frailty is associated with income [24].

Chronic diseases have been associated with frailty [25]. In our study, only hypertension was statistically significantly associated with the number of frailty indicators. This is in line with previous studies conducted among older adults [2, 12]. Diabetes, myocardial infarction, angina pectoris, and arterial obstruction were not associated. Compared to these factors, hypertension was much more prevalent in our study population and it is therefore possible that we lacked power to detect associations for these less frequent factors.

Both BMI and waist-to-hip ratio were negatively associated with the number of frailty indicators. Frailty is conceptualized as a wasting disorder and sarcopenia is one of frailty major pathophysiological features. Therefore our results are concordant with the frailty syndrome. Yet, some previous studies found BMI and waist circumference to be positively associated with frailty [11, 26]. This relationship remains to be better determined.

We found an inverse relationship between total cholesterol and frailty. The relationships between lipid profiles and frailty have rarely been explored [11]. In a study on 637 hospitalized old patients, Ranieri et al. concluded that lower serum cholesterol levels were an independent hematologic marker of frailty [27]. Low cholesterol level is a marker of malnutrition and could therefore be noncausally associated with frailty status. More recently, Schupf et al. also concluded that low cholesterol level is a robust predictor of mortality in nondemented old adults and may be a surrogate of frailty or subclinical disease [28].

When interpreting the findings of this study, one has to keep in mind its limitations. While four of the five frailty indicators were collected using standard procedures, information on walking speed was missing and conventional definition of frailty syndrome (including prefrail and frail status) could not be used. Also using the conventional definition of frailty syndrome, having only one frailty indicator could perhaps predict who would be frail in the future but does not identify them as frail. All participants were assumed to have normal walking speed and the prevalence of frailty is therefore likely to be actually underestimated. Grip strength test was performed on the right hand. While, for left-handed persons, grip strength is considered equivalent in both hands, for right-handed persons the dominant hand possesses 10% greater grip strength than the nondominant hand [29]. Although significant efforts are made to avoid selection bias (e.g., random sampling, multiple means to contact potential participants, multiple recruitment sites including outside the hospital using a mobile examination unit, and no financial incentive), we cannot exclude that participants differ from nonparticipants with respect to some attributes that may potentially influence the presence or absence of frailty indicators. Several participant characteristics were determined by the use of questionnaires. By nature of its reliance on self-reported data, this is a source of possible bias. Due to the nature of information collected in the "Bus Santé" study (that collects information on cardiovascular risk factors in the Canton of Geneva), only diabetes and cardiovascular risk factors could be considered and not other health conditions potentially associated with frailty, such as other respiratory illnesses, arthritis, neurological disorders, depression/mental health, and cognitive impairment. Given the representativeness of the study sample, these conditions are likely to be prevalent and may therefore confound some of the associations reported. Also, we lack information on education level, which may play an important role in frailty, and cannot exclude that some of the associations reported are explained—at least in part—by education level.

5. Conclusions

In a Swiss region with universal healthcare coverage, frailty indicators are frequently encountered in both older and middle-aged adults from the general population. Frailty is partly reversible in its initial phase. This study identified determinants of frailty that can help in identifying vulnerable adults who could benefit from interventions to prevent adverse health outcomes and disability.

Conflict of Interests

The authors declare that there is no conflict of interests regarding the publication of this paper.

Acknowledgment

The Bus Santé study is funded by the Geneva University Hospitals through the General Directorate of Health (Canton of Geneva).

References

[1] D. B. Hogan, C. MacKnight, and H. Bergman, "Models, definitions, and criteria of frailty," *Aging Clinical and Experimental Research*, vol. 15, no. 3, pp. 1–29, 2003.

[2] L. P. Fried, C. M. Tangen, J. Walston et al., "Frailty in older adults: evidence for a phenotype," *Journals of Gerontology Series A: Biological Sciences and Medical Sciences*, vol. 56, no. 3, pp. M146–M156, 2001.

[3] J. Garre-Olmo, L. Calvó-Perxas, S. López-Pousa, M. de Gracia Blanco, and J. Vilalta-Franch, "Prevalence of frailty phenotypes and risk of mortality in a community-dwelling elderly cohort," *Age and Ageing*, vol. 42, no. 1, pp. 46–51, 2013.

[4] T. M. Gill, E. A. Gahbauer, H. G. Allore, and L. Han, "Transitions between frailty states among community-living older persons," *Archives of Internal Medicine*, vol. 166, no. 4, pp. 418–423, 2006.

[5] R. M. Collard, H. Boter, R. A. Schoevers, and R. C. Oude Voshaar, "Prevalence of frailty in community-dwelling older persons: a systematic review," *Journal of the American Geriatrics Society*, vol. 60, no. 8, pp. 1487–1492, 2012.

[6] B. Santos-Eggimann, P. Cuénoud, J. Spagnoli, and J. Junod, "Prevalence of frailty in middle-aged and older community-dwelling Europeans living in 10 countries," *Journals of Gerontology Series A: Biological Sciences and Medical Sciences*, vol. 64, no. 6, pp. 675–681, 2009.

[7] M. Cesari, G. Gambassi, G. A. Van Kan, and B. Vellas, "The frailty phenotype and the frailty index: different instruments for different purposes," *Age and Ageing*, vol. 43, no. 1, pp. 10–12, 2014.

[8] S. L. Szanton, C. L. Seplaki, R. J. Thorpe Jr., J. K. Allen, and L. P. Fried, "Socioeconomic status is associated with frailty: the Women's Health and Aging Studies," *Journal of Epidemiology and Community Health*, vol. 64, no. 1, pp. 63–67, 2010.

[9] J. Woo, W. Goggins, A. Sham, and S. C. Ho, "Social determinants of frailty," *Gerontology*, vol. 51, no. 6, pp. 402–408, 2005.

[10] H. Syddall, H. C. Roberts, M. Evandrou, C. Cooper, H. Bergman, and A. A. Sayer, "Prevalence and correlates of frailty among community-dwelling older men and women: findings from the Hertfordshire Cohort Study," *Age and Ageing*, vol. 39, no. 2, Article ID afp204, pp. 197–203, 2009.

[11] C. S. Blaum, Q. L. Xue, E. Michelon, R. D. Semba, and L. P. Fried, "The association between obesity and the frailty syndrome in older women: the Women's Health and Aging Studies," *Journal of the American Geriatrics Society*, vol. 53, no. 6, pp. 927–934, 2005.

[12] B. E. Alvarado, M.-V. Zunzunegui, F. Béland, and J.-M. Bamvita, "Life course social and health conditions linked to frailty in latin American older men and women," *Journals of Gerontology Series A: Biological Sciences and Medical Sciences*, vol. 63, no. 12, pp. 1399–1406, 2008.

[13] I. Guessous, M. Bochud, J.-M. Theler, J.-M. Gaspoz, and A. Pechère-Bertschi, "1999–2009 trends in prevalence, unawareness, treatment and control of hypertension in Geneva, Switzerland," *PLoS ONE*, vol. 7, no. 6, Article ID e39877, 2012.

[14] M. Bernstein, D. Sloutskis, S. Kumanyika, A. Sparti, Y. Schutz, and A. Morabia, "Data-based approach for developing a physical activity frequency questionnaire," *The American Journal of Epidemiology*, vol. 147, no. 2, pp. 147–154, 1998.

[15] R. Daniels, E. Van Rossum, L. de Witte, G. I. J. M. Kempen, and W. van den Heuvel, "Interventions to prevent disability in frail community-dwelling elderly: a systematic review," *BMC Health Services Research*, vol. 8, article 278, 2008.

[16] E. Y. Shim, S. H. Ma, S. H. Hong et al., "Correlation between frailty level and adverse health-related outcomes of community-dwelling elderly, one year retrospective study," *Korean Journal of Family Medicine*, vol. 32, no. 4, pp. 249–256, 2011.

[17] S. H. Ma, K. Y. Jeung, S. H. Hong et al., "Correlation between frailty level and disability of the elderly and frailty related factors," *Korean Journal of Family Medicine*, vol. 30, no. 8, pp. 588–597, 2009.

[18] J. Woo, R. Chan, J. Leung, and M. Wong, "Relative contributions of geographic, socioeconomic, and lifestyle factors to quality of life, frailty, and mortality in elderly," *PLoS ONE*, vol. 5, no. 1, Article ID e8775, 2010.

[19] C. Hirsch, M. L. Anderson, A. Newman et al., "The association of race with frailty: the cardiovascular health study," *Annals of Epidemiology*, vol. 16, no. 7, pp. 545–553, 2006.

[20] N. F. Woods, A. Z. LaCroix, S. L. Gray et al., "Frailty: emergence and consequences in women aged 65 and older in the Women's Health Initiative observational study," *Journal of the American Geriatrics Society*, vol. 53, no. 8, pp. 1321–1330, 2005.

[21] R. I. Casale-Martínez, A. P. Navarrete-Reyes, and J. A. Ávila-Funes, "Social determinants of frailty in elderly Mexican community-dwelling adults," *Journal of the American Geriatrics Society*, vol. 60, no. 4, pp. 800–802, 2012.

[22] I. A. Lang, R. E. Hubbard, M. K. Andrew, D. J. Llewellyn, D. Melzer, and K. Rockwood, "Neighborhood deprivation, individual socioeconomic status, and frailty in older adults," *Journal of the American Geriatrics Society*, vol. 57, no. 10, pp. 1776–1780, 2009.

[23] P. Jürschik, C. Nunin, T. Botigué, M. A. Escobar, A. Lavedán, and M. Viladrosa, "Prevalence of frailty and factors associated with frailty in the elderly population of Lleida, Spain: the FRALLE survey," *Archives of Gerontology and Geriatrics*, vol. 55, no. 3, pp. 625–631, 2012.

[24] O. Theou, T. D. Brothers, M. R. Rockwood, D. Haardt, A. Mitnitski, and K. Rockwood, "Exploring the relationship between national economic indicators and relative fitness and frailty in middle-aged and older europeans," *Age and Ageing*, vol. 42, no. 5, Article ID aft010, pp. 614–619, 2013.

[25] C. O. Weiss, "Frailty and chronic diseases in older adults," *Clinics in Geriatric Medicine*, vol. 27, no. 1, pp. 39–52, 2011.

[26] R. E. Hubbard, I. A. Lang, D. J. Llewellyn, and K. Rockwood, "Frailty, body mass index, and abdominal obesity in older people," *Journals of Gerontology—Series A Biological Sciences and Medical Sciences*, vol. 65, no. 4, pp. 377–381, 2010.

[27] P. Ranieri, R. Rozzini, S. Franzoni, P. Barbisoni, and M. Trabucchi, "Serum cholesterol levels as a measure of frailty in elderly patients," *Experimental Aging Research*, vol. 24, no. 2, pp. 169–179, 1998.

[28] N. Schupf, R. Costa, J. Luchsinger, M. X. Tang, J. H. Lee, and R. Mayeux, "Relationship between plasma lipids and all-cause mortality in nondemented elderly," *Journal of the American Geriatrics Society*, vol. 53, no. 2, pp. 219–226, 2005.

[29] P. Petersen, M. Petrick, H. Connor, and D. Conklin, "Grip strength and hand dominance: challenging the 10% rule," *The American Journal of Occupational Therapy*, vol. 43, no. 7, pp. 444–447, 1989.

15

Families, Friends, and the Neighborhood of Older Adults: Evidence from Public Housing in Singapore

Treena Wu and Angelique Chan

Health Services & Systems Research, Duke-NUS Graduate Medical School, Level 4, 8 College Road, Singapore 169857

Correspondence should be addressed to Treena Wu, soctwsl@nus.edu.sg

Academic Editor: Lindy Clemson

Introduction. This empirical paper examines how the Housing Development Board (HDB) public housing neighborhood influences older urban Singaporeans' social interactions and ameliorates social isolation. *Methods.* Using 4,542 observations of noninstitutionalized urban adults aged 60 and above, ordered logistic regressions are run to determine the predictors of isolation while controlling for physical health and demographics. *Results.* 87% of older Singaporeans reside in public housing apartments while 13% reside in private market housing. The main predictor of social isolation is living alone and the second main predictor is coresidence with adult children. The relationship between coresidence with adult children and isolation is mediated when controlling for older adult functional limitations. The public apartment neighborhood and daily participation in public neighborhood events have substantial effects on reducing the risk of isolation. Older adult contact with friends alleviates isolation more than contact with non-coresiding relatives. *Conclusion.* Findings suggest that the public neighborhood-built environment in Singapore plays a positive role in the social interactions of the elderly. Knowledge of the factors that decrease the risk of social isolation will have implications for studying morbidity and mortality among the elderly.

1. Introduction

In newly industrialized economies (NIE) in Asia, economic growth and demographic changes are leading to longer life and smaller family size. In Asia, given the Confucian beliefs of filial piety, it has been traditionally expected that the younger members of the family provide time, money, goods, and instrumental and emotional support for older adults. However, with later marriage and lower fertility, it is now more likely that older adults in Asian NIE have smaller families and a higher likelihood of living alone. As a consequence elders in urban settings may have fewer social interactions as they age. However it is not necessarily the case that late life is characterized by social isolation.

Individuals can adapt to the aging process with changes in their behavior and the environment. Older adults may compensate for a loss of social interaction when their families become smaller by interacting more with friends and neighbors who are in close physical proximity. This may especially be the case for the oldest old with functional limitations who may not only be neighborhood-based but neighborhood-bound. We hypothesize that in the Singapore densely populated city state the built neighborhood environment contributes to older adult social interactions and ameliorates social isolation. Using state Housing Development Board (HDB) policy, we examine social interactions in the neighborhoods of older urban Singaporeans aged 60 and above.

Scholars studying the aging process have wrestled with the assumption that, in later life, an individual gradually disengages from society and inevitably becomes isolated [1]. However, it is posited that an older adult can choose to adapt the size of the social network and the quality of each contact. The composition and the extent of the social network of the spouse, children, friends, and neighbors can possibly change and be refined; this can vary for the young old and oldest old. To test our hypothesis, we are guided by the psychology theory of socioemotional selectivity by Carstensen et al. [2].

Most studies of social relationships in later life focus on the amount (e.g., number of individuals, frequency of contact) or content (practical help, advice) of social contact, not on individuals' perceived social isolation [3]. Isolation is often linked to a higher risk of worse health such as the risk of all-cause mortality, increased morbidity, depression, and cognitive decline [4]. Subjective interpretations of social relationships are likely to be a key to understanding the impact of actual social connections on older adult health and well-being.

Based on the social-psychology disengagement theory of aging by Cumming and Henry [1], there is decreased interaction between the aging individual and others in the social system; but when disengagement is complete, the equilibrium which existed in middle age between the individual and his society will give way to a new equilibrium characterized by a greater distance and an altered type of relationship. This altered state is arguably isolation where the aged individual may be without any form of support. In contrast, socioemotional selectivity theory [2] states that as resources and energy decline in late life, older adults shed less intimate or rewarding relationships and increase their emotional investments in relationships that are more intimate or rewarding. In applying this theory to social networks, we argue that older Singaporeans can be motivated to selectively and actively engage with others in the social system. Disengagement and withdrawal from society in late life may not necessarily occur.

There are several aspects of social network connectedness that contribute to the ease of late life transitions and a lessening of isolation. One of these aspects is the number of direct ties to people and where some types of social ties may be more beneficial than others. There is the value of ties with kin members, who are likely to provide unconditional instrumental and emotional support [5, 6]. Another aspect is the value of close-knit social contacts in which the older person's contacts in a network know each other. This makes for a social network that enables the older adult's contacts to provide instrumental and emotional support, share caregiving duties, and pool resources.

For older adults especially the oldest old, due to debilitating health problems, neighbor interaction and neighborhood attachment may play a large role in their social networks. Older adults may be more vulnerable to the influence of their residential environment as they tend to travel outside their own neighborhoods less often than do younger adults and children who travel for work and school and tend to have a longer duration of exposure to neighborhood influences than younger individuals [7]. Being neighborhood-bound can then affect the older person's perceptions of the neighborhood. In a British cross-sectional population survey of people aged 65 plus living at home, Bowling and Stafford [8] find that individual perceptions of the area as neighborly and having good facilities are independently associated with lower likelihood of low social activities. Within the context of the city in the US, Subramanian et al. [9] find that a neighborhood with residential stability and a concentration of elders is positively associated with older person self-rated health.

2. Methods

We carried out an ordered logit estimation using the Singapore Social Isolation, Health, and Lifestyles Survey (SIHLS) 2009 cross-sectional data of 5,000 noninstitutionalized urban Singaporeans aged 60 and above. The SIHLS provides information on the older adult's extent of social isolation; health status and well-being; income, social engagement, housing, network support, and loneliness. The nationally representative survey data was collected using face-to-face interviews with older adults. Almost 90% of Singaporeans reside in HDB public apartment housing. The remaining 10% with higher household incomes reside in private housing.

The state agency HDB was established in Singapore to provide guarantees of housing for its citizens. The unchallengeable right to housing in the densely populated city state was achieved through the construction of affordable urban public housing which began in 1960. Public housing works started in 1960 when Singapore was still a British colony. In 1965, Singapore achieved Independence. From the 1980s, the HDB shifted its focus to building communities within self-contained towns. In spatial terms, because of close proximity, each HDB apartment building has become a neighborhood block; a cluster of neighborhood blocks has become an urban community equipped with social support services for the elderly and children and public spaces such as playgrounds, markets, and cafés, all with the aim of building a sense of place and community [10]. As life expectancy now for men is approximately 79 years and for women 84 years [11], there are increased interventions that promote aging-in-place such as day care and home care support services at the ground level of a HDB apartment block; apartments for the elderly with activities of daily living (ADL) limitations retrofitted with alarm buttons for emergency assistance; communal living for the oldest old without spouses or children; state subsidized senior activity centers that provide organized group activities. Based on HDB population level household survey interviews [12, 13] with residents, it is found that the longer the residence in the same neighborhood block and community, the greater the sense of belonging. This is especially for residents aged 55 and above with a length of residence that is 10 years or more. Thus, the older adult is likely able to maintain an intimate social network or build a stronger social network of family, friends, and neighbors.

HDB manages the public housing stock. This consists of approximately 90% of the total housing stock in the market. The monthly income of the household head that is below SGD$8,000 (Singapore Dollar $1 = US$0.81) and the family size form the criteria of housing assignment to a given apartment. But this rule does not apply to the secondary or resale market. On the basis of this income threshold, each family is then allocated to a HDB apartment building block which consists of different built-up area sizes. Within each HDB neighborhood block, there is variation in household income from the lowest monthly income group of <SGD$500 to the SGD$8,000 threshold. The lowest income group resides in one-room HDB apartments, and the highest income group resides in four-room or five-room HDB apartments. Adult children starting their own homes have preferential access to an apartment that is in close physical proximity to their parents' apartment, which can then enable frequent contact.

Beyond this SGD$8,000 monthly income threshold, individuals then purchase housing from the private housing stock which makes up the remaining 10% of the total stock. While higher socioeconomic status individuals aspire to switch from public housing to private housing, the vast majority of individuals particularly the younger age groups upgrade from smaller size HDB apartments to five-room HDB apartments [10]. The private housing stock consists of condominiums (gated communities with security and key card access), private apartments, bungalow houses, semidetached houses, terrace houses, and townhouses. Geographically, public housing and private housing are mixed because of land shortage in the island state. Public apartment buildings can be located next to private apartment buildings. However, public housing and state subsidized social activity centers are geographically concentrated. The care support services and social activity centers are within close walking distance for the elderly in public housing.

2.1. Data. Table 1 shows a description of the key variables that we used from SIHLS such as the outcome variable social isolation; residential type, composition, and size of the social network; age and covariates including physical health and demographics.

For the outcome variable of perceived isolation, respondents were asked "How often do you feel isolated from others?" This subjective measure is on a scale of 1–5, 1 = lowest level, and 5 = highest level. In our analysis, we study the social network as an interaction between the social network and feelings of isolation change. As physical health is an age-related factor, we wanted to control for physical health and assess whether the association between the social network and isolation holds. The physical health measures that we used were difficulties with activities of daily living (ADLs) which refer to self-care tasks and instrumental activities of daily living (IADLs) which refer to the ability to carry out activities associated with maintaining a household. For ADL limitations, respondents were asked the number of difficulties they had with the following activities: (1) take a bath/shower, (2) dress up, (3) eat, (4) transfer stand up from a bed/chair, (5) walk around the house, (6) walk outside of the house, (7) use a squatting toilet, and (8) use a sitting toilet. For IADL limitations, respondents were asked the number of difficulties they had with the following activities: (1) prepare own meals, (2) leave the home to purchase necessary items or medication, (3) take care of financial matters such as paying utilities, (4) use the phone, (5) light housework, (6) take public transport to leave home, and (7) take medication as prescribed.

2.2. Empirical Specification. The aim is to understand how social interactions taking place within the HDB neighborhood environment may decrease isolation. The relationship between the HDB-built environment and perceived isolation may be operating through the older adult's perception of the neighborhood. Bowling and Stafford [8] found that individual perceptions of the area as neighborly and having good facilities are independently associated with lower likelihood of low social activities. In our empirical specifications, we included the explanatory variable of daily participation in HDB neighborhood events as a proxy for neighborhood perception.

Using our cross-sectional data, we first start by gaining an understanding of the distribution of social interactions with non-coresiding kin members and nonkin members. We would like to understand how the elderly choose to interact with social contacts outside of the home and how this changes with age. If contacts outside of the home are intimate and rewarding relationships, we hypothesize that the elderly will make more of an effort to stay connected. We then compared this with the distribution of social interactions for older adults in private housing. For these distributions, we used locally weighted bivariate regressions and we did not control for health. From these bivariate regressions, we then explored in depth the composition of the social network consisting of family within the home and non-coresiding relatives, friends, and neighbors outside of the home using multivariate regression.

Multivariate regression techniques were used for generating estimates of perceived isolation. We first regressed the measure of perceived isolation on the variables, HDB residence, participation in HDB neighborhood events, household size, whether the older adult is widowed, whether the older adult lives alone or coresides with a child/children, and age. The focus is on how the older adult's relationships with the family within the home and residence area vary with isolation. The explanatory variable, participation in HDB neighborhood activity is a proxy for the older adult's neighborhood perception. If the older adult perceives the neighborhood favorably, then there is a high likelihood of participation in social activity within the neighborhood. Because of data limitations we were unable to add a variable for length of residence in the same neighborhood.

We then proceeded to factor in the social network of non-coresiding relatives including children, friends, and neighbors who are outside of the home. The social connectedness of non-coresiding relatives and friends was specified as the interaction between the number of individuals connected and the frequency of contact each month. Types of contact include face-to-face visits in the home and outside of the home and phone calls. We did not specify such an interaction for neighbor connectedness because of data limitations. The covariates used were physical health, income, gender, and ethnicity. Physical health is an age-related factor in terms of functional limitations that deteriorate with age. We present a likelihood ratio test to determine if the covariates make a difference to the outcome when not included.

3. Results

Using kernel regressions, Figures 1 and 2 show the age for distributions of social interaction among non-coresiding relatives, friends, and neighbors by HDB housing and private market housing. They provide useful information on the pattern of social interactions outside of the home which is important to consider for the elderly with physical mobility

Table 1: Description of variables.

Variable	Description	
Social isolation	"How often do you feel isolated from others?"	Never = 56.6%, Rarely = 30.7%, Occasionally = 9.5%, Fairly Often = 2.3%, Always = 1%
Residence in HDB housing	The respondent resides in HDB public housing	Yes = 87.3%, No = 12.7%
Daily participation in a HDB neighborhood event		Yes = 78.1%, No = 21.9%
Network Composition and size	The respondent is widowed	Yes = 35.5%, No = 64.5%
	The respondent lives alone	Yes = 5.8%, No = 94.2%
	The respondent lives with children	Yes = 69.6%, No = 30.4%
	"If you live with your children, what is the household size?"	Mean = 4.2, SD = 1.6
	"Among all your relatives not living with you (including children and grandchildren), how many relatives do you see or hear from at least once a month?"	0 relatives = 14.7%, 1 relative = 4.1%, 2 relatives = 12.5%, 3-4 relatives = 26.9%, 5–8 relatives = 23.9%, ≥9 relatives = 17.9%
	"Among all your friends including those who live in your neighborhood, how many friends do you see or hear from at least once a month?"	0 friends = 14.7%, 1 friend = 3.6%, 2 friends = 14.1%, 3-4 friends = 30.7%, 5–8 friends = 14.9%, ≥9 friends = 22%
	"Among all your neighbors including those you consider your friend, how many neighbors do you see or hear from at least once a month?"	0 neighbors = 11.1%, 1 neighbor = 10.1%, 2 neighbors = 21.8%, 3-4 neighbors = 36%, 5–8 neighbors = 12.4%, ≥9 neighbors = 8.6%
Frequency of Contact within Network	"How often do you see or hear from relatives with whom you have the most contact?"	Never = 5%, Seldom = 11.6%, Sometimes = 25%, Often = 36.9%, Very Often = 12.5%, Always = 9%
	"How often do you see or hear from friends including those who live in your neighborhood with whom you have the most contact?"	Never = 13.2%, Seldom = 12.6%, Sometimes = 27.7%, Often = 32.8%, Very Often = 7.7%, Always = 6%
	There is no question in the survey on the frequency of contact with neighbors including those considered as friends	
Age		Min = 60, Max = 101 Mean = 72.8, SD = 8.1
Income	Household monthly income (Singapore Dollar $1 = US$0.81)	Less than S$500 = 9.5%, S$500–S$999 = 14.6%, S$1,000 to S$1,999 = 24.6%, S$2,000 to S$2,999 = 15.9%, S$3,000 to S$3,999 = 6.2%, S$4,000 to S$4,999 = 2.8%, ≥S$5,000 = 3.2%, refuse to respond = 3.2%, do not know = 20%

TABLE 1: Continued.

Variable	Description	
Physical health	Self-rated difficulties with the following eight ADLs: (1) take a bath/shower, (2) dress up, (3) eat, (4) transfer stand up from a bed/chair, (5) walk around the house, (6) walk outside of the house, (7) use a squatting toilet, and (8) use a sitting toilet	0 ADL difficulty = 62.7% 1 ADL difficulty = 13.6% 2-3 ADL difficulties = 12.7% ≥4 ADL difficulties = 11%
	Self-rated difficulties with the following seven IADLs: (1) prepare own meals, (2) leave the home to purchase necessary items or medication, (3) take care of financial matters such as paying utilities, (4) use the phone, (5) light housework, (6) take public transport to leave home, and (7) take medication as prescribed	0 IADL difficulty = 82.5% 1-2 IADL difficulties = 8.5% ≥3 IADL difficulties = 9%
Gender	The respondent is female	Female = 54.9%, Male = 45.1%
Ethnicity		Chinese = 71.52%, Malay = 17.08%, Indian = 10.22%, Other ethnicities = 1.18%

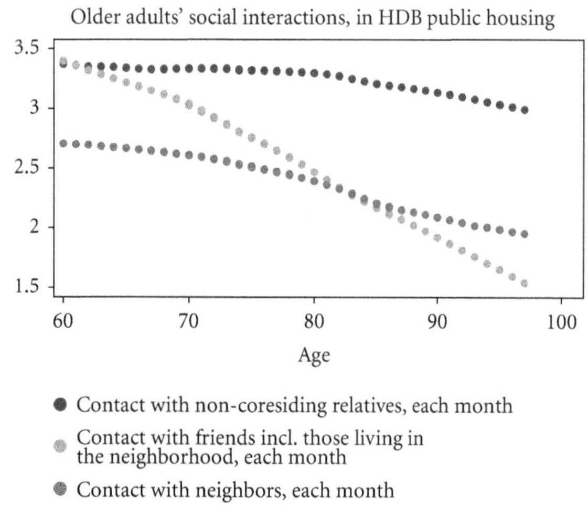

FIGURE 1: These locally weighted bivariate regressions do not control for health.

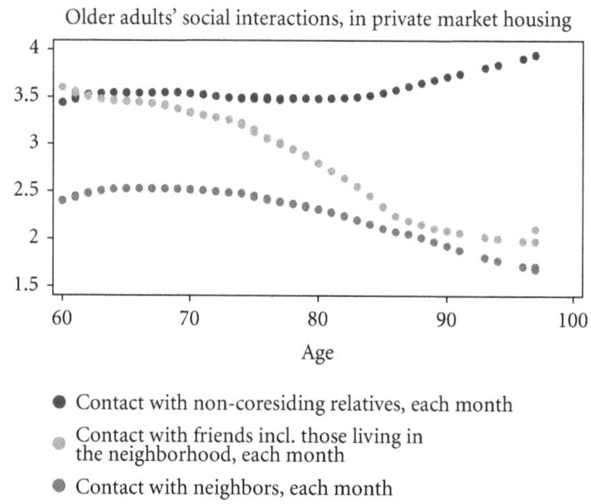

FIGURE 2: These locally weighted bivariate regressions do not control for health.

that deteriorates with age. Contact with non-coresiding relatives remains at relatively high levels across age. A decline of contact with friends and neighbors starts within the range of age 70 and 80, and the decline is sharpest for contact with friends, including those who live in the same neighborhood. The decline is sharper for those in a HDB neighborhood than for those in private housing. However, Figure 2 shows that for individuals from the mid 80s to 100, contact with neighbors in HDB housing falls at a slower rate than contact with friends. The oldest old in public housing appears to substitute neighbors for friends.

From Table 1, mean age of respondents is 72.8 years and 54.9% of them are women. 12.7% report suffering from isolation occasionally, fairly often, or always. 35.5% are widowed, and 5.8% live alone. 87.3% reside in HDB public housing, and 78.1% report daily participation in HDB neighborhood events. 76.7% report that they have monthly contact with three or more relatives. 58.2% report that they often, fairly often, or always see or hear from close relatives. 67.5% report that they have monthly contact with three or more friends including friends who live in the same neighborhood. 46.6% report that they often, fairly often, or always see or hear from friends. 56.9% report that they have monthly contact with three or more neighbors who may not necessarily be friends.

Table 2 provides the predictors for perceived social isolation using ordered logistic regressions. The predictors are expressed as coefficient effect sizes, β. The first model (1) does not include the social network outside the home or covariates. (2), (3), (4), and (5) include the social network outside the home and covariates. The different contacts that make up the social network are added stepwise across (3), (4), and (5). In the first model, (1) which excludes the social network outside the home, the strongest predictor of isolation is living alone ($\beta = 0.683$, $P < 0.01$). Similarly when household size is smaller, there is a higher likelihood

TABLE 2: Marginal effect coefficients from ordered logistic regression models predicting older adult perceived social isolation.

	(1)	(2)	(3)	(4)	(5)
Residence in HDB	−.169** (.086)	−.162* (.087)	−.186** (.087)	−.209** (.088)	−.219** (.088)
Daily participation in HDB neighborhood events	.008 (.006)	−.114 (.070)	−.100 (.070)	−.164** (.071)	−.160** (.071)
Living arrangements					
Household size	−.165*** (.022)	−.140*** (.022)	−.138*** (.022)	−.139*** (.022)	−.139*** (.022)
Widowed	.137* (.071)	.210** (.079)	.200** (.079)	.197** (.080)	.199** (.080)
Residing alone	.683*** (.134)	.680*** (.134)	.615*** (.135)	.652*** (.135)	.655*** (.135)
Coresiding with adult children	.332*** (.082)	.247** (.083)	.248** (.083)	.234** (.084)	.230** (.084)
Social network					
Relatives incl. non-coresiding children			−.023*** (.004)	−.010** (.005)	−.012** (.005)
Friends				−.035*** (.005)	−.037*** (.005)
Neighbors					.040 (.024)
Age	.011** (.004)	.003 (.004)	.003 (.004)	−.0007 (.0044)	−.0006 (.004)
Covariates	No	Yes	Yes	Yes	Yes
Observations	4,542	4,542	4,542	4,542	4,542

Notes: $^{***}P < 0.01$, $^{**}P < 0.05$ and $^{*}P < 0.10$. The covariates are physical health limitations—ADL and IADL, income, gender, and ethnicity. The likelihood ratio test for the restricted model without the covariates and the unrestricted model with covariates shows that there is no variation in the main coefficients of interest—HDB residence, daily participation in HDB neighborhood events, family living arrangements, and the social network. LR $\text{Chi}^2(4) = 336.02$. Prob > $\text{Chi}^2 = 0.0000$.

of perceived isolation ($\beta = -0.165$, $P < 0.01$). From this model the second strongest predictor of isolation is whether the older adult coresides with adult children ($\beta = 0.332$, $P < 0.01$). However, when physical health and demographic controls were added, the effect of coresidence with adult children on increasing isolation weakens ($\beta = 0.247$, $P < 0.05$).

In terms of whether isolation increases with age, we found a relatively small positive effect ($\beta = 0.011$, $P < 0.05$) in the first model (1). The effect size of age remains very small even when the social network is incorporated and even after controlling for physical health, income, and demographics. See models (2), (3), (4), and (5).

Next, we focused on predictors of lower isolation. From model (1) in Table 2, older adult residence in HDB public housing ameliorates the likelihood of perceived isolation ($\beta = -0.169$, $P < 0.05$). The HDB coefficient effect size remains strong and statistically significant across models (2), (3), (4), and (5). We attempt to explain the relationship between HDB neighborhood and isolation through older adult daily participation in HDB neighborhood social activities via models (4) and (5) when contact with friends is added. From (4), daily participation in social activities in the HDB neighborhood has a substantial effect on lessening isolation ($\beta = -0.164$, $P < 0.05$). There is a similar coefficient effect size in (5). From (4) controlling for other variables, contact with friends has a positive effect on lessening isolation ($\beta = -0.035$, $P < 0.01$). There is a similar coefficient effect size in (5).

4. Discussion

The results show that the strongest predictor of isolation in old age is living alone. Unexpectedly, the second main predictor of isolation is coresidence with children. This result is somewhat surprising as it is traditional Singaporean practice for older adults to coreside with children and to some extent grandchildren. The positive association between coresidence with adult children and isolation has some similarity to studies on the determinants of older adult subjective well-being. In a review of sociological and psychological studies on aging and well-being, George [14] finds that interacting with adult children appears to have a weak or nonexistent relationship with subjective well-being. But from our findings, the relationship between living with adult children in old age and isolation is mediated when there is consideration for the older adult's functional limitations. The extent of ADL and IADL limitations may increase their dependency on coresiding children for instrumental support and assuage perceived isolation.

The strongest predictors for decreasing the likelihood of isolation are in order, residence in HDB public housing and daily social participation in HDB neighborhood events. The elderly are very likely to view their HDB neighborhood favorably because of the availability of social care and support services and public spaces for social interaction. The HDB built environment may then be perceived as conducive for social contact for the elderly who are neighborhood-based and neighborhood-bound. In contrast, growing old in private condominiums which are gated communities or bungalow houses that are fenced off may inadvertently create a sense of being cut off from society.

The social network of non-coresiding relatives and the elders' friends also has influence on reducing isolation. In comparing the relationship between the different social contact types, contact with friends has a far more positive effect on alleviating isolation compared to contact with non-coresiding relatives including children. Contact with neighbors does not have any effect on perceived isolation. From the literature on elderly subjective well-being, George [14] summarizes studies that show that friends are generally more important for subjective well-being in later life than are relationships with children or other relatives. Friendships that are sustained in late life may be more intimate as the elderly grow old together and reminisce about the rapid modernization of Singapore over the span of 46 years.

Following the application of socioemotional selectivity theory to social networks, we have provided some understanding about the predictors for reduced social isolation among Singaporean elderly. The HDB neighborhood environment plays a positive role in the social interactions of the elderly who are neighborhood-based and neighborhood-bound. Knowledge of the factors that decrease the risk of social isolation will have implications for studying morbidity and mortality in old age. But the cross-sectional nature of the data limits our analyses in that we are unable to directly assess how individuals transition into late life and how behavioral adaptation and isolation vary as the young old become the oldest old. Also, we are unable to make clear arguments for causal relationships or to fully distinguish between age and cohort effects.

Acknowledgments

This paper was completed with grant funding from the Tsao Foundation Aging Research Initiative at NUS. Access to the Singapore Social Isolation, Health and Lifestyles Survey 2009 was provided by the Ministry of Community Development, Youth and Sports.

References

[1] E. Cumming and W. Henry, *Growing Old: The Process of Disengagement*, Basic Books, New York, NY, USA, 1961.

[2] L. L. Carstensen, D. M. Isaacowitz, and S. T. Charles, "Taking time seriously: a theory of socioemotional selectivity," *The American Psychologist*, vol. 54, no. 3, pp. 165–181, 1999.

[3] M. E. Hughes, L. J. Waite, L. C. Hawkley, and J. T. Cacioppo, "A short scale for measuring loneliness in large surveys," *Research on Aging*, vol. 26, no. 6, pp. 655–672, 2006.

[4] J. T. Cacioppo and L. C. Hawkley, "Social isolation and health, with an emphasis on underlying mechanisms," *Perspectives in Biology and Medicine*, vol. 46, no. 3, pp. S39–S52, 2003.

[5] T. Antonucci and H. Akiyama, "Convoys of social relations: family and friendships within a life span context," in *Handbook of Aging and the Family*, R. Blieszner and V. H. Bedford, Eds., pp. 355–371, Greenwood, Westport, Conn, USA, 1995.

[6] J. S. Hurlbert, V. A. Haines, and J. J. Beggs, "Core networks and tie activation: what kinds of routine networks allocate resources in nonroutine situations?" *American Sociological Review*, vol. 65, no. 4, pp. 598–618, 2000.

[7] T. A. Glass and J. L. Balfour, "Neighborhoods, aging, and functional limitations," in *Neighborhoods and Health*, I. Kawachi and L. F. Berkman, Eds., pp. 303–334, Oxford University Press, New York, NY, USA, 2003.

[8] A. Bowling and M. Stafford, "How do objective and subjective assessments of neighbourhood influence social and physical functioning in older age? Findings from a British survey of ageing," *Social Science & Medicine*, vol. 64, no. 12, pp. 2533–2549, 2007.

[9] S. V. Subramanian, L. Kubzansky, L. Berkman, M. Fay, and I. Kawachi, "Neighborhood effects on the self-rated health of elders: uncovering the relative importance of structural and service-related neighborhood environments," *The Journals of Gerontology B*, vol. 61, no. 3, pp. S153–S160, 2006.

[10] P. Teo and S. Huang, "A sense of place in public housing: a Case Study of Pasir Ris, Singapore," *Habitat International*, vol. 20, no. 2, pp. 307–325, 1996.

[11] Department of Statistics Singapore http://www.singstat.gov.sg/.

[12] Housing Development Board (HDB), *Public Housing in Singapore: Well-Being of Communities, Families and the Elderly*, 2003.

[13] Housing Development Board (HDB), *Public Housing in Singapore: Well-Being of Communities, Families and the Elderly*, 2008.

[14] L. K. George, "Still happy after all these years: research frontiers on subjective well-being in later life," *Journals of Gerontology B*, vol. 65, no. 3, pp. 331–339, 2010.

16

Genetic Risk Score Predicts Late-Life Cognitive Impairment

Mariegold E. Wollam,[1] Andrea M. Weinstein,[1,2] Judith A. Saxton,[3] Lisa Morrow,[4] Beth Snitz,[3] Nicole R. Fowler,[5] Barbara L. Suever Erickson,[1] Kathryn A. Roecklein,[1,2] and Kirk I. Erickson[1,2]

[1]*Department of Psychology, University of Pittsburgh, Sennott Square, 3rd Floor, 210 South Bouquet Street, Pittsburgh, PA 15260, USA*
[2]*Center for the Neural Basis of Cognition, University of Pittsburgh, 4400 Fifth Avenue, Suite 115, Pittsburgh, PA 15213, USA*
[3]*Department of Neurology, University of Pittsburgh, 811 Kaufmann Medical Building, 3471 Fifth Avenue, Pittsburgh, PA 15213, USA*
[4]*Department of Psychiatry, University of Pittsburgh, Thomas Detre Hall, 3811 O'Hara Street, Pittsburgh, PA 15213, USA*
[5]*Division of General Internal Medicine and Geriatrics, Indiana University, Fifth Third Faculty Building, 720 Eskenazi Avenue, Indianapolis, IN 46202, USA*

Correspondence should be addressed to Kirk I. Erickson; kiericks@pitt.edu

Academic Editor: Elke Bromberg

Introduction. A family history of Alzheimer's disease is a significant risk factor for its onset, but the genetic risk associated with possessing multiple risk alleles is still poorly understood. *Methods.* In a sample of 95 older adults (Mean age = 75.1, 64.2% female), we constructed a genetic risk score based on the accumulation of risk alleles in *BDNF, COMT,* and *APOE*. A neuropsychological evaluation and consensus determined cognitive status (44 nonimpaired, 51 impaired). Logistic regression was performed to determine whether the genetic risk score predicted cognitive impairment above and beyond that associated with each gene. *Results.* An increased genetic risk score was associated with a nearly 4-fold increased risk of cognitive impairment (OR = 3.824, $P = .013$) when including the individual gene polymorphisms as covariates in the model. *Discussion.* A risk score combining multiple genetic influences may be more useful in predicting late-life cognitive impairment than individual polymorphisms.

1. Introduction

A family history of late-life cognitive impairment is a well-recognized risk factor for the development of Alzheimer's disease (AD) and its preclinical stage of Mild Cognitive Impairment [1] (MCI). Twin studies report the heritability of AD to be between 58 and 79% [2], prompting a persistent search for genetic variants that influence susceptibility for AD and cognitive decline. The primary genetic risk factor for late-onset AD (LOAD) is widely considered to be the ε4 allele of the apolipoprotein E (*APOE*) gene, which has been consistently identified by genome-wide association studies (GWAS) of AD [3]. In the brain, apolipoprotein E serves a vital function in neuronal activity by regulating cholesterol metabolism [4]. Approximately 40% of all Caucasian adults who develop AD possess at least one ε4 allele [5], and ε4 carriers exhibit more precipitous cognitive decline [6, 7].

In addition to *APOE*, other genetic variants have been identified as risk factors for cognitive decline because they influence biological pathways involved in memory and executive function, which exhibit the earliest deficits during the progression of AD [8]. For example, the *BDNF* gene codes for brain-derived neurotrophic factor, a protein secreted by neurons that promotes neurogenesis and synaptic plasticity and transmission in the central nervous system; BDNF is particularly critical for learning and memory processes because it facilitates long-term potentiation in hippocampal neurons [9]. AD has been associated with decreased BDNF levels in the temporal and parietal cortices [10]. BDNF also circulates and can be measured in the periphery. Decreased

Table 1: Genotypes of *BDNF*, *COMT*, and *APOE* SNPs.

SNP	Primer sequence	Primer concentration	Amplicon length	Melt range (°C)
BDNF rs6265	FW 5′-GCTTGACATCATTGGCTGAC-3′ RV 5′-TACTGAGCATCACCCTGGAC-3′	375 nM	129	70.0–92.0
COMT rs4680	FW 5′-TCATCACCATCGAGATCAACC-3′ RV 5′-TTTTTCCAGGTCTGACAACG-3′	300 nM	112	70.0–91.0
APOE rs429358/rs7412	FW 5′-GGCACGGCTGTCCAAGGA-3′ RV 5′-GCCCCGGCCTGGTACAC-3′	200 nM	228	80.0–98.0

levels of serum BDNF have been associated with AD [11]. Age-related reductions in serum BDNF levels have also been related to smaller hippocampal volume and poorer memory function even in healthy older adults [12]. In the human *BDNF* gene, variation in the protein's function has been attributed to a single nucleotide polymorphism (SNP, rs6265, *Val66Met*) resulting in a *valine* (*Val*) to *methionine* (*Met*) substitution at codon 66. The *Met*-substituted product is associated with impaired intracellular trafficking and secretion of BDNF, poorer performance in declarative memory [13] and executive function [14], and reduced hippocampal volume and function [13–16]. Despite these convincing links with AD, weak association between this SNP and AD has been identified by GWAS [17] and candidate gene studies yield inconsistent results regarding whether the *Met* allele confers an increased risk of AD [18, 19], suggesting a need for further investigation of its role as a contributing, but not sole, risk factor.

In addition to *APOE* and *BDNF*, the catechol-o-methyltransferase (*COMT*) gene codes for an enzyme responsible for catalysis and inactivation of catecholamine neurotransmitters such as dopamine, norepinephrine, and epinephrine [20]. A common SNP of *COMT* (rs4680, *Val158Met*) involves a substitution of *Val* by *Met* at codon 158, the product of which is four times less metabolically active than the homozygous *Val* allele product [21]. Slower enzymatic activity of COMT delays inactivation of dopamine in the synaptic cleft in the prefrontal cortex, resulting in enhanced executive function for *Met* carriers relative to *Val* homozygotes [22]. Although association between the *COMT* polymorphism and AD has not been confirmed by GWAS or meta-analysis [23], studies have demonstrated that throughout adulthood the *Val* allele is associated with characteristics of cognitive decline and dementia such as poorer performance on tasks of executive functioning and working memory [24], declarative memory [25], and slower processing speed [26]. As in the case of BDNF *Val66Met*, the COMT *Val158Met* SNP is likely an under-recognized contributing genetic risk factor in the development of AD.

These and other genetic polymorphisms likely contribute relatively small independent effects to collectively predispose one to develop a complex disease such as AD. Studies have begun to investigate how multiple genetic influences can be aggregated into a single risk profile to predict the prevalence or course of a given pathology, either by summing the total number of risk alleles possessed or by obtaining a weighted sum including each risk allele multiplied by its associated effect size. Rodríguez-Rodríguez et al. [27] constructed a genetic risk score to predict progression from MCI to AD that combined genotype information across 8 non-*APOE* genetic variants (16 total alleles) identified by GWAS of AD risk, with each allele weighted by its AD risk odds ratio. Although the weighted genetic risk score was not significant, the authors found that subjects who possessed a total of six or more risk alleles progressed from MCI to AD twice as quickly as those who possessed fewer than six risk alleles. While the accumulation of risk alleles was a significant predictor for rate of progression to AD (OR = 1.89, $P < .047$, and 95% C.I. = 1.01, 3.56), each individual genetic polymorphism did not have significant predictive power by itself, with the exception of one marginally significant gene (*CD2AP*, OR = 1.69, $P < .051$). Similar risk scores have been employed to predict other pathologies such as age-related macular degeneration, multiple sclerosis, and type II diabetes [28–30]. These studies indicate that incorporating multiple SNPs pertinent to a given phenotype into a genetic risk score is more useful in predicting the prevalence or progression of a disease than considering polymorphisms individually.

In this genetic risk score study, we took a candidate gene approach by targeting genetic variants that have either been identified as having a clear link with risk for AD (i.e., *APOE*) or that have an important role in cognitive and brain functions in late adulthood and have a relatively common minor allele frequency (i.e., *BDNF*, *COMT*) but may have been previously undetected by GWAS due to small individual effect sizes. To test whether the combination of these three risk genotypes was collectively predictive of late-life cognitive impairment, we created a cumulative genetic risk score by summing the possession or absence of each SNP's risk allele. We predicted that a higher genetic risk score would correspond to an increased risk of cognitive impairment above and beyond that of the individual gene polymorphisms.

2. Methods

2.1. Participants. Data for this study were collected as part of a larger study examining the utility of providing cognitive testing of older adults in primary care physician (PCP) offices [31, 32]. Participants included 109 adults who were consented into the parent study. The parent study recruited participants from eleven PCP practices in the greater Pittsburgh and surrounding areas. Participants were eligible to participate if they were 65 years or older, had no medical chart diagnosis of dementia, had no acute illness, and were not residing in a nursing home. They were excluded if initial screening revealed the presence of sensory deficits that would preclude computerized and paper and pencil neuropsychological testing. Additionally, they were excluded if initial screening revealed the presence of dementia as indicated by a score of ≤18 on the Mini-Mental State Examination [33].

One participant was removed due to incorrectly recorded cognitive data. Since distributions of allelic frequencies differ between races, 4 African American participants were removed from the analysis to minimize confounding by genetic admixture. Age, gender, and years of education were self-reported. All participants signed a consent form approved by the University of Pittsburgh Institutional Review Board and were remunerated $20 for participation.

2.2. Cognitive Assessment and Group Classification. Each participant completed a comprehensive neuropsychological test battery assessing five primary cognitive domains: memory, executive function, spatial ability, language, and attention/psychomotor speed. Measures of memory were the Consortium to Establish a Registry for Alzheimer's Disease (CERAD) Word List Learning Test with delayed recall [34], the Wechsler Memory Scale-Revised Logical Memory I and II [35], and the modified Rey-Osterrieth figure for immediate and delayed recall [36]. Tests of executive function were the Wechsler Adult Intelligence Scale-Revised (WAIS-R) Backward Digit Span [37], the controlled oral word association test (FAS) [38], Part B of the Trail-Making Test [39], the WAIS-R Digit Symbol [37], and the Clock Drawing Test [38]. Tests of spatial ability were the modified Rey-Osterrieth Copy [36] and the modified WAIS-R Block Design [37]. Language tests consisted of the Boston Naming Test [40] and semantic fluency (animals) [38]. Tests of attention/psychomotor speed were the WAIS-R Digit Span Forward [37] and Part A of the Trail-Making Test [39]. Participants were also administered the Center for Epidemiologic Studies Depression (CES-D) Scale[41] for assessment of depression symptomatology, the Activities of Daily Living (ADL) Scale [42], and the Instrumental Activities of Daily Living (IADL) Scale [43].

A clinical adjudication panel of three expert neuropsychologists (all licensed psychologists) determined cognitive status: normal, mild cognitive impairment (MCI), or dementia. Classifications were done according to the criteria from the University of Pittsburgh Alzheimer's Disease Research Center [44, 45]. Dementia range = scores ≥ 2SD below age norms on two cognitive domains, one of which must be memory; MCI range = at least two scores 1-2SD below age norms; normal cognition = individuals not included in ranges for either dementia or MCI. The final diagnosis took into account the cognitive test scores as well as demographic, functional, behavioral, and medical information. Adjudications were conducted blind to study group status of the parent study. Final cognitive status categories consisted of cognitively nonimpaired (n = 44), Mild Cognitive Impairment (MCI, n = 47), or dementia (n = 4). Because of the low number of individuals with dementia, those with either Mild Cognitive Impairment or dementia were combined into a single group labeled "cognitive impairment" (n = 51).

2.3. Genotype Collection, Coding, and Risk Score Computation. Genomic DNA was collected with the Oragene-DNA Self-Collection Kit OG-500 (DNA Genotek Inc., Ontario, Canada). Extraction and purification of DNA were completed using the laboratory protocol from Oragene-DNA. DNA was diluted with TE buffer to 10 ng/μL and stored at −20°C.

Participants were genotyped for rs6265 (*Val66Met*) in *BDNF*, rs4680 (*Val158Met*) in *COMT*, and rs429358/rs7412 in *APOE* (*ApoE2*, *ApoE3*, and *ApoE4*). Genotype analysis was performed by high-resolution melting (HRM) analysis. Each polymerase chain reaction (PCR) was performed on a CFX96 real-time PCR system (Bio-Rad, Hercules, CA) using 1x Precision Melt Supermix (Bio-Rad, Hercules, CA). The reaction volume was 20 μL and contained 50 ng of genomic DNA. See Table 1 for primer sequence, primer concentration, amplicon length, and melt range. The running conditions for *BDNF* were 1 cycle of 95°C for 2 min and 65 cycles of 95°C for 10 s, and 56.6°C for 30 sec. The running conditions for *COMT* were 1 cycle of 95°C for 2 min and 65 cycles of 95°C for 10 s, and 60.1°C for 30 sec. The conditions for *APOE* were 1 cycle of 95°C for 2 min and 60 cycles of 95°C for 10 s, 63.8°C for 30 s, and 72°C for 30 sec. The melting range varied per SNP (see Table 1) but all began with a heteroduplex formation of 95°C for 30 seconds and 60°C for 1 min. The temperature increment for melting analysis for all three genotypes was 0.2°C per 10 sec. The melting curve was analyzed using Bio-Rad Precision Melt Analysis 1.2 software. Negative and positive controls were included on each run to ensure genotyping accuracy. Greater than 50% of samples were run in duplicate.

For the individual genotype analyses, *BDNF* genotype groups consisted of *Val* homozygotes, *Val* heterozygotes, and *Met* homozygotes; *COMT* genotype groups similarly consisted of *Val* homozygotes, *Val* heterozygotes, or *Met* homozygotes; *APOE* genotype groups included ε2/ε3, ε2/ε4, ε3/ε3, ε3/ε4, or ε4/ε4. See Table 2 for genotype frequencies.

The genetic risk score was then computed for each participant by summing the presence or the absence of risk genotypes. That is, each genotype was assigned either "0" for minimally associated genetic risk with cognitive deficits or "1" for a putative association with cognitive deficits. This scoring criterion was based on the literature for each of the three polymorphisms. For *APOE*, the ε4 allele is widely considered to be a risk allele for cognitive deficits and decline; so its possession warranted "1" towards the risk score and its absence "0". For *BDNF*, the *Met* allele is associated with decreased cognitive function; so possession of a *Met* allele resulted in "1" and its absence "0". For *COMT*, the *Val* allele is considered to be most strongly associated with cognitive deficits, conferring "1" for its possession and "0" in its absence.

In effect, the risk score combines *BDNF Met* carriers into one group to be compared with *Val* homozygotes due to our interest in possession of the *Met* allele at either locus. In a similar fashion, homozygous and heterozygous *COMT Val* carriers were grouped and compared with *Met* homozygotes. Following convention established by the *APOE* literature, ε4 allele carriers were grouped and compared with all non-ε4

Table 2: Frequencies of *BDNF*, *COMT*, and *APOE* genotypes and risk allele carriers.

Gene	Genotype	*n*	Risk allele carrier status	*n*
BDNF	Val/Val	61	*Met* carriers (risk score value = 1)	34
	Val/Met	33	*Val* homozygotes (risk score value = 0)	61
	Met/Met	1		
COMT	Val/Val	23	*Val* carriers (risk score value = 1)	63
	Val/Met	40	*Met* homozygotes (risk score value = 0)	32
	Met/Met	32		
APOE	ε2/ε3	12	ε4 carriers (risk score value = 1)	22
	ε2/ε4	1	Non-ε4 carriers (risk score value = 0)	73
	ε3/ε3	61		
	ε3/ε4	18		
	ε4/ε4	3		

Table 3: Participant demographics.

Characteristic	All participants ($n = 95$)	Nonimpaired ($n = 44$)	Impaired ($n = 51$)
Age (mean years [SD])	75.1 (5)	73.9 (4.2)	76.1 (5.4)
Completed education (mean years [SD])	14.4 (3.2)	15.1 (2.9)	13.8 (3.3)
Gender (% female)	64.2	70.5	58.8
MMSE (mean [SD])	28.1 (2.1)	28.9 (1.2)	27.5 (2.4)

carriers. See Table 2 for risk genotype frequencies for each gene.

The sum of these three component risk genotypes for all three polymorphisms yielded a risk score with a scale of genetic risk values between 0 and 3. An overall risk score value of "0" translates into the absence of any risk genotypes and represents the lowest genetic risk category for decline in cognitive status; "1" represents possession of only one risk genotype, "2" represents possession of two risk genotypes, and "3" represents possession of all 3 risk genotypes and is proposed to represent the highest genetic risk category for decline in cognitive status.

2.4. Statistics. First, in order to determine whether any of the three genotypes were individually predictive of cognitive status, hierarchal logistic regression analyses were performed (SPSS Version 22). The demographic variables, consisting of age, gender, and years of education, comprised the 1st block while *BDNF*, *COMT*, and *APOE* genotype were each entered as the 2nd block in separate regression models. In these analyses, the *BDNF* genotype was coded as "1" for *Val/Val*, "2" for *Val/Met*, or "3" for *Met/Met*. In a similar fashion, the *COMT* genotype was coded as "1" for *Val/Val*, "2" for *Val/Met*, or "3" for *Met/Met*. Based on the literature, the independent effect of *APOE* genotype on cognitive status was determined by assigning "1" for non-ε4 carriers and "2" for the possession of at least one ε4 allele; for subsequent risk score analyses, the *APOE* genotype variable reflects all possible genotypes, coded as "23" for ε2/ε3, "24" for ε2/ε4, "33" for ε3/ε3, "34" for ε3/ε4, and "44" for ε4/ε4. These genotype variables were subsequently used as the individual genotype covariates in the genetic risk score analyses.

Hierarchal logistic regression was then performed to determine whether the composite genetic risk score variable (entered as the 3rd block) predicted cognitive status (nonimpaired versus impaired) above and beyond the individual genotypes (all three comprising the 2nd block) and the demographic variables (the 1st block). We report odds ratios (OR) and confidence intervals (C.I.) resulting from these analyses and report *P* values below 0.05.

3. Results

3.1. Demographics and Covariates. Nine participants were excluded (7 were missing genotype information for all three genes while an additional 2 were missing *APOE* genotype, resulting in an overall failure rate of 7.37% and error rate of 0%). Our final sample size of $n = 95$ was 64.2% female with a mean age of 75.1 years. Allelic frequencies did not significantly differ from Hardy-Weinberg equilibrium for any of the three genes. Table 3 shows demographic information and MMSE scores for the overall sample as well as between the nonimpaired and impaired participants. Cognitive status (the presence or absence of impairment) was significantly associated with age (OR = 1.113, $P = .025$, and 95% C.I. = 1.014, 1.222) and years of education (OR = .861, $P = .038$, and 95% C.I. = .748, .992) such that higher age and fewer years of education were associated with a higher risk of impairment. Gender was not significantly associated with an increased risk of impairment (OR = .537, $P = .177$, and 95% C.I. = .217, 1.324), but there were a higher proportion of men in the cognitively impaired group and there is evidence of sexual dimorphism of both *BDNF* and *APOE* on risk for AD [46, 47]. Therefore, we included age, gender, and years of education as covariates in all analyses to isolate the effects of *BDNF*, *COMT*, and *APOE* genotype or the genetic risk score on cognitive status. See Table 3.

3.2. Association between Individual SNPs and Risk for Cognitive Impairment. Consistent with the literature, *APOE* ε4 carrier status was significantly predictive of an increased risk of cognitive impairment (OR = 3.561, $P = .032$, and 95% C.I. = 1.116, 11.365) after controlling variation from age, gender, and education. Neither *BDNF* nor *COMT* genotype was related to cognitive status (*BDNF*, OR = 1.149, $P = .755$, and 95% C.I. = .479, 2.759; *COMT*, OR = 1.074, $P = .808$, and 95% C.I. = .606, 1.903).

3.3. Association between Genetic Risk Score and Risk for Cognitive Impairment. Table 4 shows the frequencies for each genetic risk score value. Each additional point towards the genetic risk score was significantly associated with a nearly 4-fold increased risk of cognitive impairment (OR = 3.824,

TABLE 4: Genetic risk score frequencies.

Risk score value	n
0	16
1	46
2	26
3	7
Total	95

TABLE 5: Results of genetic risk score controlling individual genotypes.

Variable	OR	p value	95% C.I.
BDNF	0.369	0.145	0.096–1.410
COMT	2.147	0.061	0.966–4.773
APOE	0.9	0.093	0.796–1.018
Risk score	3.824	0.013	1.333–10.973

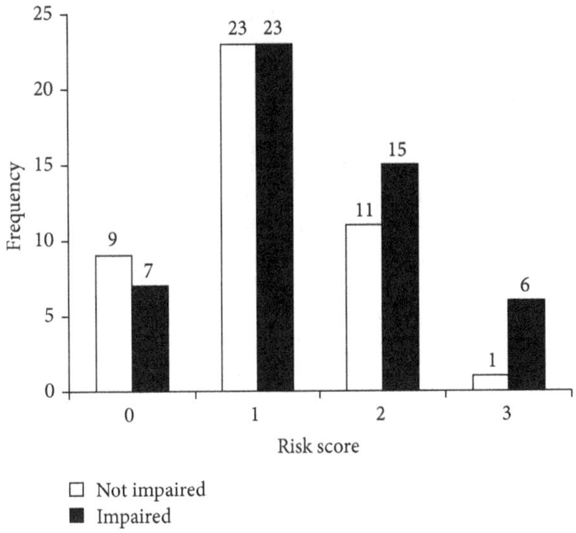

FIGURE 1: Risk score frequencies between cognitive status categories.

P = .013, and 95% C.I. = 1.333, 10.973) even after including all of the individual gene polymorphisms in the model (see Table 5). Consistent with our hypothesis, a higher genetic risk score representing an increasing number of risk genotypes was predictive of an increased risk of cognitive impairment above and beyond the variation attributable to individual polymorphisms. Figure 1 shows the distribution of risk scores between cognitive status categories.

Follow-up analyses were performed to determine whether the 4 individuals with dementia were driving the association between the genetic risk score and cognitive impairment. After removing the 4 individuals with dementia from the analysis, the risk score remained significant (OR = 3.138, P = .039, and 95% C.I. = 1.059, 9.302) while the individual genotypes remained nonsignificant in the full model, with the exception of *COMT* which reached nominal significance (*BDNF*, OR = .446, P = .248, and 95% C.I. = .113, 1.755; *COMT*, OR = 1.977, P = .095, and 95% C.I. = .889, 4.396; *APOE*, OR = .899, P = .105, and 95% C.I. = .790, 1.022).

4. Discussion

We created a genetic risk score to represent the accumulation of risk genotypes of polymorphisms in *BDNF*, *COMT*, and *APOE* to test whether the risk score predicted the presence of late-life cognitive impairment above and beyond that of each individual gene polymorphism. Consistent with our predictions, a higher genetic risk score significantly predicted a higher risk of having cognitive impairment (OR = 3.824, P = .013, and 95% C.I. = 1.333, 10.973) when controlling individual polymorphisms in *BDNF*, *COMT*, and *APOE* (see Tables 4 and 5). Congruent with the literature, *BDNF* and *COMT* genotype were not independently predictive of cognitive status, whereas *APOE* ε4 carrier status was predictive of cognitive status (OR = 3.561, P = .032, and 95% C.I. = 1.116, 11.365). These results demonstrate that the aggregation of multiple risk genotypes into one total risk score predicted the presence or absence of impairment to a higher degree than any of the individual polymorphisms.

The genes under consideration for this study were chosen due to their involvement in general neural function (*APOE*) as well as in processes known to present the earliest deficits in AD such as learning, memory, and executive function (*BDNF* and *COMT*). Polymorphisms in these genes (*BDNF*, rs6265; *COMT*, rs4680; and *APOE*, rs429358/rs7412) have been associated with differential protein function, with possession of each SNP's risk allele (*Met*, *Val*, and ε4, resp.) associated with poorer cognitive performance. Our findings support the use of a single genetic risk score to represent the accumulation of genetic influences affecting multiple domains of cognition and brain health in relation to AD, which may be more important in determining cognitive decline than testing individual genotypes. When considered individually, these same genetic polymorphisms contribute small or negligible effects and remain largely undetected by previous GWAs (except *APOE*) but may still represent influential aspects of AD pathology. These results beg the question of the importance of other risk genotypes not assessed here that could also contribute to risk of AD. Additionally, our results complement previous reports of significant interaction between *COMT Val158Met* and *APOE* ε4 on risk for AD [48], additive effects of *BDNF Val66Met* and *APOE* ε4 on hippocampal activity in healthy older adults [49], and interaction between *BDNF Val66Met* and *APOE* ε4 on episodic memory in cognitively healthy older adults [50].

Our study represented a unique population of older adults who underwent a comprehensive cognitive assessment and diagnosis. However, one limitation is the relatively small sample size of our study (n = 95). In genetic association studies, hundreds of subjects are genotyped in order to achieve sufficient power to reliably test specific genetic interactions or confirm epistatic effects between genes. However, we still detected an association between higher risk scores and increased odds of being cognitively impaired (Figure 1). Future studies will need to expand these results to larger samples with a higher proportion of cognitively impaired individuals. This will help verify the associations to more clearly examine potential interactions between these gene polymorphisms as well as assess effect sizes and dose-dependent effects of possessing one, both, or no risk allele(s) for each gene considered. The genetic risk score reported here was unable to account for and examine the effects of possessing either one or both risk alleles for each gene without further reducing the number of participants in each risk score category and diminishing the statistical power and interpretation of the results. Finally, an additional limitation of the current study is that we included only individuals of European descent to avoid confounding by population admixture. Future studies should recruit from various racial and ethnic backgrounds to determine whether the genetic and phenotypic trends observed here are present in other races and ethnicities while adequately accounting for population stratification.

In summary, we found that a cumulative genetic risk score across three genes related to cognition, brain function, and risk for dementia (*BDNF*, *COMT*, and *APOE*) significantly predicted late-life cognitive impairment. The risk score was significant above and beyond the effects of each individual genotype. Our findings demonstrate the effectiveness of genetic risk scores and their potential utility as predictors of more genetic variation in cognitive outcomes such as AD than polymorphisms considered individually.

Conflict of Interests

All authors declare that there is no conflict of interests regarding the publication of this paper.

Authors' Contribution

Mariegold Wollam performed data analysis and interpretation and preparation of paper. Andrea Weinstein helped in data acquisition and preparation of paper. Judith Saxton helped in data acquisition and preparation of paper. Lisa Morrow helped in data acquisition and preparation of paper. Beth Snitz helped in data acquisition and preparation of paper. Nicole Fowler helped in data acquisition and preparation of paper. Barbara Suever Erickson helped in genotyping procedures and preparation of paper. Kathryn Roecklein helped in genotyping procedures, data analysis and interpretation, and preparation of paper. Kirk Erickson helped in study concept and design, data analysis and interpretation, and preparation of paper.

Acknowledgment

This study was supported by grants from the National Institutes of Health (R01 DK095172 and R01 AG023129).

References

[1] Alzheimer's Association, "2014 Alzheimer's disease facts and figures," *Alzheimer's & Dementia*, vol. 10, no. 2, pp. e47–e92, 2014.

[2] M. Gatz, C. A. Reynolds, L. Fratiglioni et al., "Role of genes and environments for explaining Alzheimer disease," *Archives of General Psychiatry*, vol. 63, no. 2, pp. 168–174, 2006.

[3] K. D. Coon, A. J. Myers, D. W. Craig et al., "A high-density whole-genome association study reveals that APOE is the major susceptibility gene for sporadic late-onset Alzheimer's disease," *Journal of Clinical Psychiatry*, vol. 68, no. 4, pp. 613–618, 2007.

[4] R. E. Pitas, J. K. Boyles, S. H. Lee, D. Hui, and K. H. Weisgraber, "Lipoproteins and their receptors in the central nervous system. Characterization of the lipoproteins in cerebrospinal fluid and identification of apolipoprotein B,E(LDL) receptors in the brain," *The Journal of Biological Chemistry*, vol. 262, no. 29, pp. 14352–14360, 1987.

[5] L. A. Farrer, L. A. Cupples, J. L. Haines et al., "Effects of age, sex, and ethnicity on the association between apolipoprotein E genotype and Alzheimer disease. A meta-analysis. APOE and Alzheimer Disease Meta Analysis Consortium," *The Journal of the American Medical Association*, vol. 278, no. 16, pp. 1349–1356, 1997.

[6] D. C. Whitehair, A. Sherzai, J. Emond et al., "Influence of apolipoprotein e $\varepsilon 4$ on rates of cognitive and functional decline in mild cognitive impairment," *Alzheimer's and Dementia*, vol. 6, no. 5, pp. 412–419, 2010.

[7] S. Cosentino, N. Scarmeas, E. Helzner et al., "APOE $\varepsilon 4$ allele predicts faster cognitive decline in mild Alzheimer disease," *Neurology*, vol. 70, no. 19, pp. 1842–1849, 2008.

[8] National Institutes of Health, National Institute on Aging, and Human Services Department, *Alzheimer's Disease: Unraveling the Mystery*, Government Printing Office, 2011.

[9] D. K. Binder and H. E. Scharfman, "Brain-derived neurotrophic factor," *Growth Factors*, vol. 22, no. 3, pp. 123–131, 2004.

[10] J. Lee, H. Fukumoto, J. Orne et al., "Decreased levels of BDNF protein in Alzheimer temporal cortex are independent of BDNF polymorphisms," *Experimental Neurology*, vol. 194, no. 1, pp. 91–96, 2005.

[11] M. Ventriglia, R. Zanardini, C. Bonomini et al., "Serum brain-derived neurotrophic factor levels in different neurological diseases," *BioMed Research International*, vol. 2013, Article ID 901082, 7 pages, 2013.

[12] K. I. Erickson, R. S. Prakash, M. W. Voss et al., "Brain-derived neurotrophic factor is associated with age-related decline in hippocampal volume," *The Journal of Neuroscience*, vol. 30, no. 15, pp. 5368–5375, 2010.

[13] J. P. Kambeitz, S. Bhattacharyya, L. M. Kambeitz-Ilankovic, I. Valli, D. A. Collier, and P. McGuire, "Effect of BDNF val^{66}met polymorphism on declarative memory and its neural substrate: a meta-analysis," *Neuroscience and Biobehavioral Reviews*, vol. 36, no. 9, pp. 2165–2177, 2012.

[14] Y. Y. Lim, V. L. Villemagne, S. M. Laws et al., "BDNF Val66Met, Aβ amyloid, and cognitive decline in preclinical Alzheimer's disease," *Neurobiology of Aging*, vol. 34, no. 11, pp. 2457–2464, 2013.

[15] R. A. Honea, C. Cruchaga, R. D. Perea et al., "Characterizing the role of brain derived neurotrophic factor genetic variation in Alzheimer's disease neurodegeneration," *PLoS ONE*, vol. 8, no. 9, Article ID e76001, 2013.

[16] L. Pezawas, B. A. Verchinski, V. S. Mattay et al., "The brain-derived neurotrophic factor val66met polymorphism and variation in human cortical morphology," *The Journal of Neuroscience*, vol. 24, no. 45, pp. 10099–10102, 2004.

[17] G. Laumet, V. Chouraki, B. Grenier-Boley et al., "Systematic analysis of candidate genes for Alzheimer's disease in a French, genome-wide association study," *Journal of Alzheimer's Disease*, vol. 20, no. 4, pp. 1181–1188, 2010.

[18] R. Huang, J. Huang, H. Cathcart, S. Smith, and S. E. Poduslo, "Genetic variants in brain-derived neurotrophic factor associated with Alzheimer's disease," *Journal of Medical Genetics*, vol. 44, no. 2, article e66, 2007.

[19] Á. Fehér, A. Juhász, Á. Rimanóczy, J. Kálmán, and Z. Janka, "Association between BDNF Val66Met polymorphism and alzheimer disease, dementia with lewy bodies, and pick disease," *Alzheimer Disease and Associated Disorders*, vol. 23, no. 3, pp. 224–228, 2009.

[20] B. Bertocci, V. Miggiano, M. Da Prada, Z. Dembic, H.-W. Lahm, and P. Malherbe, "Human catechol-O-methyltransferase: cloning and expression of the membrane-associated form," *Proceedings of the National Academy of Sciences of the United States of America*, vol. 88, no. 4, pp. 1416–1420, 1991.

[21] P. T. Männistö and S. Kaakkola, "Catechol-O-methyltransferase (COMT): biochemistry, molecular biology, pharmacology, and clinical efficacy of the new selective COMT inhibitors," *Pharmacological Reviews*, vol. 51, no. 4, pp. 593–628, 1999.

[22] R. M. Bilder, J. Volavka, H. M. Lachman, and A. A. Grace, "The catechol-O-methyltransferase polymorphism: relations to the tonic-phasic dopamine hypothesis and neuropsychiatric phenotypes," *Neuropsychopharmacology*, vol. 29, no. 11, pp. 1943–1961, 2004.

[23] J. H. Barnett, L. Scoriels, and M. R. Munafò, "Meta-analysis of the cognitive effects of the catechol-O-methyltransferase gene Val158/108Met polymorphism," *Biological Psychiatry*, vol. 64, no. 2, pp. 137–144, 2008.

[24] G. E. Bruder, J. G. Keilp, H. Xu et al., "Catechol-O-methyltransferase (COMT) genotypes and working memory: associations with differing cognitive operations," *Biological Psychiatry*, vol. 58, no. 11, pp. 901–907, 2005.

[25] C. M. de Frias, K. Annerbrink, L. Westberg, E. Eriksson, R. Adolfsson, and L.-G. Nilsson, "COMT gene polymorphism is associated with declarative memory in adulthood and old age," *Behavior Genetics*, vol. 34, no. 5, pp. 533–539, 2004.

[26] J. M. Starr, H. Fox, S. E. Harris, I. J. Deary, and L. J. Whalley, "COMT genotype and cognitive ability: a longitudinal aging study," *Neuroscience Letters*, vol. 421, no. 1, pp. 57–61, 2007.

[27] E. Rodríguez-Rodríguez, P. Sánchez-Juan, J. L. Vázquez-Higuera et al., "Genetic risk score predicting accelerated progression from mild cognitive impairment to Alzheimer's disease," *Journal of Neural Transmission*, vol. 120, no. 5, pp. 807–812, 2013.

[28] L. G. Fritsche, W. Chen, M. Schu et al., "Seven new loci associated with age-related macular degeneration," *Nature Genetics*, vol. 45, no. 4, pp. 433–439, 2013.

[29] P. L. De Jager, L. B. Chibnik, J. Cui et al., "Integration of genetic risk factors into a clinical algorithm for multiple sclerosis susceptibility: a weighted genetic risk score," *The Lancet Neurology*, vol. 8, no. 12, pp. 1111–1119, 2009.

[30] M. C. Cornelis, L. Qi, C. Zhang et al., "Joint effects of common genetic variants on the risk for type 2 diabetes in U.S. men and women of European ancestry," *Annals of Internal Medicine*, vol. 150, no. 8, pp. 541–550, 2009.

[31] B. E. Snitz, L. A. Morrow, E. G. Rodriguez, K. A. Huber, and J. A. Saxton, "Subjective memory complaints and concurrent memory performance in older patients of primary care providers," *Journal of the International Neuropsychological Society*, vol. 14, no. 6, pp. 1004–1013, 2008.

[32] L. A. Morrow, B. E. Snitz, E. G. Rodriquez, K. A. Huber, and J. A. Saxton, "High medical co-morbidity and family history of dementia is associated with lower cognitive function in older patients," *Family Practice*, vol. 26, no. 5, pp. 339–343, 2009.

[33] N. R. Fowler, L. A. Morrow, L. Tu et al., "Association between cognitive decline in older adults and use of primary care physician services in Pennsylvania," *Journal of Primary Care & Community Health*, vol. 3, no. 3, pp. 201–209, 2012.

[34] J. C. Morris, A. Heyman, R. C. Mohs et al., "The Consortium to Establish a Registry for Alzheimer's Disease (CERAD). Part I. Clinical and neuropsychological assessment of Alzheimer's disease," *Neurology*, vol. 39, no. 9, pp. 1159–1165, 1989.

[35] D. Wechsler, *Wechsler Memory Scale—Revised*, The Psychological Corporation, New York, NY, USA, 1987.

[36] M.-S. Shin, S.-Y. Park, S.-R. Park, S.-H. Seol, and J. S. Kwon, "Clinical and empirical applications of the Rey-Osterrieth Complex Figure Test," *Nature Protocols*, vol. 1, no. 2, pp. 892–899, 2006.

[37] D. Wechsler, *Wechsler Adult Intelligence Scale—Revised Manual*, The Psychological Corporation, New York, NY, USA, 1981.

[38] O. Spreen and E. Strauss, *A Compendium of Neuropsychological Tests*, Oxford University Press, New York, NY, USA, 1998.

[39] R. M. Reitan, "Validity of the trail-making tests as an indication of organic brain damage," *Perceptual and Motor skills*, no. 8, pp. 271–276, 1958.

[40] E. Kaplan, H. Goodglass, and S. Weintraub, *Boston Naming Test*, Lippincott Williams & Wilkins, Philadelphia, Pa, USA, 2nd edition, 2001.

[41] L. S. Radloff, "The CES-D Scale: a self-report depression scale for research in the general population," *Applied Psychological Measurement*, vol. 1, no. 3, pp. 385–401, 1977.

[42] I. McDowell and C. Newell, *Measuring Health: A Guide to Rating Scales and Questionnaires*, Oxford University Press, Oxford, UK, 1987.

[43] D. Galasko, D. Bennett, M. Sano et al., "An inventory to assess activities of daily living for clinical trials in Alzheimer's disease," *Alzheimer Disease & Associated Disorders*, vol. 11, no. 2, pp. S33–S39, 1997.

[44] M. Ganguli, J. Gilby, E. Seaberg, and S. Belle, "Depressive symptoms and associated factors in a rural elderly population: the MoVIES project," *The American Journal of Geriatric Psychiatry*, vol. 3, no. 2, pp. 144–160, 1995.

[45] O. L. Lopez, J. T. Becker, W. Klunk et al., "Research evaluation and diagnosis of possible Alzheimer's disease over the last two decades: II," *Neurology*, vol. 55, no. 12, pp. 1863–1869, 2000.

[46] N. Fukumoto, T. Fujii, O. Combarros et al., "Sexually dimorphic effect of the Val66Met polymorphism of BDNF on susceptibility to Alzheimer's disease: new data and meta-analysis," *American Journal of Medical Genetics, Part B: Neuropsychiatric Genetics*, vol. 153, no. 1, pp. 235–242, 2010.

[47] J. S. Damoiseaux, W. W. Seeley, J. Zhou et al., "Gender modulates the APOE epsilon4 effect in healthy older adults: convergent evidence from functional brain connectivity and spinal fluid tau levels," *The Journal of Neuroscience*, vol. 32, no. 24, pp. 8254–8262, 2012.

[48] M. F. Martínez, X. E. Martín, L. G. Alcelay et al., "The COMT Val158 Met polymorphism as an associated risk factor for Alzheimer disease and mild cognitive impairment in APOE 4 carriers," *BMC Neuroscience*, vol. 10, article 125, 2009.

[49] K. Kauppi, L.-G. Nilsson, J. Persson, and L. Nyberg, "Additive genetic effect of APOE and BDNF on hippocampus activity," *NeuroImage*, vol. 89, pp. 306–313, 2014.

[50] D. D. Ward, M. J. Summers, N. L. Saunders, P. Janssen, K. E. Stuart, and J. C. Vickers, "APOE and BDNF Val66Met polymorphisms combine to influence episodic memory function in older adults," *Behavioural Brain Research*, vol. 271, pp. 309–315, 2014.

17

An Open-Label Trial of Memantine for Cognitive Impairment in Patients with Posttraumatic Stress Disorder

Sriram Ramaswamy,[1,2] Jayakrishna Madabushi,[3] John Hunziker,[1,2] Subhash C. Bhatia,[1,2] and Frederick Petty[4,5]

[1]*Department of Mental Health and Behavioral Sciences, VA Nebraska-Western Iowa Health Care System, 4101 Woolworth Avenue, Omaha, NE 68105, USA*
[2]*Department of Psychiatry, Creighton University School of Medicine, 3528 Dodge Street, Omaha, NE 68131, USA*
[3]*Baptist Health System, 3201 4th Avenue South, Birmingham, AL 35222, USA*
[4]*Mental Health Service, Orlando VA Medical Service, 5201 Raymond Street, Orlando, FL 32803, USA*
[5]*Department of Psychiatry, University of Central Florida College of Medicine, 6850 Lake Nona Boulevard, Orlando, FL 32827, USA*

Correspondence should be addressed to Sriram Ramaswamy; sriram.ramaswamy@va.gov

Academic Editor: Elke Bromberg

Background. Studies using standard neuropsychological instruments have demonstrated memory deficits in patients with PTSD. We evaluated the efficacy and safety of the N-methyl-D-aspartate antagonist memantine in veterans with PTSD and cognitive impairment. *Methods.* Twenty-six veterans with PTSD and cognitive impairment received 16 weeks of memantine in an open-label fashion. Cognition was assessed using the Spatial Span, Logical Memory I, and Letter-Number Sequencing subtests of the Wechsler Memory Scale III and the Repeatable Battery for the Assessment of Neuropsychological Status (RBANS). RBANS measures attention, language, visuospatial skills, and immediate and delayed memories. The Clinician Administered PTSD Scale (CAPS), Hamilton Depression Scale (HAM-D), Hamilton Anxiety Scale (HAM-A), Quality of Life Enjoyment and Satisfaction Questionnaire (Q-LES-Q), and Sheehan Disability Scale (SDS) were secondary outcome measures. *Results.* There was a significant improvement in RBANS, both total and subscale scores ($P < 0.05$), over time. There was a reduction in total CAPS scores, avoidance/numbing symptoms (CAPS-C) and hyperarousal symptoms (CAPS-D), HAM-D, Q-LES-Q, and SDS scores. However, there was no reduction in reexperiencing (CAPS-B) and HAM-A scores. Memantine was well tolerated. *Conclusions.* Memantine improved cognitive symptoms, PTSD symptoms, and mood in veterans with PTSD. Randomized double-blind studies are needed to validate these preliminary observations.

1. Background

Posttraumatic stress disorder (PTSD) is a major public health problem with lifetime prevalence rate of up to 8% [1]. PTSD is more frequent after combat exposure and about 20–30% of Vietnam War veterans developed PTSD [2]. Prevalence among veterans returning from Iraq and Afghanistan is found to be as high as 17% [3] and is associated with debilitating psychological symptoms and poor quality of life.

In addition to amnesia for trauma-related stimuli, several studies have demonstrated cognitive deficits in different areas in individuals with PTSD. Deficits in verbal memory [4, 5], working memory and attention [6–10], processing speed [6], and nonverbal memory [11, 12] have been reported. A study reported short delay and long delay memory deficits in PTSD [13]. It may be argued that the comorbidities associated with PTSD could contribute to associated cognitive symptoms. However, even after controlling for confounding factors like head injury, depressive symptoms, and alcohol, significant cognitive impairment was reported in individuals with postwar PTSD [14, 15]. The neurobiology of cognitive impairment associated with PTSD has not been well elucidated. Available literature suggests involvement of the hypothalamic-pituitary-adrenal (HPA) axis leading to corticotrophin-releasing factor (CRF) dysregulation in PTSD. Variation in cortisol levels has been reported in PTSD, with most of the data suggesting hypocortisolemia as a long-term effect [16]. Some data suggest that acute stress induces elevations in endogenous corticosteroids, which may cause hippocampal damage, which in turn might be associated with memory impairment in PTSD [17, 18]. The glutamatergic system also plays a role in stress response, which is mediated by cortisol dysregulation. Glutamate and CRF appear to modulate each other's expression. Rats exposed to immobilization stress show increased expression of the N-methyl-D-aspartate (NMDA) receptor subunit in the paraventricular nucleus in the hypothalamus [19, 20]. Open-label trials of lamotrigine, an antiglutamatergic medication, in PTSD support the role of glutamatergic abnormalities in PTSD [21].

Currently, the only FDA approved medications available for the treatment of PTSD are sertraline (Zoloft) and paroxetine (Paxil). Unfortunately, many patients with PTSD are unresponsive, have only moderate or marginal responses, or have troubling side effects of first-line selective serotonin reuptake inhibitor (SSRI) treatment. As a result, there has been considerable interest in alternative pharmacological treatments for PTSD, including medications to target cognitive symptoms of PTSD. Memantine is an NMDA glutamate receptor antagonist that is approved by the US Food and Drug Administration (FDA) for treatment of dementia, and it has also been used off-label for a variety of psychiatric disorders such as major depression, bipolar disorder, schizophrenia, and anxiety disorders (for reviews, see [22–24]). While there have been no controlled studies examining the effects of memantine on PTSD, there is evidence from animal research that memantine can reduce anxiety and improve cognition [25], and case studies in humans suggest that memantine may help to treat cognitive symptoms in patients with combat-related PTSD [26, 27]. Further study is needed, however, to establish the safety and efficacy of memantine in this population. We conducted a prospective open-label study to test the hypothesis that memantine's antiglutamatergic activity could improve cognitive functioning and overall symptoms of PTSD. The secondary aim of this study was to find out usefulness of memantine for core PTSD symptoms and comorbid depressive symptoms.

2. Design and Methodology

Participants were recruited from the Omaha Veterans Affairs Medical Center following local IRB approval. We obtained written consent from all the subjects who were recruited in the study. Twenty-six veterans (25 males, 1 female) between the ages of 19 and 65 years (M = 56.4; SD = 4.5) with chronic PTSD (diagnosis for >6 months) attributable to military combat exposure were included in the study. Patients were required to be clinically stable on their psychotropic medication regimen for at least three months prior to study entry. In addition to meeting DSM-IV criteria for PTSD and endorsing subjective complaints of memory difficulties, patients had to score at least one standard deviation below the mean performance of a standardized, age- and sex-matched population on the Spatial Span, Logical Memory I, and Letter-Number Sequencing subtests of the Wechsler Memory Scale III (third edition) for study entry. Patients with a history of dementia, schizophrenia, bipolar disorder, traumatic brain injury, and seizure were excluded. Patients with any history of alcohol or illicit drug abuse or dependence within the past one month were excluded. Patients requiring concomitant treatment with drugs with potential effects on the glutamatergic system, such as amantadine, dextromethorphan, or carbonic anhydrase inhibitors, were excluded.

Subjects initially received memantine of 5 mg once daily, which was increased weekly by 5 mg/day in divided doses to a dose of 20 mg/day. Memory was assessed using the Repeatable Battery for the Assessment of Neuropsychological Status (RBANS) [28] using both forms A and B at baseline, end of week 8, and end of week 16. The RBANS is composed of 10 subtests that yield a total score and five index scores: immediate memory, visuospatial/constructional, language, attention, and delayed memory. Each index score has a normal mean of 100 and standard deviation of 15 based on the performance of a standardization sample matched to the U.S. Census on sex, ethnicity, and level of education. Alternative forms of the RBANS (forms A and B) were used to avoid bias due to practice effects. We administered Clinician Administered PTSD Scale (CAPS), Hamilton Depression Scale (HAM-D), Hamilton Anxiety Scale (HAM-A), Quality of Life Enjoyment and Satisfaction Questionnaire (Q-LES-Q), and Sheehan Disability Scale (SDS) to assess the secondary measures. Changes in the scores over time with repeated measures were estimated with mixed-effects models. The primary outcome measures of interest were index and percentile scores in RBANS total and subscale scores. The repeated measures model included visit (as a categorical variable) as a fixed effect. An unstructured covariance matrix was used to fit the within patient repeated measures effect. Tukey's method was used to compare pairwise means.

Secondary outcome measures, CAPS, HAM-A, HAM-D, Q-LES-Q, and SDS, were analyzed similarly to the RBANS with repeated measures models. P values less than 0.05 are considered to be statistically significant. SAS software version 9.1 (SAS Institute, Cary, NC) was used for the analysis.

3. Results

A total of 26 patients were included in the study. Participants were compliant with their appointments; only three patient visits during the entire study were missed. Significant change was found in RBANS total and subscale scores during the follow-ups at baseline, end of week 8, and end of week 16 (Table 1). For RBANS, the total score and subscales all changed significantly over time, whether looking at index scores or percentiles (all $P < 0.01$). Figures 1 and 2 illustrates changes in RBANS index scores and percentile scores respectively over time. Table 3 illustrates the estimated means and standard errors for secondary outcome scores at each visit. Age and gender were not contributing factors to the results. This is not surprising since almost all subjects were males and the age ranges very small.

Table 1: Demographic and baseline characteristics.

	N (%)
Ethnicity	
African American	3
White	23 (76)
Hispanic	0
Asian	0
Other	0
Gender	
Male	24 (92)
Female	2 (8)
Age (mean/SD)	56.88 years (3.9)

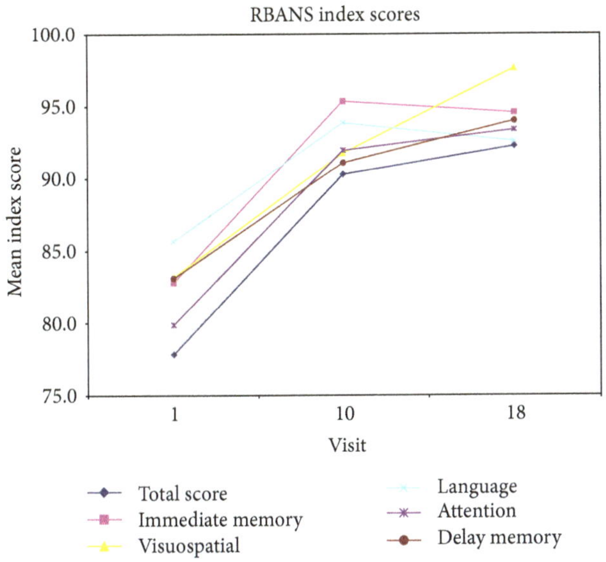

Figure 1: This figure illustrates changes in Repeatable Battery for the Assessment of Neuropsychological Status index scores over time.

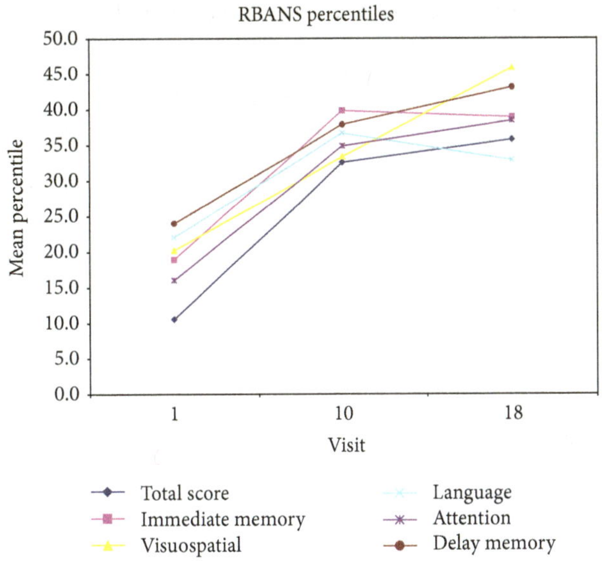

Figure 2: This figure illustrates changes in Repeatable Battery for the Assessment of Neuropsychological Status percentile scores over time.

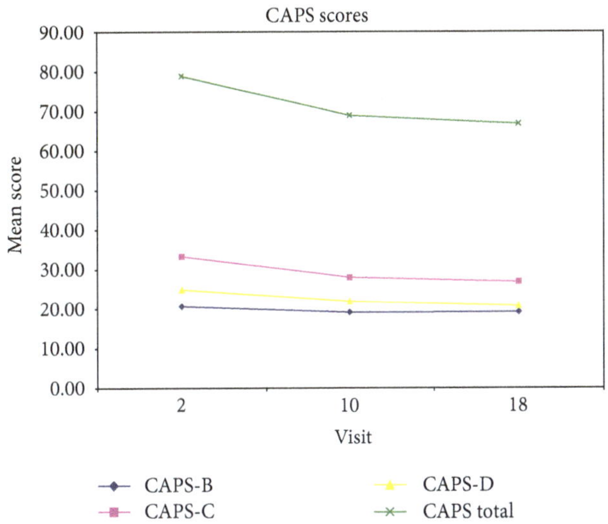

Figure 3: This figure illustrates changes in Clinician Administered PTSD Scale scores over time.

4. Secondary Outcome Measures

Secondary outcomes for this study included CAPS, HAM-A, HAM-D, Q-LES-Q, and SDS. Table 2 shows the results of the repeated measures, mixed-effects (ME) model for secondary outcomes. CAPS-C, CAPS-D, CAPS total, HAM-D, Q-LES-Q, and SDS all changed significantly over time (all $P < 0.05$). CAPS-B and HAM-A showed no overall change over time.

Adverse effects were mild in nature. There were no serious adverse effects in the trial. Two subjects were lost to follow-up after completing the baseline visit. One subject experienced constipation, so the drug was not increased above 10 mg in that particular subject. Figures 3, 4, and 5 illustrate changes in CAPS, HAM-A, HAM-D scores over time. Figure 5 illustrates changes in Quality of Life Enjoyment and Satisfaction Questionnaire scores over time.

5. Discussion

Chronic PTSD is associated with cognitive dysfunction [4, 6, 11]. Dysregulations in the hypothalamic-pituitary-adrenal (HPA) axis, cortisol system, and glutamate pathways are associated with PTSD symptoms. Limited data is available regarding the neurobiology of cognitive symptom in PTSD. Glutamate and its subreceptors are intrinsically linked to memory process by their involvement in long-term potentiation (LTP) and long-term desensitization (LTD), mechanisms underlying learning and memory. However, the role of the glutamatergic system in cognitive dysfunction associated with PTSD is not well elucidated. It has been shown that stress can affect the glutamatergic system, presumably through the cortisol pathway [21]. There is a dearth of studies looking at pharmacological interventions for cognitive symptoms of PTSD.

Table 2: Change in RBANS scores during repeated measures.

	Visit	Mean	SE	*P* value
Total score	Baseline	77.8	2.0	<0.0001
	Week 8	90.3	2.6	
	Week 16	92.2	2.7	
Total score percentile	Baseline	10.6	1.6	<0.0001
	Week 8	32.6	4.9	
	Week 16	35.8	5.4	
Immediate memory	Baseline	82.8	2.5	<0.0001
	Week 8	95.3	2.3	
	Week 16	94.6	2.7	
Immediate memory percentile	Baseline	18.9	4.4	<0.0001
	Week 8	39.8	5.3	
	Week 16	38.9	5.8	
Visuospatial index score	Baseline	83.2	2.6	0.0001
	Week 8	91.8	2.9	
	Week 16	97.6	3.1	
Visuospatial percentile	Baseline	20.2	3.8	0.0002
	Week 8	33.4	5.6	
	Week 16	45.8	5.9	
Language	Baseline	85.7	2.2	0.0024
	Week 8	93.9	1.9	
	Week 16	92.6	1.7	
Language percentile	Baseline	22.0	3.7	0.0006
	Week 8	36.7	3.5	
	Week 16	32.9	3.7	
Attention	Baseline	79.9	2.7	0.0017
	Week 8	92.0	3.0	
	Week 16	93.4	3.3	
Attention percentile	Baseline	16.0	3.1	0.0009
	Week 8	34.9	5.9	
	Week 16	38.4	6.3	
Delayed memory	Baseline	83.1	3.5	0.0003
	Week 8	91.1	3.6	
	Week 16	94.0	3.5	
Delayed memory percentile	Baseline	24.0	4.4	0.0003
	Week 8	37.9	5.6	
	Week 16	43.1	5.5	

There was significant improvement in all RBANS scores, including language, attention, and immediate and delayed memory from baseline, week 8, and week 16.

Table 3: Estimated means and standard errors for secondary outcome scores at each visit (from ME model).

	Week	Mean	SE	*P* value
CAPS-B	Baseline	20.65	1.73	0.52
	End of week 8	19.10	1.62	
	End of week 16	19.17	1.60	
CAPS-C	Baseline	33.31	1.54	0.0055
	End of week 8	27.98	2.08	
	End of week 16	26.92	1.97	
CAPS-D	Baseline	24.88	0.97	0.023
	End of week 8	21.88	1.58	
	End of week 16	20.75	1.44	
CAPS total score	Baseline	78.85	3.79	0.027
	End of week 8	68.92	4.72	
	End of week 16	66.80	4.45	
HAM-A	Baseline	25.04	1.71	0.056
	End of week 8	20.76	1.99	
	End of week 16	20.18	1.74	
HAM-D	Baseline	19.96	1.17	0.013
	End of week 8	14.57	1.36	
	End of week 16	15.53	1.54	
Q-LES-Q	Baseline	40.27	1.79	0.0076
	End of week 8	47.07	2.25	
	End of week 16	46.81	2.21	
SDS	Baseline	7.02	0.31	0.020
	End of week 8	6.20	0.66	
	End of week 16	5.73	0.50	

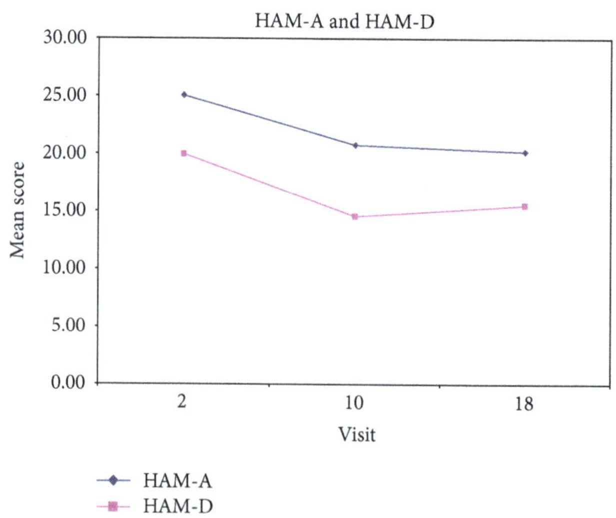

Figure 4: This figure illustrates changes in Hamilton Depression Scale and Hamilton Anxiety Scale scores over time.

Memantine, which has actions on the glutamatergic system, has been approved by the FDA for dementia. In a pilot study [26], memantine was reported to be useful for delayed recall measure of memory, variable reduction of depressive symptoms, and variable reduction in hyperarousal symptoms. Results of our study demonstrate improvement in cognitive symptoms in PTSD patients following therapy with memantine for 16 weeks. Improvement in memory was observed as early as 8 weeks, reflected by improvement in RBANS total score and subscales over time in both index scores and percentiles.

This is consistent with the results in Alzheimer's disease studies, where differences between memantine and

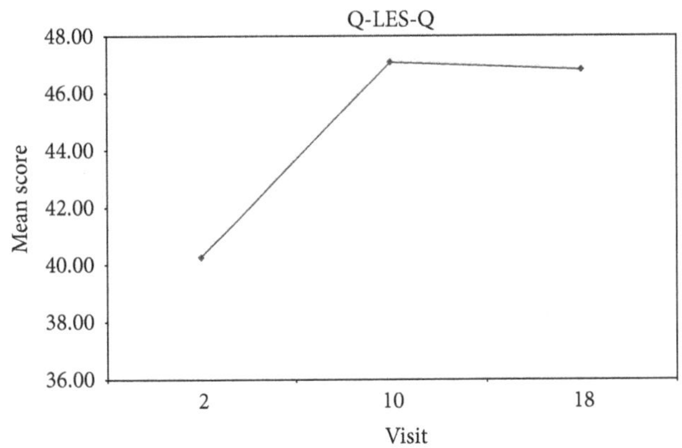

Figure 5: This figure illustrates changes in Quality of Life Enjoyment and Satisfaction Questionnaire scores over time.

placebo in cognition were observed after 8 weeks [29]. Except for the visuospatial percentile scores, the remainder of our scores demonstrated improvement beyond 8 weeks. There was an increase in the proportion of subjects who attained normal scores of attention, visuospatial skills, and immediate and delayed memories with memantine at subsequent visits compared to the initial visit. In our study memantine was associated with significant improvement across all RBANS subscales. This is in contrast to several negative studies of memantine in cognitive dysfunction associated with schizophrenia. The neurobiology of both PTSD and schizophrenia cognitive impairment is not fully known although there is stronger evidence for cholinergic dysfunction in schizophrenia than in PTSD. The robust effect in our study might be explained by a strong placebo response, a task learning effect, or merely confirmatory of glutamatergic abnormalities in chronic PTSD. Nevertheless, the results were surprising and support investigation with larger controlled trials.

Improvement was also noticed in PTSD symptoms, including hyperarousal, avoidance, and depressive symptoms, as demonstrated by improvement in CAPS scores and HAM-D scores. Memory disturbances are predominant in the presentation of posttraumatic stress disorder (PTSD) and are part of the diagnostic criteria. There was no improvement in the reexperiencing set of symptoms (CAPS-B). The reexperiencing symptom criteria of PTSD include intrusive memories of the traumatic event. It is plausible that a true effect of memantine on this subset of PTSD symptoms might have been missed secondary to its effect on improving overall declarative memory.

To summarize, we observed improvement in memory, core symptoms of PTSD, and depression in combat veterans with PTSD following open-label treatment with memantine. Our study was limited by the nature of its open-label, non-placebo controlled study design and small sample size. The open-label design was chosen for its advantages for a proof of concept study such as simplicity, ease of patient recruitment and retention. Memory performance has been associated with education on the RBANS. [30] Also, the relationship between chronicity of PTSD and cognitive decline has to be borne in mind especially since there is data that prolonged PTSD that may have cumulative adverse effects on hippocampal volume [31]. Our study did not look at the effect of education and chronicity of PTSD on the outcome variables. Future studies should control for these important variables. Despite the limitations our data are the best currently available and provide useful insights into the management of cognitive impairment associated with PTSD. Larger, double-blind, placebo-controlled, randomized, and controlled trials are warranted to validate the findings of this study.

Conflict of Interests

The authors declare that they have no conflict of interests.

Acknowledgment

This work was supported by an Investigator-Initiated grant from Forest Research Institute.

References

[1] R. C. Kessler, P. Berglund, O. Demler, R. Jin, K. R. Merikangas, and E. E. Walters, "Lifetime prevalence and age-of-onset distributions of DSM-IV disorders in the national comorbidity survey replication," *Archives of General Psychiatry*, vol. 62, no. 6, pp. 593–602, 2005.

[2] D. D. Blake, T. M. Keane, P. R. Wine, C. Mora, K. L. Taylor, and J. A. Lyons, "Prevalence of PTSD symptoms in combat veterans seeking medical treatment," *Journal of Traumatic Stress*, vol. 3, no. 1, pp. 15–27, 1990.

[3] C. W. Hoge, C. A. Castro, S. C. Messer, D. McGurk, D. I. Cotting, and R. L. Koffman, "Combat duty in Iraq and Afghanistan, mental health problems, and barriers to care," *The New England Journal of Medicine*, vol. 351, no. 1, pp. 13–22, 2004.

[4] B. M. Elzinga and J. D. Bremner, "Are the neural substrates of memory the final common pathway in posttraumatic stress disorder (PTSD)?" *Journal of Affective Disorders*, vol. 70, no. 1, pp. 1–17, 2002.

[5] M. D. Horner and M. B. Hamner, "Neurocognitive functioning in posttraumatic stress disorder," *Neuropsychology Review*, vol. 12, no. 1, pp. 15–30, 2002.

[6] D. Brandes, G. Ben-Schachar, A. Gilboa, O. Bonne, S. Freedman, and A. Y. Shalev, "PTSD symptoms and cognitive performance in recent trauma survivors," *Psychiatry Research*, vol. 110, no. 3, pp. 231–238, 2002.

[7] T. Gil, A. Calev, D. Greenberg, S. Kugelmass, and B. Lerer, "Cognitive functioning in post-traumatic stress disorder," *Journal of Traumatic Stress*, vol. 3, no. 1, pp. 29–45, 1990.

[8] M. W. Gilbertson, T. V. Gurvits, N. B. Lasko, S. P. Orr, and R. K. Pitman, "Multivariate assessment of explicit memory function in combat veterans with posttraumatic stress disorder," *Journal of Traumatic Stress*, vol. 14, no. 2, pp. 413–432, 2001.

[9] J. J. Vasterling, J. I. Constans, K. Brailey, and P. B. Sutker, "Attention and memory dysfunction in posttraumatic stress disorder," *Neuropsychology*, vol. 12, no. 1, pp. 125–133, 1998.

[10] J. J. Vasterling, L. M. Duke, K. Brailey, J. I. Constans, A. N. Allain Jr., and P. B. Sutker, "Attention, learning, and memory performances and intellectual resources in Vietnam veterans: PTSD and no disorder comparisons," *Neuropsychology*, vol. 16, no. 1, pp. 5–14, 2002.

[11] L. Jelinek, D. Jacobsen, M. Kellner et al., "Verbal and nonverbal memory functioning in posttraumatic stress disorder (PTSD)," *Journal of Clinical and Experimental Neuropsychology*, vol. 28, no. 6, pp. 940–948, 2006.

[12] G. E. Johnsen, P. Kanagaratnam, and A. E. Asbjørnsen, "Memory impairments in posttraumatic stress disorder are related to depression," *Journal of Anxiety Disorders*, vol. 22, no. 3, pp. 464–474, 2008.

[13] R. S. MacKin, J. A. Lesselyong, and K. Yaffe, "Pattern of cognitive impairment in older veterans with posttraumatic stress disorder evaluated at a memory disorders clinic," *International Journal of Geriatric Psychiatry*, vol. 27, no. 6, pp. 637–642, 2012.

[14] J. J. Vasterling, S. P. Proctor, P. Amoroso, R. Kane, T. Heeren, and R. F. White, "Neuropsychological outcomes of army personnel following deployment to the Iraq War," *Journal of the American Medical Association*, vol. 296, no. 5, pp. 519–529, 2006.

[15] P. B. Sutker, J. J. Vasterling, K. Brailey, and A. N. Allain Jr., "Memory, attention, and executive deficits in POW survivors: contributing biological and psychological factors," *Neuropsychology*, vol. 9, no. 1, pp. 118–125, 1995.

[16] R. Yehuda, "Sensitization of the hypothalamic-pituitary-adrenal axis in posttraumatic stress disorder," in *Psychobiology of Posttraumatic Stress Disorder (Annals of the New York Academy of Sciences)*, A. C. McFarlane and R. Yehuda, Eds., vol. 821, pp. 57–75, Academy of Sciences, New York, NY, USA, 1997.

[17] T. V. Gurvits, M. E. Shenton, H. Hokama et al., "Magnetic resonance imaging study of hippocampal volume in chronic, combat-related posttraumatic stress disorder," *Biological Psychiatry*, vol. 40, no. 11, pp. 1091–1099, 1996.

[18] N. Kitayama, V. Vaccarino, M. Kutner, P. Weiss, and J. D. Bremner, "Magnetic resonance imaging (MRI) measurement of hippocampal volume in posttraumatic stress disorder: a meta-analysis," *Journal of Affective Disorders*, vol. 88, no. 1, pp. 79–86, 2005.

[19] D. R. Ziegler, W. E. Cullinan, and J. P. Herman, "Organization and regulation of paraventricular nucleus glutamate signaling systems: N-methyl-D-aspartate receptors," *The Journal of Comparative Neurology*, vol. 484, no. 1, pp. 43–56, 2005.

[20] J. Nair and S. S. Ajit, "The role of the glutamatergic system in posttraumatic stress disorder," *CNS Spectrums*, vol. 13, no. 7, pp. 585–591, 2008.

[21] M. A. Hertzberg, M. I. Butterfield, M. E. Feldman et al., "A preliminary study of lamotrigine for the treatment of posttraumatic stress disorder," *Biological Psychiatry*, vol. 45, no. 9, pp. 1226–1229, 1999.

[22] H. Kavirajan, "Memantine: a comprehensive review of safety and efficacy," *Expert Opinion on Drug Safety*, vol. 8, no. 1, pp. 89–109, 2009.

[23] G. Sani, G. Serra, G. D. Kotzalidis et al., "The role of memantine in the treatment of psychiatric disorders other than the dementias: a review of current preclinical and clinical evidence," *CNS Drugs*, vol. 26, no. 8, pp. 663–690, 2012.

[24] K. Zdanys and R. R. Tampi, "A systematic review of off-label uses of memantine for psychiatric disorders," *Progress in Neuro-Psychopharmacology and Biological Psychiatry*, vol. 32, no. 6, pp. 1362–1374, 2008.

[25] R. Minkeviciene, P. Banerjee, and H. Tanila, "Cognition-enhancing and anxiolytic effects of memantine," *Neuropharmacology*, vol. 54, no. 7, pp. 1079–1085, 2008.

[26] M. A. Battista, R. Hierholzer, H. R. Khouzam, A. Barlow, and S. O'Toole, "Pilot trial of memantine in the treatment of posttraumatic stress disorder," *Psychiatry*, vol. 70, no. 2, pp. 167–174, 2007.

[27] M. P. Chopra, K. M. Trevino, and N. W. Kowall, "Memantine for posttraumatic stress disorder in an older veteran," *Journal of Clinical Psychopharmacology*, vol. 31, no. 6, pp. 787–788, 2011.

[28] C. Randolph, *Repeatable Battery for the Assessment of Neuropsychological Status (RBANS)*, Harcourt, The Psychological Corporation, San Antonio, Tex, USA, 1998.

[29] E. R. Peskind, S. G. Potkin, N. Pomara et al., "Memantine treatment in mild to moderate Alzheimer disease: a 24-week randomized, controlled trial," *American Journal of Geriatric Psychiatry*, vol. 14, no. 8, pp. 704–715, 2006.

[30] W. W. Beatty, J. W. Mold, and S. T. Gontkovsky, "RBANS performance: influences of sex and education," *Journal of Clinical and Experimental Neuropsychology*, vol. 25, no. 8, pp. 1065–1069, 2003.

[31] K. Felmingham, L. M. Williams, T. J. Whitford et al., "Duration of posttraumatic stress disorder predicts hippocampal grey matter loss," *NeuroReport*, vol. 20, no. 16, pp. 1402–1406, 2009.

18

Living on the Edge: Social Exclusion and the Receipt of Informal Care in Older People

Lena Dahlberg[1,2] **and Kevin J. McKee**[1]

[1]*School of Education, Health and Social Studies, Dalarna University, Dalarna, Sweden*
[2]*Aging Research Center, Karolinska Institutet & Stockholm University, Stockholm, Sweden*

Correspondence should be addressed to Lena Dahlberg; ldh@du.se

Academic Editor: Barbara Shukitt-Hale

Older people have been identified as being at risk of social exclusion. However, despite the fact that care is commonly required in later life and the majority of that care is provided by informal carers, a connection between social exclusion and informal care-receipt has rarely been considered. The aim of this study was to examine how informal care-receipt is related to social exclusion. A face-to-face questionnaire survey on social exclusion and informal care-receipt was carried out among older people (n = 1255) living in Barnsley, United Kingdom. Multivariable analyses examined the association between social exclusion and categories of informal care-receipt: care-receiver; assurance-receiver; nonreceiver with no need; and nonreceiver with need. Compared to being a nonreceiver with no need, participants were more likely to be care-receivers or assurance-receivers if they had higher levels of social exclusion. The highest level of social exclusion, however, was found in nonreceivers with need. Despite a lack of informal care and support, formal practical support and personal care were also low in this latter group. Findings are discussed in relation to the conceptualisation of care-receipt and how contact with medical services could be an opportunity for identification and appropriate referral of nonreceivers with need.

1. Introduction

A policy agenda at the European level is the reduction of social exclusion [1–3], defined as a "process whereby certain individuals are pushed to the edge of society and prevented from participating fully" [4]. Social exclusion is associated with reduced quality of life and health deterioration [5, 6]. Older people have been identified as a population subgroup at particular risk of social exclusion (e.g., [7]). Every second older person in England is experiencing social exclusion [8] and in deprived urban areas in England two-thirds of older people experience social exclusion [9]. While social exclusion has been explored in relation to a number of factors, including income, health, and disability, it has rarely been considered in relation to informal care-receipt. This is despite the fact that with increasing age older people require greater amounts of care and support and that informal care comprises the majority of this care [10]. Furthermore, research has shown that the transition to requiring care can reinforce social exclusion (cf. [11]). This paper considers how dimensions of, as well as risk factors for, social exclusion are linked to informal care-receipt in older people.

Social exclusion is a multifaceted concept covering dimensions such as production activity, financial activities, social relations, social activity, and political/civic activity [12, 13]. Lack of participation in or access to activities/services specified by these dimensions can be seen as indicators of social exclusion. Within social exclusion research concerning older people Scharf and colleagues [6] propose that older people may experience social exclusion on the following dimensions: social relationships; civic activities; basic services; neighbourhoods; and material resources. By comparison a United Kingdom (UK) government report [8] defines social exclusion of older people in terms of exclusion on the following dimensions: social relationships; cultural and leisure activities; civic activities; basic services; neighbourhoods; financial products; and material goods. As can be seen, although there are different operationalisations there is consensus around core dimensions of social exclusion for older people. What is apparent is that in social exclusion research on older people there is less emphasis on production activity and more emphasis on the importance of neighbourhood, also often discussed in terms of community. Many older people have spent a substantial period of their lives in a particular neighbourhood, have strong emotional investments in the surrounding community, increasingly rely on neighbourhood relationships for support in old age, and also tend to spend more time than younger people in the immediate neighbourhood [14].

Research exploring risk factors for social exclusion among older people has identified an enhanced risk of social exclusion with increasing age and ethnic minority origin and, among those living alone, having no children, and being on low income [6, 8]. Poor health, long-standing illness, and depression have also been found to increase the risk of social exclusion ([6, 8, 15], cf. [16]). Negative consequences of poor health can to some extent be compensated for by access to social and health care [17], thereby helping to prevent social exclusion. A few studies have focused on access to formal care in relation to social exclusion [11, 18–20], but research on access to *informal* care (i.e., care provided by friends and family) in the context of social exclusion is very limited. This is surprising, since as noted previously the majority of all care for older people in the community is informal and recent research indicates that the level of informal care is increasing [21, 22].

As people age, a reduction in functional capacity occurs that increases their need for help with activities of everyday life [23]. While the level of care received by an older person might be expected to map onto their need for care (due to, e.g., functional limitation and frailty), there are many factors that can disrupt this mapping resulting in unmet need for care in a significant minority of older people [24–26]. Unmet need can have serious consequences for an older person including increased mortality risk [27] and also prevent them from participating fully in society. Thus, unmet need for care could arguably place an older person at risk of social exclusion.

The relationship between care-receipt and social exclusion could be hypothesised to take different forms. It could be argued that the level of care-receipt if directly mapping onto the level of need in the older person would be a marker for his/her level of social exclusion, given that higher levels of care received would be in response to higher levels of illness or frailty, that is, risk factors for social exclusion. Yet care-receipt is linked to indicators of social *inclusion* such as the availability of, as well as access to, social networks, so an alternative hypothesis is that higher levels of contact with family and friends as a result of being a care-receiver might serve to reduce social exclusion. There is also the critical issue of where the level of care-receipt is not appropriate to need: where need for care exists but care is not received, is the degree of social exclusion particularly high?

This paper aims to examine the relationship between social exclusion and the receipt of informal care and reports the analysis of relevant data from the Barnsley Social Exclusion in Old Age Study, which sought to explore social exclusion among older people via a survey of over 1,000 respondents (see also [28]).

2. Materials and Methods

2.1. Design and Sampling. A questionnaire survey was carried out in the metropolitan area of Barnsley, England, UK. Barnsley was selected as the study site since it encompasses both urban and rural areas, allowing the exploration of how social exclusion processes might differ in such contrasting areas. To ensure adequate cell size at subgroup level for specific analyses, a sample of $n = 600$ for each of the two areas (i.e., $N = 1200$) was proposed, providing good statistical power for the analyses reported in this paper. Sampling occurred from seven electoral wards with an urban profile and from 16 electoral wards with a rural profile. Within each electoral ward households (which included supported accommodation) were randomly selected via local electoral registers. With oversampling of households required in order to obtain sufficient participants, a total of 11,035 households were sampled.

2.2. Participants. Potential participants were ineligible if they were under 65 years of age and were excluded from the study if their physical and/or mental health was too poor to allow them to complete an interview or respond to questions reliably; 59 individuals were excluded from the study as a result of this latter criterion. Only one older person was recruited per household regardless of whether more than one older person resided at a given address. In total 1,255 older people participated in the study, of whom 6.5% were recruited from supported accommodation. The response rate was 68.1% and did not differ significantly between urban and rural areas.

2.3. Materials. A questionnaire was developed that addressed a range of indicators of, as well as risk factors for, social exclusion, together with the topic of care-receipt. Given the potential frailty of some respondents, the need to keep the questionnaire concise meant that brevity was a key criterion during instrument selection. On occasion items and scales were adapted to more precisely address the study population or agenda.

An item used in the EUROFAMCARE study [29] to identify informal carers was adapted to produce a categorical variable of *informal care-receipt*: "Do you rely on a friend or relative (including your partner or other people in your household) to provide you with care or support for four hours per week or more?" (response categories: *yes*/*no*). Those participants responding "yes" were categorised as *care-receivers*. Participants who responded "no" were asked: "Do you have someone who looks in on you to see if 'everything is all right'?" (cf. [30]) (the three response categories were *yes*; *no, no need*; and *no, despite need*). Those participants responding "yes" were categorised as *assurance-receivers*; those responding "no, no need" were categorised as *nonreceivers without need*; those responding "no, despite need" were categorised as *nonreceivers with need*. This procedure therefore produced a four-category variable of care-receipt.

In this article, the following dimensions of social exclusion were considered: financial resources; social relationships; community; and social engagement.

Financial resources were operationalised via the following item measuring income discomfort: "Which of these descriptions comes closest to how you feel about your household's income nowadays?" with response options ranging from *very comfortable on present income* (1) to *very difficult on present income* (5) [31].

Social relationships were measured via items on social contacts, informal caregiving, and loneliness. For data on social contacts a question asked "how often do you meet and spend time with any of the following people?" Independent responses were required for family members (six categories), neighbours, and friends [32, 33]. For family member contact responses were coded as *weekly contact or more* (1) or *less than weekly contact* (0) for each category and items summed to indicate overall level of contact (scores ranging from 0 to 6, high scores indicating high contact). For the two categories of nonfamily members responses were combined and coded for analysis as *no contact* (0), *at least twice weekly contact with friends or neighbours* (1), or *at least twice weekly contact with friends and neighbours* (2).

The informal care item in the EUROFAMCARE study mentioned above was used in its original form for measuring informal caregiving, that is, "Have you a friend or relative (including your partner or other people in your household) who relies on you to provide them with care or support for four hours per week or more?" (response categories: *yes/no*).

Loneliness was measured by the De Jong Gierveld Loneliness Scale, in which respondents indicate the extent to which 11 statements relating to loneliness apply to their situation and the way they feel now, with response options *yes*, *more or less*, and *no*. The items are scored in relation to two subscales: Emotional Loneliness (scale range 0–6, sample Cronbach α = .81) and Social Loneliness (scale range 0–5, sample Cronbach α = .76) [34].

Respondents were asked to what extent they agreed with each of 13 statements about their local community, defined as "within 20 minutes' walk or about a mile from home." Example items are "I feel really part of this area"; "Vandalism and graffiti are a big problem in this area" (response scale from *strongly agree* (1) to *strongly disagree* (4) [7, 8, 35]).

For data on social engagement participants were asked, first, to consider for "how often, if at all, do you engage in the following activities?" and record a response for twenty different activities. Example activities are "Go out for a meal"; "Attend leisure activities (e.g., dancing, bingo or attend a social club)"; "Tend to the garden or allotment" (response scale *several times a week* (6) to *never* (0)) and, second, to indicate for each applicable activity if it is performed *usually with somebody* (3), *sometimes with somebody* (2), or *usually alone* (1) [32, 33]. The product of participants' engagement scores and socializing scores resulted in a single "social engagement" score for each activity.

This study considered the following risk factors for social exclusion: sociodemographic characteristics; health; and well-being. The questionnaire contained standard items addressing sociodemographic characteristics: age; gender; marital and coresident status; ethnicity; and duration of local residence. Education was measured by an item with six response categories, merged into two broader categories for analysis: "low education" (highest level, *completed school, no qualification/certificate*) and "medium to high education" (lowest level, *completed school with qualification/certificate*).

Self-reported health was assessed via the item: "In general, would you say your health is..." [31] measured on a five-point scale (*excellent* (1) to *very poor* (5)). Psychological well-being was measured using the World Health Organisation-5 Well-being Index [36] (WHO-5; scale range 0–25 (high score = high well-being); sample Cronbach α = .87).

Finally information on formal care-receipt was gathered via items asking if the participant had in the last month received medical care, personal care (e.g., from a district nurse), or practical support (e.g., from social services, home help, and warden); response categories for all items were *yes/no*.

2.4. Procedure. In order to ensure standardisation of data collection procedures and maximise interviewer sensitivity to reliability issues (e.g., physical or mental health problems in respondents, the influence of people present during interviews), interviewers were provided with training commensurate with their prior experience. Training therefore amounted to a few hours (for experienced interviewers) to two days (for inexperienced interviewers).

Upon selection, a household was sent a letter presenting the purpose of the study. An interviewer subsequently visited the address to establish whether anybody in the household was 65 years or older and, if so, whether this person was willing to participate in an interview. Each interview lasted on average 50 minutes. Seventy-eight percent of the interviews were conducted alone with the interviewee, while the rest were carried out with the interviewee accompanied, usually by a family member.

Interviewers completed several items at the end of the questionnaire as a quality check addressing whether or not the respondent had tried to answer the questions to the best of his or her ability; whether the respondent understood the questions; and whether anyone was present during the interview that could have interfered with the interview. There was also an option for the interviewer to write additional information about the interview. Where data drawn from these items indicated a problem with the interview, researchers discussed the problem with the interviewer, and if there was a suggestion that the reliability of the data could be suspected, the interview was excluded from the study.

2.5. Data Analysis. Data were analysed using the IBM Statistical Package for Social Science (SPSS) 22.0 for Windows.

Scale development occurred for items on perception of the local community and social engagement, utilizing principle components analysis and reliability (Cronbach α) analyses with item trial removal. Three subscales of perceptions of the local community were developed: Perceived Community Trust (3 items, M = 11.4, SD = 1.89, and α = .68); Perceived Community Integration (4 items, M = 15.6, SD = 2.39, and α = .69); and Perceived Community Security (3 items,

TABLE 1: Care-receipt status and sociodemographic characteristics of the sample (N = 1255).

Variable	
Care-receipt status: n (%)	
Care-receiver	269 (21.8)
Assurance-receiver	297 (24.1)
Nonreceiver with need	68 (5.5)
Nonreceiver without need	599 (48.6)
Age: M (SD), range	75.7 (7.29), 65–101
Gender: n (%)	
Women	776 (61.8)
Men	479 (38.2)
Marital status: n (%)	
Married, cohabiting	557 (44.6)
Single, divorced, separated, and never married	148 (11.8)
Widowed	545 (43.6)
Education level: n (%)	
Low	931 (74.2)
Medium to high	324 (25.8)
Area of residence: n (%)	
Urban area	627 (50.0)
Rural area	628 (50.0)

Note. Due to missing data n = 1250 for age; n = 1253 for coresident status.

M = 9.53, SD = 3.27, and α = .80). Two reliable subscales of social engagement were developed: Social, Cultural and Leisure Activity (7 items, M = 26.14, SD = 18.42, and α = .65) and Sport and Outdoor Activity (5 items, M = 12.40, SD = 13.06, and α = 0.56).

Bivariate analyses identified significant associations between the dependent variable (DV; the categorical care-receipt variable) and independent variables (IVs; indicators of and risk factors for social exclusion and other assessed variables). One-way ANOVA was performed for continuous IVs, with Hochberg's GT2 and Games-Howell tests as appropriate for post hoc analysis of group differences; Chi-square procedures were used for categorical IVs. A multinomial logistic regression was then performed to determine those IVs that predicted membership of the categories of care-receipt in a multivariable model. No adjustment to experimental alpha was made for multiple testing; significance for each test was set at $p < .05$. Given also the substantial sample size significant tests should be regarded cautiously and with thought to effect size.

3. Results

Care-receipt status and sample characteristics are summarised in Table 1. Regarding care-receipt 21.8 percent of the respondents were care-receivers and 24.1 percent were assurance-receivers, while 5.5 percent were nonreceivers with need and 48.6 percent were nonreceivers without need.

3.1. Bivariate Analysis. A brief summary of the bivariate analyses is described below, with a full presentation of the results of the analyses in Table 2. For the sake of concision IVs with nonsignificant associations with the DV are not presented.

At the top of the table bivariate associations between care-receipt status and social exclusion dimensions are presented. In post hoc tests nonreceivers without need had significantly lower dissatisfaction with household income than care-receivers and nonreceivers with need. Post hoc tests also showed that family contact was significantly lower, and Social Loneliness and Emotional Loneliness was significantly higher in nonreceivers with need compared to the three care-receipt categories, and the lowest proportion of older people with contact with friends and neighbours was also found in this group. Post hoc tests also indicated that nonreceivers without need were significantly lower on both Social and Emotional Loneliness than care-receivers and lower on Emotional Loneliness than assurance-receivers.

Other post hoc tests indicated that nonreceivers with need scored significantly lower on Perceived Community Integration than older people in the other three care-receipt categories. For Perceived Community Trust and Perceived Community Security post hoc tests indicated significantly lower scores for nonreceivers with need and care-receivers compared to assurance-receivers and nonreceivers without need. Finally, post hoc tests indicated that nonreceivers without need had significantly higher scores on Social, Cultural and Leisure Activity and Sport and Outdoor Activity than older people in the other three care-receipt categories.

In the next part of Table 2 analyses of risk factors of social exclusion are presented. Of the categorical IVs gender, coresident status, education, and place of residence were all significantly associated with care-receipt. Of the continuous IVs, in post hoc tests, nonreceivers without need were significantly younger than those in the other three categories. Post hoc tests determined that duration of local residence was significantly greater in care-receivers and nonreceivers

Table 2: Associations between care-receipt and social exclusion dimensions, risk factors of social exclusion, and formal care receipt (N = 1233).

	Care-receivers (n = 269)	Assurance-receivers (n = 297)	Nonreceivers with need (n = 68)	Nonreceivers without need (n = 599)	Test statistics, significance
Social Exclusion Variables					
Income comfort: M (SD) (high score = low comfort)	2.72 (0.80)	2.63 (0.87)	2.93 (1.00)	2.53 (0.81)	$F(3, 1218) = 6.79$, $p < .001$
Family contact: M (SD)	1.87 (1.08)	1.86 (1.18)	1.13 (1.13)	1.67 (1.17)	$F(3, 1189) = 9.01$, $p < .001$
Nonfamily contact: *n* (%)					
None	78 (29.3)	93 (31.4)	27 (39.7)	180 (30.3)	
Friends or neighbours	105 (39.5)	107 (36.1)	30 (44.1)	247 (41.5)	$\chi^2(6) = 9.34$, $p = .156$
Friends and neighbours	83 (31.2)	96 (32.4)	11 (16.2)	168 (28.2)	
Caregiving: *n* (%)	34 (12.7)	30 (10.1)	5 (7.4)	81 (13.6)	$\chi^2(3) = 3.82$, $p = .282$
Social Loneliness: M (SD)	1.69 (1.58)	1.38 (1.58)	2.79 (2.04)	1.26 (1.50)	$F(3, 1217) = 21.2$, $p < .001$
Emotional Loneliness: M (SD)	1.95 (1.91)	1.86 (2.00)	2.85 (2.29)	1.23 (1.68)	$F(3, 1206) = 22.8$, $p < .001$
Perceived Community Trust: M (SD)	10.9 (2.17)	11.7 (1.59)	10.4 (2.36)	11.6 (1.71)	$F(3, 1217) = 18.6$, $p < .001$
Perceived Community Integration: M (SD)	15.4 (2.56)	15.8 (2.20)	14.3 (3.18)	15.8 (2.22)	$F(3, 1218) = 9.49$, $p < .001$
Perceived Community Security: M (SD)	8.08 (3.79)	9.79 (2.75)	7.88 (3.69)	10.2 (2.94)	$F(3, 1215) = 34.5$, $p < .001$
Social, Cultural and Leisure Engagement: M (SD)	18.0 (16.7)	25.7 (17.0)	15.9 (14.5)	31.6 (18.3)	$F(3, 1128) = 43.9$, $p < .001$
Sport and Outdoor Engagement: M (SD)	5.19 (8.35)	11.4 (12.2)	7.36 (9.00)	16.9 (13.8)	$F(3, 1161) = 60.5$, $p < .001$
Risk Factors for Social Exclusion					
Age: M (SD)	77.6 (7.98)	76.9 (7.32)	77.4 (7.67)	74.1 (6.47)	$F(3, 1225) = 21.2$, $p < .001$
Female gender: *n* (%)	184 (68.4)	206 (69.4)	41 (60.3)	334 (55.8)	$\chi^2(3) = 21.5$, $p < .001$
Living alone: *n* (%)	138 (51.3)	206 (69.6)	53 (77.9)	231 (38.6)	$\chi^2(3) = 97.3$, $p < .001$
Low education level: *n* (%)	238 (88.5)	224 (75.4)	54 (79.4)	399 (66.6)	$\chi^2(3) = 47.9$, $p < .001$
Living in urban area: *n* (%)	174 (64.7)	149 (50.2)	47 (69.1)	247 (41.2)	$\chi^2(3) = 51.6$, $p < .001$
Duration of local residence: M (SD)	63.0 (21.7)	55.3 (26.4)	65.9 (17.3)	55.5 (22.3)	$F(3, 1222) = 10.5$, $p < .001$
Self-reported health: M (SD) (high score = poor health)	3.74 (0.83)	3.16 (0.84)	3.45 (0.84)	2.83 (0.83)	$F(3, 1212) = 75.7$, $p < .001$
Well-being: M (SD) (high score = high well-being)	12.0 (6.55)	13.5 (6.39)	12.7 (6.77)	16.0 (5.86)	$F(3, 1219) = 29.5$, $p < .001$
Medical care-receipt: *n* (%)	202 (75.1)	185 (62.3)	53 (77.9)	312 (52.1)	$\chi^2(3) = 50.9$, $p < .001$
Formal care-receipt:					
Personal care-receipt: *n* (%)	54 (20.2)	31 (10.5)	6 (8.82)	34 (5.68)	$\chi^2(3) = 42.9$, $p < .001$
Practical support-receipt: *n* (%)	44 (16.4)	28 (9.5)	3 (4.41)	4 (0.66)	$\chi^2(3) = 82.5$, $p < .001$

Note. Due to missing data on individual variables, *n* will vary across bivariate analyses.

with need than among assurance-receivers and nonreceivers without need. For measures of self-rated health and well-being post hoc tests indicated that nonreceivers without need differed significantly from those in the other three categories, having better self-reported health and better well-being. In addition, post hoc tests indicated that care-receivers had poorer self-reported health and well-being than assurance-receivers.

At the bottom of Table 2 associations between care-receipt and formal care use are presented. The highest level of medical care receipt was found among nonreceivers with need, with the lowest level in nonreceivers without need. This pattern differed in comparison with formal personal care-receipt and formal practical support-receipt as care-receivers and assurance-receivers were those with the highest proportion in receipt of these formal services.

3.2. Multivariable Analysis. The *nonreceivers without need* category was used as the reference category for the DV in the multinomial logistic regression. IVs entered into the regression consisted of those established through bivariate analysis to be significantly associated with care-receipt. The IV Social, Cultural and Leisure Activity was recoded from a 5-point to a 3-point scale to reduce the number of cells in the model. Following trial runs best model fit statistics were obtained when nonfamily contact and Perceived Community Security were deleted. Due to missing data model $n = 980$ (see Table 3).

In comparison to a constant-only model the model was reliable ($\chi^2(51) = 488.68$, $p < .001$), with good model fit (model $\chi^2(2886) = 2905.15$ $p > .05$, Nagelkerke $R^2 = .43$). Table 3 presents for all variables in the model the Wald test for significance of each coefficient and the odds ratio with 95% confidence intervals for each of the three comparisons between the three care-receipt categories and the reference category.

We consider first the prediction of membership in the *care-receiver* category relative to being in the reference category. Starting with social exclusion variables, a unit increase in Perceived Community Trust and Social, Cultural and Leisure Activity corresponded to 0.87 and 0.98 odds of being a care-receiver, and participants at the lowest and middle levels of Sport and Outdoor Activity had, respectively, 4.79 and 1.93 odds of being a care-receiver compared with participants at the highest level. Regarding risk factors of social exclusion, a unit increase in age corresponded to a 1.06 increase in the likelihood of being a care-receiver; participants in the rural group had 0.38 odds of being a care-receiver compared to the urban group; a unit increase in (poor) self-reported health corresponded to a 2.54 increase in the likelihood of being a care-receiver. Regarding formal care use, participants who had received medical care had 2.81 odds of being a care-receiver compared to those who had not received medical care.

Next we consider prediction of membership in the *assurance-receiver* category relative to the reference category. Regarding social exclusion variables, one-unit increase in family contact and Emotional Loneliness corresponded, respectively, to 1.21 and 1.16 increases in the likelihood of being assurance-receivers, while participants at the lowest and middle levels of Sport and Outdoor Activity had, respectively, 1.85 and 1.71 odds of being assurance-receivers compared with participants at the highest level. Regarding social exclusion risk factors, a unit increase in age corresponded to a 1.05 increase in the likelihood of being an assurance-receiver; male participants had 0.63 odds of being assurance-receivers compared to female participants; participants in the rural group had 0.49 odds of being assurance-receivers compared to the urban group; a unit increase in duration of local residence corresponded to 0.99 odds of being assurance-receivers; a unit increase in (poor) self-rated health corresponded to a 1.30 increase in the likelihood of being assurance-receivers. Finally, participants who had received medical care had 1.51 odds of being assurance-receivers compared to those who had not received medical care.

Lastly, we considered prediction of membership in the *nonreceivers with need* category relative to being in the category nonreceiver without need. Regarding social exclusion dimensions, analyses show that a unit increase in Social Loneliness corresponded to a 1.39 increase in the likelihood of being nonreceivers with need. Regarding risk factors of social exclusion, a unit increase in age corresponded to a 1.07 increase in the likelihood of being nonreceivers with need; participants in the rural group had 0.26 odds of being nonreceivers with need compared to the urban group. Finally, participants who had received medical care had 5.82 odds of being nonreceivers with need compared to those who had not received medical care.

4. Discussion

Our multivariable analysis produced a significant model that predicted older people's membership of care-receipt categories on the basis of social exclusion dimensions and a range of risk factors for social exclusion. The pattern of associations in the model had face validity. Greater age, recent contact with medical care, and poorer health, all being meaningful indicators of frailty and/or need for support in an older person, increased participants' likelihood of being an assurance-receiver and were associated with an even greater likelihood of being a care-receiver, relative to being a nonreceiver with no need. Greater age and poorer health are established risk factors for social exclusion [8]. Another variable significant in the model, Sport and Outdoor Activity, is included in the social exclusion dimension social engagement. The picture that emerges from the model is that older people with higher scores on dimensions of and risk factors for social exclusion were significantly more likely to be in receipt of assurance and care. Membership of the nonreceivers with need category was also predicted by indicators of frailty (greater age, recent contact with medical services) and an indicator of social exclusion (greater Social Loneliness). If one examines the pattern of bivariate associations between the IVs and the care-receipt variable, nonreceivers with need in comparison to older people in the other categories demonstrated the highest levels of Social and Emotional Loneliness and the lowest levels of income comfort, social contact (with family members, friends and

Table 3: Summary of multinomial logistic regression analysis of variables predicting membership of category of care-receipt[a] ($n = 980$).

Category: Variable:	Care-receivers Odds ratio (95% CI)	Assurance-receivers Odds ratio (95% CI)	Nonreceivers with need Odds ratio (95% CI)
Income comfort (low comfort)	0.78 (0.61, 1.01)	0.89 (0.71, 1.11)	1.10 (0.73, 1.64)
Family contact	1.19 (0.99, 1.43)	1.21 (1.03, 1.42)*	0.82 (0.61, 1.10)
Social Loneliness	1.08 (0.94, 1.25)	0.97 (0.85, 1.11)	1.39 (1.12, 1.72)*
Emotional Loneliness	0.99 (0.87, 1.11)	1.16 (1.04, 1.29)*	1.18 (0.99, 1.41)
Perceived Community Trust	0.87 (0.77, 0.99)*	1.04 (0.91, 1.18)	0.86 (0.72, 1.03)
Perceived Community Integration	1.09 (0.99, 1.21)	1.04 (0.95, 1.14)	0.97 (0.85, 1.12)
Social, Cultural and Leisure Engagement	0.98 (0.97, 1.00)*	1.00 (0.99, 1.01)	0.98 (0.96, 1.00)
Sport and Outdoor Engagement (0)	4.79 (2.46, 9.34)*	1.85 (1.06, 3.24)*	1.10 (0.37, 3.25)
Sport and Outdoor Engagement (1)	1.93 (1.05, 3.56)*	1.71 (1.10, 2.67)*	1.06 (0.42, 2.70)
Age	1.06 (1.03, 1.09)*	1.05 (1.03, 1.08)*	1.07 (1.02, 1.12)*
Gender (female)	0.77 (0.51, 1.16)	0.63 (0.43, 0.90)*	0.68 (0.35, 1.29)
Education Level	1.54 (0.86, 2.74)	0.98 (0.63, 1.51)	0.99 (0.42, 2.35)
Area of residence (rural)	0.38 (0.24, 0.59)*	0.49 (0.31, 0.67)*	0.26 (0.12, 0.56)*
Duration of local residence	1.00 (0.99, 1.01)	0.99 (0.98, 0.99)*	1.01 (0.99, 1.02)
Self-reported health (poor)	2.54 (1.88, 3.43)*	1.30 (1.01, 1.67)*	1.10 (0.73, 1.64)
Well-being	0.99 (0.95, 1.03)	0.97 (0.94, 1.01)	1.00 (0.94, 1.06)
Medical care-receipt	2.81 (1.85, 4.28)*	1.51 (1.06, 2.15)*	5.82 (2.68, 12.67)*

[a]Reference category = nonreceivers without need. * $p < .05$.

neighbours), social engagement (Social, Cultural and Leisure Engagement), Perceived Community Integration, Trust, and Security, indicating that these older people experienced the highest levels of social exclusion. If the categories of care-receipt are considered as a continuum with nonreceivers without need as one end of the continuum, then nonreceivers with need would exist at the other end: the odds ratios for greater age and recent contact with medical services are larger for this category than for care-receivers and assurance-receivers.

However, other variables uniquely contributed to membership of different care-receipt categories, suggesting that nonreceivers with need, care-receivers, and assurance-receivers might differ as social positions or roles not just in terms of degree. A continuum model of care-receipt might therefore be insufficient. Lower Perceived Community Trust and Social, Cultural and Leisure Activity increased the likelihood that a participant was a care-receiver; being female, greater family contact, and greater Emotional Loneliness increased the likelihood that a participant was an assurance-receiver; and greater Social Loneliness increased the likelihood that a participant was a nonreceiver with need. When seeking to conceptualise care-receipt in older people, therefore, one model would be that the experience of care-receipt is a progression through increasing levels of support and care until in many cases the informal care network breaks down. A different model would be that whether one is a care-receiver or an assurance-receiver or a nonreceiver with need is not about the current occupation of one role within a progression of care-receipt, but rather an outcome of that role being more likely when other factors are true, for example, as where being female and having recent contact with one's family increase the odds that one is an assurance-receiver. Our findings suggest that both models coexist in later life.

4.1. Social Exclusion and Care-Receipt. An Irish study of care-receipt among older people [37] reported that 49% of older people received care over a 12-month period. The study used a broad definition of care-receipt, including people receiving care once weekly or less. This corresponds in our study to those participants in the care-receipt and assurance-receipt categories combined, which comprised 46% of our sample, a similar figure. The present study's focus on the concept of assurance-receipt is relatively unique: most studies explore the issue of caregiving among burdened carers, that is, those providing many hours of care each week, with few focusing on "light" carers, and by extension older people in receipt of only a few hours of care (cf. [38]).

A question posed in the introduction to this paper was whether being a care-receiver might be associated with lower levels of social exclusion, as care-receipt is almost by definition linked to contact with friends and family, an indicator of social *inclusion*. Our findings offered little evidence to support this conjecture. Being a care-receiver was not significantly associated in the multivariable model with greater contact with friends or greater contact with family. Furthermore care-receipt was predicted by lower Perceived Community Trust, suggesting that care-receipt might be linked to a poorer relationship with one's neighbourhood, another indicator of social exclusion. While one predictor of being an assurance-receiver was greater contact with one's family, this indicator of inclusion has a counterbalance in the association between being an assurance-receiver and greater Emotional Loneliness. Similar results have been found in research on formal care-receipt. Barrett et al. [11] argue that home-based formal care contributes to a disconnectedness of the care-receiver from self, family, home, and the broader community, thereby contributing to social exclusion (see also [20]).

In the multivariable analysis one of the key predictors of membership in the different care-receipt categories was place of residence with care-receipt being more common in urban areas. There is a lack of research on rural/urban patterns of informal care-receipt, and the findings from the existing research are contradictory. For example, in line with our findings, it has been suggested that American urban older residents are more likely to have informal support from kin and to have children living nearby, as there is a general pattern of outmigration of children from rural areas and an in-migration of older people to rural areas [39]. On the other hand, Canadian research indicates that informal care-receipt is more common among rural residents [40]. With regard to our findings, since several demographic, health, and social variables were controlled for in our analysis, we suggest it is likely a complex interaction of personal, demographic, and social factors related to residence in urban environments that produced high levels of care-receipt and an unmet need for assurance, relative to residence in rural areas. More research is needed in order to obtain a deeper understanding of the mechanisms behind rural/urban care-receipt patterns.

4.2. Policy and Practice Implications. One Spanish study on older people in need of help with activities of daily living identified a group of older people (5.9% among women, 7.9% among men) who did not receive help [26], and a Canadian study [25] found that approximately 2% of older people outside institutions experienced unmet care needs. In our study such a group was represented by the nonreceivers with need, which comprised 5.5% of our sample. This group was found to score highly on several dimensions of and risk factors for social exclusion (cf. [9]). Of interest is the fact that we found that older people with higher levels of care-receipt received more formal personal care and formal practical support. The exception to the pattern was the nonreceivers with need, where despite a lack of informal care and assurance there were also low levels of formal personal care and formal practical support. However, this group had the highest level of recent contact with medical services, a relationship also found in the Spanish study mentioned above [26]. Similarly, recent research has found that lonely older people have a higher use of health care services than nonlonely people [41] and that loneliness and social isolation are a common nonmedical problem presented by noncritically ill older people in emergency departments ([42], for a review, see [43]). One interpretation of this finding is that, in the absence of informal care and in the presence of need, older people will turn to medical services (perhaps primary care practitioners) in order to address their unmet need. Whatever the contributory factors, an opportunity exists during contact with medical care providers whereby identification and assessment could offer a route into referral for appropriate formal personal care and/or formal practical support. This recommendation is in line with previous calls for integrated care and joined-up services for older people [44], and programmes have been targeted at referral of medical care patients to social services (e.g., [45]). Potential savings in medical care services that follow such referrals might compensate for increased costs to the social care budget. There is therefore a need for more emphasis on the issue of unmet need in older people within the education of medical and nursing practitioners and their own significant role in appropriate onward referral.

4.3. Conclusions. This study provides valuable insights into the personal, interpersonal, and social factors related to informal care-receipt in older people, a topic that has received relatively little attention. The experience of care-receipt can last for a substantial amount of an older person's life and its nature and content impact significantly on quality of life. The present study indicates that the need for and receipt of informal care in an older person is connected to dimensions of, as well as risk factors for, social exclusion. In our model, as older people's scores on dimensions of and risk factors for social exclusion increased so did the odds of them being care-receivers, or being nonreceivers with need. Very little evidence emerged that the receipt of care or assurance was associated with social inclusion. Our findings suggest that access to informal care is important to consider when studying social exclusion processes, in that the receipt of informal care may be a marker of social exclusion, that is, that older people relying on informal care may not be integrated into society and may have unmet social needs.

Disclosure

This research was undertaken in collaboration between Age UK, Sheffield Hallam University (SHU), Dalarna Research Institute, and Dalarna University. Phil Wormald at Age UK and Tamsin-Bowers Brown, Maria Burton, Rachel Ibbotson, Dot Biggin, Martin Hyde, and interviewers at SHU contributed to the research.

Competing Interests

The authors declare that there is no conflict of interests regarding the publication of this article.

References

[1] European Commission, Directorate general for employment and social affairs and equal opportunities, *Joint Report on Social Protection and Social Inclusion*, 2010.

[2] M. O'Brien and S. Penna, "Social exclusion in Europe: some conceptual issues," *International Journal of Social Welfare*, vol. 17, no. 1, pp. 84–92, 2008.

[3] European Commission, *Europe 2020: A Strategy for European Union Growth*, 2013.

[4] Council of European Union, *Joint Report by the Commission and the Council on Social Inclusion*, 2004.

[5] E. Cambois and F. Jusot, "Contribution of lifelong adverse experiences to social health inequalities: findings from a population survey in France," *European Journal of Public Health*, vol. 21, no. 5, pp. 667–673, 2011.

[6] T. Scharf, C. Phillipson, and A. E. Smith, "Social exclusion of older people in deprived urban communities of England," *European Journal of Ageing*, vol. 2, no. 2, pp. 76–87, 2005.

[7] Office of the Deputy Prime Minister, *A Sure Start to Later Life: Ending Inequalities for Older People. A Social Exclusion Unit Final Report*, Office of the Deputy Prime Minister, Department of Health, and Department of Work and Pensions, London, UK, 2006.

[8] M. Barnes, A. Blom, K. Cox, and C. Lessof, *The social exclusion of older people: evidence from the first wave of the English Longitudinal Study of Ageing (ELSA)*, Final Report, Office of the Deputy Prime Minister, Social Exclusion Unit, London, UK, 2006.

[9] T. Scharf, C. Phillipson, and A. E. Smith, *Multiple Exclusion and Quality of Life amongst Excluded Older People in Disadvantaged Neighbourhoods*, Social Exclusion Unit, London, UK, 2005.

[10] A. Kalwij, G. Pasini, and M. Q. Wu, "Home care for the elderly: the role of relatives, friends and neighbors," *Review of Economics of the Household*, vol. 12, no. 2, pp. 379–404, 2014.

[11] P. Barrett, B. Hale, and R. Gauld, "Social inclusion through ageing-in-place with care?" *Ageing and Society*, vol. 32, no. 3, pp. 361–378, 2012.

[12] R. Levitas, C. Pantazis, E. Fahmy, D. Gordon, E. Lloyd, and D. Patsios, *The Multi-Dimensional Analysis of Social Exclusion*, Social Exclusion Task Force, London, UK, 2007.

[13] T. Burchardt, J. Le Grand, and D. Piachaud, "Degrees of exclusion: developing a dynamic, multidimensional measure," in *Understanding Social Exclusion*, J. Hills, J. Le Grand, and D. Piachaud, Eds., pp. 30–43, Oxford University Press, Oxford, UK, 2002.

[14] T. Buffel, C. Phillipson, and T. Scharf, "Experiences of neighbourhood exclusion and inclusion among older people living in deprived inner-city areas in Belgium and England," *Ageing and Society*, vol. 33, no. 1, pp. 89–109, 2013.

[15] E. Becker and R. Boreham, *Understanding the Risks of Social Exclusion Across the Life Course: Older Age*, Cabinet Office and National Centre for Social Research, London, UK, 2009.

[16] J. Heap, C. Lennartsson, and M. Thorslund, "Coexisting disadvantages across the adult age span: a comparison of older and younger age groups in the Swedish welfare state," *International Journal of Social Welfare*, vol. 22, no. 2, pp. 130–140, 2013.

[17] B. M. Janssen, T. Van Regenmortel, and T. A. Abma, "Identifying sources of strength: resilience from the perspective of older people receiving long-term community care," *European Journal of Ageing*, vol. 8, no. 3, pp. 145–156, 2011.

[18] T. Blackman, "Social exclusion and social care," in *Social Care and Social Exclusion: A Comparative Study of Older People's Care in Europe*, T. Blackman, S. Brodhurst, and J. Convery, Eds., pp. 152–180, Palgrave Macmillan, London, UK, 2001.

[19] A. Coote, "The uneven dividend: health and well-being in later life," in *Unequal Ageing. The Untold Story of Exclusion in Old Age*, P. Cann and M. Dean, Eds., pp. 53–75, The Policy Press, Bristol, UK, 2009.

[20] A. M. Grenier and N. Guberman, "Creating and sustaining disadvantage: the relevance of a social exclusion framework," *Health and Social Care in the Community*, vol. 17, no. 2, pp. 116–124, 2009.

[21] M. Jegermalm and E. J. Grassman, "Helpful citizens and caring families: patterns of informal help and caregiving in Sweden in a 17-year perspective," *International Journal of Social Welfare*, vol. 21, no. 4, pp. 422–432, 2012.

[22] P. Ulmanen and M. Szebehely, "From the state to the family or to the market? Consequences of reduced residential eldercare in Sweden," *International Journal of Social Welfare*, vol. 24, no. 1, pp. 81–92, 2015.

[23] M. G. Parker, P. Schön, M. Lagergren, and M. Thorslund, "Functional ability in the elderly Swedish population from 1980 to 2005," *European Journal of Ageing*, vol. 5, no. 4, pp. 299–309, 2008.

[24] B. Bień, K. J. McKee, H. Döhner et al., "Disabled older people's use of health and social care services and their unmet care needs in six European countries," *European Journal of Public Health*, vol. 23, no. 6, pp. 1032–1038, 2013.

[25] K. Cranswick and D. Thomas, *Elder Care and the Complexities of Social Networks*, Statistics Canada, 2005.

[26] J. Rogero-Garcia, M.-E. Prieto-Flores, and M. W. Rosenberg, "Health services use by older people with disabilities in Spain: do formal and informal care matter?" *Ageing and Society*, vol. 28, no. 7, pp. 959–978, 2008.

[27] D. G. Blazer, N. Sachs-Ericsson, and C. F. Hybels, "Perception of unmet basic needs as a predictor of mortality among community-dwelling older adults," *American Journal of Public Health*, vol. 95, no. 2, pp. 299–304, 2005.

[28] L. Dahlberg and K. J. McKee, "Correlates of social and emotional loneliness in older people: evidence from an English community study," *Aging and Mental Health*, vol. 18, no. 4, pp. 504–514, 2014.

[29] K. J. McKee et al., "The EUROFAMCARE Common Assessment Tool (CAT): item and scale development and description," in *Family Carers of Older People in Europe: A Six-Country Comparative Study*, G. Lamura, H. Döhner, and C. Kofahl, Eds., pp. 49–73, Lit Verlag, Berlin, Germany, 2008.

[30] M. Jegermalm, "Informal care in Sweden: a typology of care and caregivers," *International Journal of Social Welfare*, vol. 15, no. 4, pp. 332–343, 2006.

[31] European Social Survey, *Source Questionnaire (Round 2, 2004/05). Final Version Amendment 03*, 2004.

[32] Stockholm University, *SWEOLD. Swedish Panel Study of Living Conditions of the Oldest Old. Code Book 1992*, Department of Social Work, Stockholm University, Stockholm, Sweden, 1998.

[33] The Institute for Fiscal Studies, *English Longitudinal Study on Ageing, Health and lifestyles of people aged 50 and over*.

[34] J. de Jong-Gierveld and F. Kamphuls, "The development of a rasch-type loneliness scale," *Applied Psychological Measurement*, vol. 9, no. 3, pp. 289–299, 1985.

[35] T. Scharf, C. Phillipson, and A. E. Smith, "Poverty and social exclusion—growing older in deprived urban neighbourhoods," in *Growing Older. Quality of Life in Old Age*, A. Walker and C. H. Hennessy, Eds., pp. 81–106, Open University Press, Maidenhead, UK, 2004.

[36] World Health Organization, WHO (Five) Well-being Index (1998 version), 1998, https://www.psykiatri-regionh.dk/who-5/Documents/WHO5_English.pdf.

[37] H. M. McGee, G. Molloy, A. O'Hanlon, R. Layte, and A. Hickey, "Older people—recipients but also providers of informal care: an analysis among community samples in the Republic of Ireland and Northern Ireland," *Health and Social Care in the Community*, vol. 16, no. 5, pp. 548–553, 2008.

[38] G. Lamura, H. Döhner, and C. Kofahl, Eds., *Family Carers of Older People in Europe: A Six-Country Comparative Study*, Lit Verlag, Berlin, Germany, 2008.

[39] N. Glasgow, "Rural/urban patterns of aging and caregiving in the United States," *Journal of Family Issues*, vol. 21, no. 5, pp. 611–631, 2000.

[40] P. Kitchen, A. Williams, R. W. Pong, and D. Wilson, "Socio-spatial patterns of home care use in Ontario, Canada: A Case Study," *Health and Place*, vol. 17, no. 1, pp. 195–206, 2011.

[41] E. Taube, J. Kristensson, M. Sandberg, P. Midlöv, and U. Jakobsson, "Loneliness and health care consumption among older people," *Scandinavian Journal of Caring Sciences*, vol. 29, no. 3, pp. 435–443, 2015.

[42] T. B. Stevens, N. L. Richmond, G. F. Pereira, C. L. Shenvi, and T. F. Platts-Mills, "Prevalence of nonmedical problems among older adults presenting to the emergency department," *Academic Emergency Medicine*, vol. 21, no. 6, pp. 651–658, 2014.

[43] N. Samaras, T. Chevalley, D. Samaras, and G. Gold, "Older patients in the emergency department: a review," *Annals of Emergency Medicine*, vol. 56, no. 3, pp. 261–269, 2010.

[44] C. Glendinning, A. Coleman, and K. Rummery, "Partnerships, performance and primary care: developing integrated services for older people in England," *Ageing and Society*, vol. 22, no. 2, pp. 185–208, 2002.

[45] R. Kue, E. Ramstrom, S. Weisberg, and M. Restuccia, "Evaluation of an emergency medical servicesbased social services referral program for elderly patients," *Prehospital Emergency Care*, vol. 13, no. 3, pp. 273–279, 2009.

19

Modeling Age-Friendly Environment, Active Aging, and Social Connectedness in an Emerging Asian Economy

Ming-Ming Lai,[1] Shi-Ying Lein,[1] Siok-Hwa Lau,[2] and Ming-Ling Lai[3]

[1]*Faculty of Management, Multimedia University, Persiaran Multimedia, 63100 Cyberjaya, Selangor, Malaysia*
[2]*Faculty of Business, Multimedia University, Jalan Ayer Keroh Lama, 75450 Bukit Beruang, Melaka, Malaysia*
[3]*Faculty of Accountancy, Universiti Teknologi MARA, Level 14, Menara SAAS, 40450 Shah Alam, Selangor, Malaysia*

Correspondence should be addressed to Ming-Ming Lai; mmlai@mmu.edu.my

Academic Editor: Arshad Jahangir

This paper empirically tested eight key features of WHO guidelines to age-friendly community by surveying 211 informal caregivers and 402 self-care adults (aged 45 to 85 and above) in Malaysia. We examined the associations of these eight features with active aging and social connectedness through exploratory and confirmatory factor analyses. A structural model with satisfactory goodness-of-fit indices (CMIN/df = 1.11, RMSEA = 0.02, NFI = 0.97, TLI = 1.00, CFI = 1.00, and GFI = 0.96) indicates that transportation and housing, community support and health services, and outdoor spaces and buildings are statistically significant in creating an age-friendly environment. We found a statistically significant positive relationship between an age-friendly environment and active aging. This relationship is mediated by social connectedness. The results indicate that built environments such as accessible public transportations and housing, affordable and accessible healthcare services, and elderly friendly outdoor spaces and buildings have to be put into place before social environment in building an age-friendly environment. Otherwise, the structural barriers would hinder social interactions for the aged. The removal of the environmental barriers and improved public transportation services provide short-term solutions to meet the varied and growing needs of the older population.

1. Introduction

Malaysia is the best place to retire in Asia and ranked third in the world according to the International Living Global Retirement Index 2014 [1]. Malaysia will be one of the aging nations by year 2030 with 15% of its population at the age of 60 and above [2]. Aging populations bring many implications that will increase the demand for long-term care rather than acute care. The elderly may have a range of disabilities, from performing daily activities to home management activities. Hence, it is imperative for Malaysia to have social policy reforms that cover areas from healthcare to building age-friendly communities for her aging society.

Effective policies that promote autonomy and enhance the quality of life among the elderly should be formed at the soonest [3]. An effective policy reformation should take into account age-friendly concepts introduced by the World Health Organization [4]. As stated by Menec et al. [5], despite WHO's [4] concept being appealing, "the research that has examined age-friendliness in diverse contexts is only starting to emerge" [5, page 15]. Prompted by these concerns, this paper is motivated to examine the associations between age-friendly environment, active aging, and social connectedness in addition to identifying the factors of aged-friendly features of the WHO [4] in Malaysia. A model with goodness-of-fit that uses structural equation modeling which integrated age-friendly features with active aging and social connectedness was built. Currently, this is a new attempt and is among the very few age-friendly environment studies. Such integration has not been investigated adequately especially in relation to the age-friendly environment, active aging, and social connectedness from the perception of middle-age adults and the above population. In particular, the significance of the eight age-friendly features of WHO [4] on active aging and social connectedness in a developing nation has yet to be fully understood in terms of the validity of a model with goodness-of-fit indices. Structural equation modeling has a higher accuracy in addressing the measurement error of variances in which the validity of the model is proven statistically through the goodness-of-fit indices [6]. This study also bridges the gaps in the current literature by examining age-friendliness with its outcomes such as social connectedness and active aging as suggested by Menec et al. [5].

The proposed structural model has contributed additional empirical evidence to the current literature for Lawton's person-environment fit [7] and Bronfenbrenner's ecological theory [8]. The findings of this study show in developing nations age-friendly domains relating to built environment where transportation and outdoor spaces and buildings need to be put in-place first before working on domains related to social interactions. It is because there are many infrastructural barriers in terms of transportation, housing, outdoor spaces, and buildings as perceived by the middle-age and older population. Accessibility and availability of modern public transportation are viewed as essential elements for social connectedness as well as participation in health and community services. An age-friendly environment "adapts its structures and services to be accessible to, and inclusive of older people with varying needs and capacities" [9, page 2].

2. Literature Review

Major studies related to aged-friendly environments, active aging, and social connectedness were reviewed. Feldman and Oberlink [10] are two of the pioneers in conceptualizing an age-friendly environment. By having 14 focus groups among individuals aged 35 and above and community leaders from various areas of the United States, they identified four domains of an age-friendly environment. The domains are identifying necessities, encouraging social and civic engagement, improving independence among the frail and disabled elderly, and optimizing physical and mental functioning and well-being.

The qualitative exploration of an age-friendly environment continued with Alley et al. [11] using the Delphi method to solicit opinions from 15 professionals in the areas of gerontology, township planning, and development. The results reveal that accessible and inexpensive transportation, housing, healthcare, safety, and prospective social involvement are the criteria for an age-friendly environment.

Subsequently, the concept of age-friendliness received global attention when WHO introduced the age-friendly cities guide [4], in which an age-friendly city "encourages active aging by optimizing opportunities for health, participation, and security in order to enhance quality of life" [4, page 1]. It is the result of an international-based study that examined the criteria of an age-friendly city by conducting focus group surveys in 33 cities involving 1,485 elderly, 250 elderly caregivers, and 515 service providers in the year 2005. The eight age-friendly environment features are outdoor spaces and buildings, transportation, housing, social participation, respect and social inclusion, civic participation and employment, communication and information, and, finally, community support and health services.

From the ecological perspective, it is important to acknowledge and integrate the social and physical environment. It is further asserted when Lui et al. [12] conducted a meta-analysis on 32 publications related to age-friendly environment and found the essentiality of the integration between physical and social environment, along with cooperation between policy makers and the elderly in building an age-friendly environment.

Emlet and Moceri [9] examined the importance of social connectedness in an age-friendly environment through focus group interviews with 23 respondents who were above 40 years of age in a community forum in the United States. The three themes of analysis were social reciprocity, meaningful interactions, and structural needs and barriers. The results reinforced the importance of social connectedness in an elder-friendly community.

Kadoya [13] explored the social interaction between the elderly and the community in Akita city, where there are a high number of elderly people in Japan. He found that living arrangement and mobility significantly affect social interactions. Those who have the ability to drive participated more in community services. He concluded that a community should not neglect social inclusion as a domain for an age-friendly environment. Menec et al. [5] conclude that the social environment is easier to address when compared to the physical environment especially in deserted areas.

The word "active aging" was first introduced by the WHO. It is defined as the "process of optimizing for health, participation and security in order to enhance quality of life as people age" [14, page 12]. The WHO proposed six determinants for active aging, namely, health and social services, behavioral determinant, personal determinant, physical environment, social determinant, and economic determinant. Active aging is perceived as the "desire and ability of older adults to integrate physical activity into daily routines" and "engagement in economic and socially productive activities" [15, page 736]. In essence, an age-friendly neighborhood design is found to be important in supporting active aging.

Bowling [16] explored active aging by surveying 337 elderly British men and women using questionnaires. The survey results revealed that the majority of the elderly described active aging as having good physical and mental health while maintaining substantial relationship with the society.

The measurement model of active aging was proposed by Paúl et al. [17]. They introduced a model that helps the elderly adjust to their disability, promote social participation, and be involved actively in a healthy lifestyle, which would improve their quality of life. An et al. [18] conducted a survey among elderly Koreans. They found that public exercise areas have a significant relationship with the elderly to be physically active which helps promote healthy and active aging.

On the other hand, social connectedness affects the elderly's health and well-being. Fratiglioni et al. [19] discovered that social engagements and participation that promote healthy and active aging are indicative of a good life among the elderly. In contrast, withdrawing from social activities may result in mental sickness. Social connectivity is viewed as

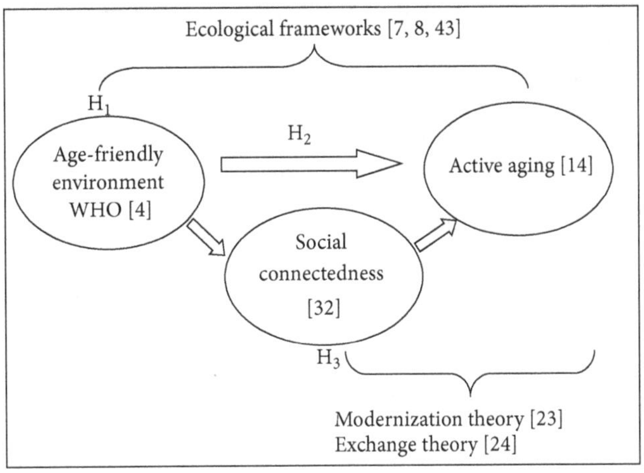

FIGURE 1: The integrated model of age-friendly environments, active aging, and social connectedness.

a major involvement in social activities and communications that may affect the well-being of the older population [20].

Cramm et al. [21] investigated the relationship between social capital, social cohesion, and well-being among 945 elderly in Rotterdam. Their findings indicated that receiving social support and having interdependent neighborhoods were important to the elderly and would enhance their well-being.

Through in-depth personal interviews, Franke et al. [22] found that self-help strategies, social connectedness, and physical environment do promote physical activities among active older adults. The findings documented evidence from an individual perspective that active older adults used their self-help strategies to promote physical activities and reciprocally physical activities benefit them in determining their self-worth. New policies in addressing social connectedness and accessibilities towards social and physical community services are highly required in supporting the mobility and independence among the aging population.

The literature review provides insights into an integrated model of an age-friendly environment, active aging, and social connectedness as shown in the theoretical framework (see Figure 1). It is believed that age-friendly environments and active aging have a substantive relationship and the relationship is mediated by social connectedness. Three hypotheses have been developed to examine the factors of age-friendly environments as well as the associations between age-friendly environments, active aging, and social connectedness. The proposed hypotheses are as follows:

H_1: the factors (outdoor spaces and buildings, transportation, housing, social participation, respect, civic participation and employment, community support and health services, and communication and information) are positively related to age-friendly environments.

H_2: an age-friendly environment is positively associated with active aging.

H_3: social connectedness mediates the association between age-friendly environment and active aging.

First, the integrated model of age-friendly environments and active aging model serves as an attempt not only to improve the status of the elderly based on modernization [23] and the exchange of resources among the old-age population [24], but also to reduce environment pressure based on the environment docility hypothesis [7]. Social connectedness is found to be an important factor to be considered in building an age-friendly environment [9, 13] as well as promoting the well-being of the elderly [20, 21]. Motivated by these, social connectedness is perceived to mediate the direct relationship between age-friendly environment and active aging.

An age-friendly environment reflects the mesosystem of Bronfenbrenner's [8] ecological theory that addresses the interactivity of an individual with his or her immediate environment. This environment enables the elderly to be mobile, preserve their health, interact, and participate in their living community. The exosystem expands from the mesosystem and is reflected by the positive relationship between age-friendly environments and active aging. When the environment is friendly to the elderly, they are able to age actively and healthily. If the elderly are active and healthy in an age-friendly environment, their connectedness and participation in social activities would increase. Active aging receives support from social connectedness as indicated by the macrosystem of Bronfenbrenner's [8] ecological theory.

3. Data and Method

At the onset, a questionnaire was designed based on the criteria of urbanization level, old-age dependency ratio, and high number of the elderly people in Malaysia. The sample of this study is gathered from the states of Penang, Perak, Selangor, Wilayah Persekutuan Kuala Lumpur, Negeri Sembilan, Melaka, and Johor. The populations of interest are self-care adults and informal caregivers who do not have apparent cognitive impairment, aged 45 and above (or those in midlife or after midlife). Self-care adults are "people looking after themselves" [14, page 37]. They live in communities and not in institutions. Informal caregivers are individuals who provide care to the elderly.

Backman and Hentinen [25] defined self-care adults as those who have the "desire to continue living as an active agent" [25, page 567]. The targeted respondents are midlife and older adults. Jaques [26] argues that these adults have come to realize their own mortality and feel the need to reassess the changes they want to make while feeling that they still have the time. Individuals aged 45 to 64 are known as prepensioners [27]. The opinions and views from those who are not yet defined as older adults are helpful as they are able to tell of future needs that are beneficial for policy planning in an age-prepared community [9, 28]. Informed and written consent were sought before conducting the survey.

The questionnaire is in English language and translated into Malay and Chinese with the help of language experts. In order to ensure accuracy, an English language expert and researchers who are familiar with both these languages verified the Malay and Chinese versions of the questionnaires. Before the actual data collection, a pilot study was conducted among 30 adults aged 45 and above in December 2013. All constructs showed high reliability with Cronbach's alpha coefficient above 0.7.

All the items, except for demographic variables, were measured based on the five-point scale. Demographic variables encompass items such as gender, nationality, age, educational background, marital status, income level, employment status, and living arrangement. Since a common instrument to assess an age-friendly environment has yet to be established, it was self-developed by adapting the findings from an activity friendly community [29], the checklist of global age-friendly cities [30], and the Internet usage scale [31].

Age-friendly environment items evaluate the perception of the respondents at the level of importance of WHO's [4] age-friendly features in the community. They are measured by the 5-point scale ranging from 1 (very unimportant) to 5 (very important). Based on past literature, a commonly used active aging scale is yet to be found. Therefore, this study has developed its own active aging scale to measure the level of active aging that reflects quality of life and well-being. On the other hand, social connectedness is measured by adapting six items of the social connectedness of Lee and Robbins [32]. The social connectedness construct measures self-perceived emotional detachment or connectedness among individuals in a society. Higher scores indicate greater social connectedness, free from social isolation. Since the items are negatively worded, they are coded in reverse. Both the active aging and social connectedness scales were measured on the 5-point agreement Likert scale ranging from 1 (strongly disagree) to 5 (strongly agree).

In the earlier stage, both Cronbach's alpha reliability and exploratory factor analyses (EFA) were performed. Since the items in the constructs were yet to be established or well known, EFA was conducted to explore and validate the measurement items before moving onto the structural equation modeling (SEM) procedures. It is advisable to perform both the exploratory and confirmatory factor analyses by using new sample sets [33, 34]. Therefore, EFA was performed by employing the data from 211 informal caregivers and subsequently with confirmatory factor analysis (CFA) on 402 self-care adults. EFA was conducted on 37 items of the factors of age-friendly environment through the principal axis factoring (PAF) and promax rotation method. Items of the constructs used in SEM are attached in Appendix.

The hypothesized model is estimated based on a two-step structural equation modeling (SEM) approach, which starts with the specification of the measurement model. The values of skewness and kurtosis for each of the items are within the threshold of absolute two and seven, respectively, indicating that that data is normally distributed [35]. In addition, the maximum likelihood method is used to estimate the structural equation modeling. After confirming the fit of the measurement model, this study proceeded to the structural model. A model has a good fit when the goodness-of-fit indices are fulfilled. The goodness-of-fit indices are shown by an insignificant p value, observed normed chi-square value (CMIN/df) lower than 3, goodness-of-fit index (GFI), adjusted goodness-of-fit index (AGFI), comparative fit index (CFI), Tucker-Lewis Index (TLI), and normed fit index (NFI) to be more than 0.9, root mean squared error (RMSEA) and standardized root mean square residual (SRMR) less than 0.08, and expected cross validation index (ECVI) to be near zero [6, 36].

To examine the validity of the model, convergent validity and discriminant validity were performed. The assessment of convergent validity involves several indicators which are standardized factor loading and average variance extracted (AVE) to be at least 0.50 and composite reliability (CR) to be at least 0.70 [37]. AVE refers to the average of variance extracted of the items in each construct [38]. The formulas to calculate AVE and CR are shown below [37]:

$$\text{Average variance extracted} = \frac{\sum \text{standardized factor loadings}^2}{\text{Number of items}};$$
$$\text{Composite reliability} = \frac{\left(\sum \text{standardized factor loadings}\right)^2}{\left(\sum \text{standardized factor loadings}\right)^2 + \left(\sum 1 - \text{standardized factor loadings}^2\right)}. \tag{1}$$

Discriminant validity was measured by using the method formulated by Fornell and Larcker [38] whereby discriminant validity is achieved when AVE is larger than the value of the square of correlation between constructs [38]. The assessment of discriminant validity ensures that variables are unique and free from multicollinearity [37]. Variables with high correlation may be redundant and, hence, reduce validity. When the constructs in the measurement model have met all the fitness values, this study proceeded to perform the structural model.

The purpose of specifying a structural model is to conduct hypothesis testing. In testing the structural model, exogenous variables remained covariates from the measurement model but the double headed arrow of endogenous variables needed to be removed and replaced with a single headed arrow as well as adding a unique variable [37].

This study further examined social connectedness as a mediator in the hypothesized model. The steps for mediation were described as below [37]. First, independent and dependent variables need to have statistical significant relationships. Second, both the independent and dependent variables need to have statistical significant relationships with the mediating variable. When the mediating variable enters the model and causes the relationship between independent and dependent variables to become statistically insignificant, this result indicates a full mediating effect. On the other hand, when mediator variable enters the model, the relationship between independent and dependent variables remains statistically significant but with a reduced magnitude, this indicates a partial mediating effect. There is no mediating effect when the relationship between independent and dependent variables remains statistically significant and with similar coefficient when the mediating variable enters the model. In examining the mediation effect, resampling statistical procedure of bootstrapping was conducted by allowing data to perform 2,000 bootstrap samples and ran the bias-corrected confidence intervals at 95% [39, 40]. Sobel test was conducted to verify the mediation effect of social connectedness [41] and was calculated through a web-calculator developed by Preacher and Leonardelli [42].

4. Results

The usable sample size from the two surveys is 613 with 402 self-care adults and 211 informal caregivers. The results of the demographic characteristics of self-care adults and informal caregivers are reported in Table 1. The results show that 71.3% are female respondents, and the sample distributions are quite even across the seven states. The self-care adults of ages greater than 65 make up 47.3%. Meanwhile 49 informal caregivers are aged less than 35 (23.3%). About 25.9% of the respondents have primary school as their highest education level.

All the variables are reliable indicated by Cronbach's alpha greater than 0.7. Two items, each from housing and active aging variables, were removed to improve Cronbach's alpha value. The results of the reliability analysis are reported in Table 2.

The results of the exploratory factor analysis (EFA) show correlation of coefficients greater than 0.30, Kaiser-Meyer-Olkin (KMO) value at 0.92 (<0.60), a significant Bartlett test of sphericity ($p = 0.00$), and factor loadings greater than 0.40. Based on Kaiser's criterion, six factors were retained, but scree plot showed five factors to be retained. In combining Kaiser's criterion and scree plot test, only five factors were retained: communication and information, transportation and housing, outdoor spaces and buildings, community support and health services, and social participation and these five factors contributed to approximately 66% of the variances.

TABLE 1: Demographic characteristics of self-care adults and informal caregivers.

Demographic characteristics	Frequency, n (%) $n = 402^a$	$n = 211^b$	$n = 613^c$
Location (states)			
Pulau Pinang	57 (14.2)	28 (13.3)	85 (13.8)
Perak	50 (12.4)	30 (14.2)	80 (13.1)
Selangor	45 (11.2)	45 (21.3)	90 (14.6)
Wilayah Persekutuan Kuala Lumpur	77 (19.2)	17 (8.1)	94 (15.3)
Negeri Sembilan	58 (14.4)	30 (14.2)	88 (14.4)
Melaka	57 (14.2)	31 (14.7)	88 (14.4)
Johor	58 (14.4)	30 (14.2)	88 (14.4)
Gender			
Male	128 (31.8)	48 (22.7)	176 (28.7)
Female	274 (68.2)	163 (77.3)	437 (71.3)
Nationality			
Malaysian	402 (100)	211 (100)	613 (100)
Age			
≤35	—	49 (23.2)	49 (8.0)
35.1–45	—	37 (17.5)	37 (6.0)
45.1–55	66 (16.4)	44 (20.9)	110 (17.9)
55.1–65	146 (36.3)	45 (21.3)	191 (31.2)
≥65.1	190 (47.3)	36 (17.1)	226 (36.9)
Race			
Malay	141 (35.1)	50 (23.7)	191 (31.1)
Chinese	240 (59.7)	138 (65.4)	378 (61.7)
Indian	20 (5.0)	21 (10.0)	41 (6.7)
Portuguese	1 (0.2)	—	1 (0.2)
Orang Asli	—	2 (0.9)	2 (0.3)
Marital status			
Single	38 (9.5)	56 (26.5)	94 (15.3)
Married	260 (64.7)	142 (67.3)	402 (65.6)
Widowed	96 (23.9)	9 (4.3)	105 (17.1)
Divorced	8 (2.0)	4 (1.9)	12 (2.0)
Highest education level attained			
No formal education	47 (11.7)	13 (6.2)	60 (9.8)
Primary school	131 (32.6)	28 (13.3)	159 (25.9)
Secondary school	82 (20.4)	23 (10.9)	105 (17.1)
SPM[d]	65 (16.2)	37 (17.5)	102 (16.6)
STPM[e]/diploma	38 (9.5)	39 (18.5)	77 (12.6)
Degree	32 (8.0)	55 (26.1)	87 (14.2)
Postgraduate	7 (1.7)	16 (7.6)	23 (3.8)
Total	*402 (100)*	*211 (100)*	*613 (100)*

Notes: [a]self-care adult respondents; [b]informal caregiver respondents; [c]self-care adult and informal caregiver respondents; [d]Sijil Pelajaran Malaysia or also known as Malaysian Certificate of Education examination is equivalent to O-Level qualification; [e]Sijil Tinggi Pelajaran Malaysia or also known as Malaysian Higher School Certificate examination which is equivalent to A-Level qualification.

Table 2: Reliability test results of self-care adults and informal caregivers.

Variables	Cronbach's alpha $n = 402^{a}$	$n = 211^{b}$	$n = 613^{c}$
Independent variables			
(1) Outdoor spaces and buildings	0.92	0.90	0.91
(2) Transportation	0.87	0.83	0.86
(3) Housing	0.91	0.89	0.90
(4) Social participation	0.84	0.89	0.86
(5) Respect and social inclusion	0.89	0.88	0.88
(6) Civic participation and employment	0.87	0.90	0.88
(7) Community support and health services	0.95	0.92	0.94
(8) Communication and information	0.98	0.96	0.97
Dependent variables			
(1) Age-friendly environment	0.95	0.95	0.95
(2) Active aging	0.86	0.85	0.85
(3) Social connectedness	0.95	0.94	0.95

Notes: [a]self-care adult respondents; [b]informal caregiver respondents; [c]self-care adult and informal caregiver respondents.

EFA showed only five factors, namely, (i) communication and information, (ii) outdoor spaces and buildings, (iii) housing and transportation, (iv) community support and health services, and (v) social participation, are significant in the Malaysian context. The results of EFA are presented in Table 3. These five factors were confirmed through CFA with the 402 self-care adults.

The initial measurement model had an unsatisfactory fit; therefore, a model modification was performed. In respecifying the measurement model, factor loadings, error terms, and modification indices were obtained to determine which items in the model should be dropped or added. This is to identify the best items of a construct before proceeding to specifying the structural model [36]. Modification indices of about four or larger indicate that model fit can be improved statistically by setting the estimated path to be free. They also indicate the possibility of cross-loadings among the problematic items [37].

During the model modification process, items with high modification indices were dropped after theoretical justification was employed. The two factors, namely, communication and information and social participation, were dropped. This is because, during the model respecification process, these two factors left with two items. Statistically, these two factors were underidentified and may be problematic in further SEM procedures [37]. The final measurement model has six constructs: outdoor spaces and buildings, transportation and housing, community support and health services, age-friendly environment, active aging, and social connectedness. The final measurement was adequately fit, indicated by $p = 0.13$, CMIN/df = 1.15, GFI = 0.96, RMSEA = 0.02, SRMR = 0.03, NFI = 0.97, TLI = 1.00, CFI = 1.00, AGFI = 0.95, and ECVI = 0.60.

The measurement model was examined using the convergent validity and discriminant validity tests. The result of convergent validity indicates that the variables achieved their convergent validity with average variance extracted greater than 0.50 as well as composite reliability greater than 0.70 (see Table 4). The results in Table 5 indicate that discriminant validity is attained when the values of average variance extracted in bold are all greater than the values of the square of correlations between variables that are not in bold.

Table 6 reports the standardized coefficient of the variables in the structural model of age-friendly environment and active aging. The structural model has adequate goodness-of-fit; hence, the hypothesized model is considered reasonably fit. The model's goodness-of-fit indices have achieved the threshold with $p = 0.18$, CMIN/df = 1.14, GFI = 0.97, RMSEA = 0.02, SRMR = 0.02, NFI = 0.98, TLI = 1.00, CFI = 1.00, AGFI = 0.96, and ECVI = 0.42. The structural model is illustrated in Figure 2.

The overall structural model with mediator is illustrated in Figure 3. The model fit values are within its threshold with $p = 0.19$, CMIN/df = 1.11, GFI = 0.96, RMSEA = 0.02, SRMR = 0.03, NFI = 0.97, TLI = 1.00, CFI = 1.00, AGFI = 0.95, and ECVI = 0.57. On the other hand, the results of mediation effect are reported in Table 7. The results verified the mediation model at 2.23 with p value of 0.03 with Sobel test [41] and through a web-calculator developed by Preacher and Leonardelli [42] (see Table 7).

The structural model shows that transportation and housing, outdoor spaces and buildings, and community support and health services represent 70.2% in total variance of an age-friendly environment. Transportation and housing factor is the most statistically significant factor in explaining an age-friendly model, followed by outdoor spaces and buildings and, lastly, community support and health services with standardized coefficient of 0.33, 0.30, and 0.30, respectively. All these three significant age-friendly features are found to be positively significantly associated with age-friendly environments. An age-friendly environment is positively significantly associated with active aging as shown by the standardized coefficient of 0.25 ($p = 0.00$), indicating that an age-friendly environment enables the elderly to age actively. Hence, H_1 and H_2 are supported.

The results show that an age-friendly environment is significantly linked to active aging and social connectedness with standardized coefficient of 0.25 and 0.13, respectively (see Table 7). Active aging is significantly related to social connectedness with standardized coefficient of 0.42. When social connectedness enters the model as a mediator, the relationship between an age-friendly environment and active aging remained statistically significant but at reduced standardized coefficient of 0.19. This is indicative of the fact that social connectedness partially mediates the relationship between an age-friendly environment and active aging, thus supporting H_3. The standardized indirect effect of an age-friendly environment on active aging is statistically significant at 0.05.

TABLE 3: Exploratory factor analysis (EFA) on the factors of age-friendly environment employing the informal caregiver respondents.

Variables	Pattern matrix				
	1	2	3	4	5
(1) Communication and information					
(a) Stay in touch with people	0.97				
(b) Feel more connected	0.94				
(c) Easier to reach people	0.92				
(d) Increases communication	0.90				
(e) Feel less isolated	0.88				
(f) Easier to meet new people	0.74				
(2) Outdoor spaces and buildings					
(a) Good street lighting		0.91			
(b) Sufficient outdoor seating		0.84			
(c) Pavements are wide		0.81			
(d) Bicycle lanes and walking trails		0.78			
(e) Traffic signals for crossing		0.68			
(f) Recreational facilities		0.67			
(g) Interesting things to look at		0.49			
(3) Transportation and housing					
(a) Neighborhood safety			0.78		
(b) Drop-off and pickup areas			0.77		
(c) Accessible public transportation			0.73		
(d) Priority seating			0.71		
(e) Taxis are with discounts			0.62		
(f) Free of pollution			0.57		
(g) Available public transportation			0.56		
(h) Accessible public toilets			0.55		
(i) Walking trail from home to public transport station			0.55		
(4) Community support and health services					
(a) Reachable health services				0.88	
(b) Affordable medical care				0.86	
(c) Adequate range of services				0.72	
(d) Physiotherapy services				0.69	
(5) Social participation					
(a) Leisure activities					0.81
(b) Social activities					0.81
(c) Lifelong learning					0.81
(d) Religion activities					0.70
KMO	0.92				
Eigenvalue	13.96	4.09	2.14	1.77	1.21
Percentage of variance (%)	41.31	11.81	5.53	4.47	2.74

5. Discussions and Implications

The overall structural model demonstrates a link between age-friendliness of the environment of an individual and active aging where the link is being partially mediated by social connectedness. The constructed structural model reflects the person-environment fit [7, 43] and is consistent with Bronfenbrenner's ecological theory [8]. Age-friendly environments enable adults to age actively. The results provide evidence that an age-friendly environment is significantly positively related to active aging [4, 12, 44]. Social participation with fair health promotes active aging [45]. The mediated model shows that 21% of active aging is explained by an age-friendly environment and social connectedness.

When adults are connected with society, emotional support received from their family and friends serves as emotional resources for them. Therefore, by increasing their social capital and gaining greater self-esteem and social status, they would be able to age actively. They further promote social connectedness that indirectly helps increase their exchange power and status in a modern society. Increase in exchange resources improves intergenerational relationships between

TABLE 4: Analysis of convergent validity of integrated model of age-friendly environment, active aging, and social connectedness.

Variables	Standardized factor loadings	Convergent validity Average variance extracted	Composite reliability	Cronbach's alpha
(1) Outdoor spaces and buildings		0.66	0.86	0.85
(a) Pavements are wide	0.78			
(b) Traffic signals for crossing	0.84			
(c) Recreational facilities	0.83			
(2) Transportation and housing		0.67	0.86	0.86
(a) Accessible public toilets	0.84			
(b) Accessible public transportation	0.84			
(c) Free of pollution	0.78			
(3) Community support and health services		0.84	0.94	0.94
(a) Physiotherapy services	0.92			
(b) Affordable medical care	0.94			
(c) Reachable health services	0.90			
(4) Age-friendly environment		0.74	0.90	0.89
(a) Age-in-place	0.78			
(b) Ease of services to be delivered	0.92			
(c) Promote participation	0.88			
(5) Active aging		0.64	0.83	0.80
(a) Satisfied with well-being	0.96			
(b) Quality of life meets my expectation	0.86			
(c) Life is good	0.51			
(6) Social connectedness		0.74	0.90	0.89
(a) Disconnected from the world around me	0.80			
(b) Distant from people	0.90			
(c) Don't feel related to anyone	0.88			

Note: values of average variance extracted and composite reliability are calculated manually through the below formulas: average variance extracted = $\sum$ standardized factor loadings^2/number of items; composite reliability = $\sum$(standardized factor loadings)^2/($\sum$(standardized factor loadings)^2 + ($\sum$ 1 − standardized factor loadings^2)).

TABLE 5: Analysis of discriminant validity of integrated model of age-friendly environment, active aging, and social connectedness.

Variables	Mean	SD	1	2	3	4	5	6
(1) Outdoor spaces and buildings	4.40	0.60	**0.66**					
(2) Transportation and housing	4.49	0.54	0.63 (0.79)	**0.67**				
(3) Community support and health services	4.50	0.56	0.43 (0.66)	0.52 (0.72)	**0.84**			
(4) Age-friendly environment	4.33	0.59	0.57 (0.76)	0.61 (0.78)	0.54 (0.74)	**0.74**		
(5) Active aging	3.82	0.67	0.03 (0.19)	0.04 (0.21)	0.02 (0.15)	0.06 (0.25)	**0.64**	
(6) Social connectedness	3.80	0.90	0.01 (0.10)	0.02 (0.12)	0.01 (0.11)	0.02 (0.12)	0.17 (0.42)	**0.74**

Notes: values in diagonal (bold) are average variance extracted (AVE) while values off-diagonal are the square of correlations between constructs; values in parentheses are correlations between constructs.

them and their families as well as with their caregivers. Negative emotions for these older adults can be eliminated by reducing the imbalance in exchange relationships [46]. Harmonious familial relationships that support the emotional well-being of the older adults are formed.

It is surprising that not all of the eight main domains of the WHO [4] age-friendly features are perceived to be important by these respondents in Malaysia. Further discussions and analyses would provide insights in explaining the age-friendly environment from the Malaysian perspectives. First, the transportation and housing domain is perceived as the most important feature in building an age-friendly environment. The age-friendly transportation and housing would enable the elderly to participate in local community social events, exercise in parks, receive adequate healthcare, and visit family and friends, which would help promote social connectedness and participation [9]. Privately owned cars have become a common mode of transportation in Malaysia

Table 6: Results of hypotheses testing.

Hypothesized path	R^2	Std. estimate[a]	CR[b]	Hypothesis supported
Variables	0.70			
Age-friendly environment				
Transportation and housing		0.33**	4.04	Yes
Community support and health services		0.30**	5.36	Yes
Outdoor spaces and buildings		0.30**	4.03	Yes
Communication and information			Variable deleted	
Social participation			Variable deleted	
Civic participation and employment			Variable deleted	
Respect and social inclusion			Variable deleted	
Age-friendly environment → active aging	0.06	0.25**	4.52	Yes

Notes: [a]Std. estimate denotes standardized estimate; [b]CR denotes critical ratio; **path is significant at $p \leq 0.01$.

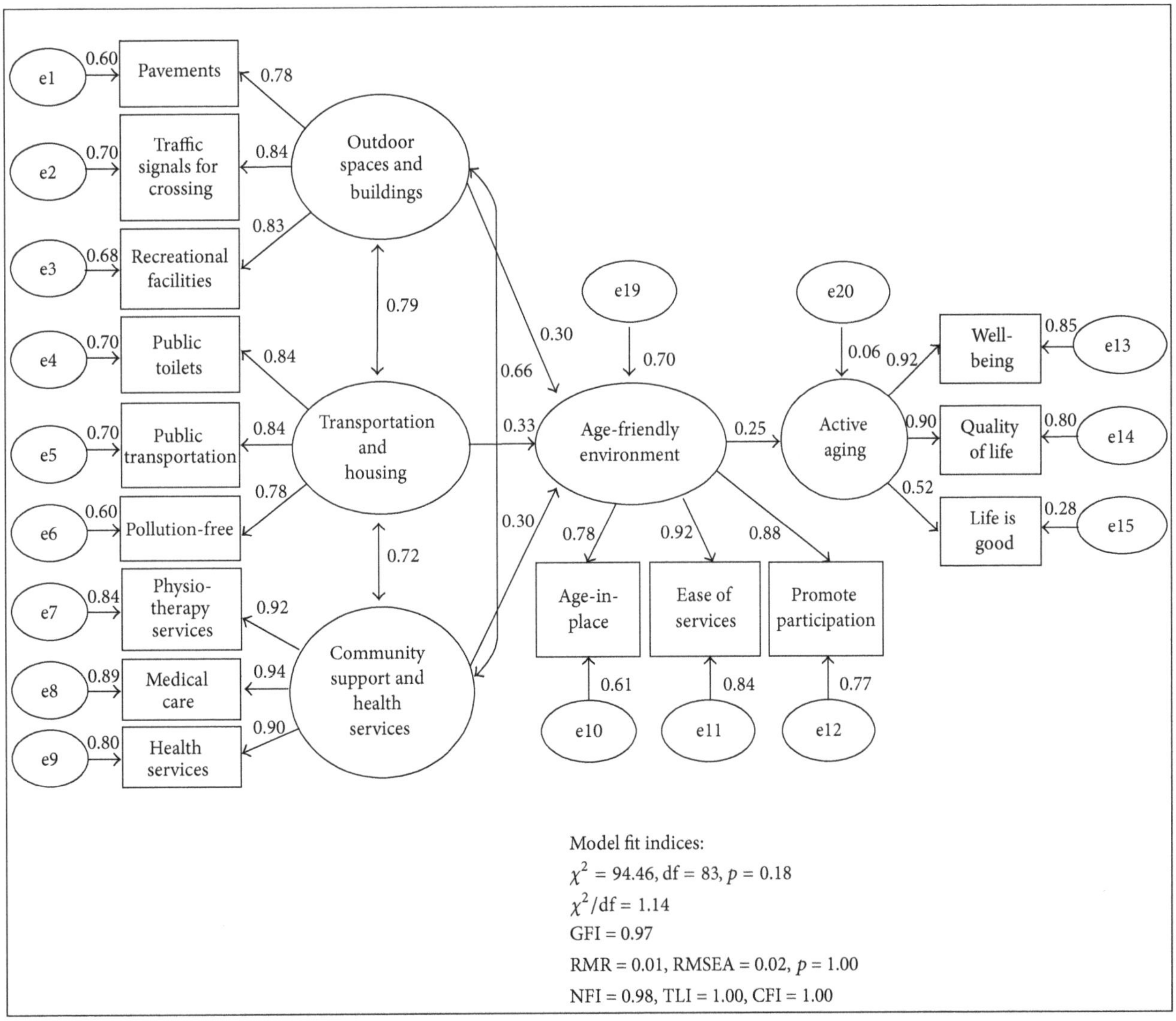

Figure 2: Structural model of age-friendly environment and active aging.

TABLE 7: Results of mediation effect.

Hypothesized path	Direct model without mediation	Standardized direct model with mediation	Standardized indirect model with mediation	CR[a]	Mediation effect	Hypothesis supported
Age-friendly environment → social connectedness	0.13*	0.13*	NA	2.34	NA	NA
Age-friendly environment → active aging	0.25**	0.19**	NA	3.89	NA	NA
Social connectedness → active aging	0.42**	0.39**	NA	7.52	NA	NA
Age-friendly environment → social connectedness → active aging	NA	NA	0.05**	NA	Yes/partial	Yes

Notes: [a]CR denotes critical ratio; NA denotes not applicable; **path is significant at $p \leq 0.01$; *path is significant at $p \leq 0.05$; Sobel test = 2.23 (p value = 0.03) calculated through a web-calculator developed by Preacher and Leonardelli [42].

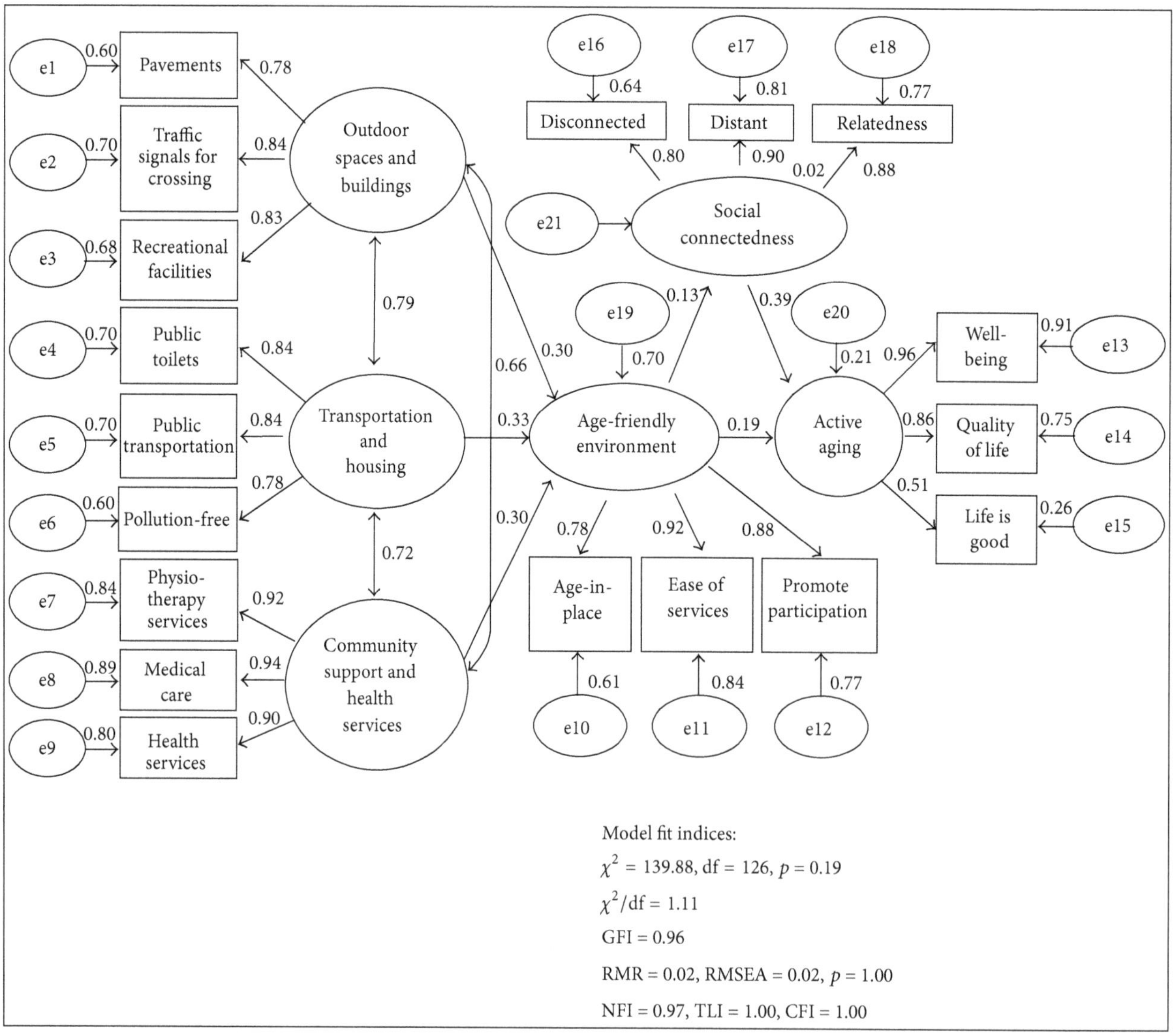

FIGURE 3: Overall structural model of age-friendly environment, active aging, and social connectedness.

[47]. Given the fact that communities in Malaysia are highly car dependent, this has created challenges when older people are no longer able to drive. The unavailability and inaccessibility of the public transport system have indirectly affected other domains such as quality of social participation and civic engagement [13]. "The ability to drive (and feeling safe while driving) is crucial to social participation" [48, page 227].

This model helps policy makers and relevant authorities to understand that a public transportation system that is accessible, safe, and convenient helps to improve mobility when a person ages. This is what Malaysia should learn from developed countries [49]. Having accessibility to community services not only improves social and physical activities, but also provides an alternative to enhance the health of the elderly [22].

Second, outdoor spaces and buildings play an important role in the adaptability of adults in their living environment. Safe outdoor spaces equipped with the appropriate facilities help ease the mobility of adults, especially older adults [4]. The safe and elder-friendly outdoor spaces and buildings are in line with the person-environment fit [7, 43] which increases the level of adaptation and reduces the burden that arises from the environment. It further promotes the concept of aging-in-place where the elderly could continue to live in their community safely and independently [20].

In order for an individual to actively age and age-in-place, outdoor spaces and buildings that have friendly built environment are essential. The findings have contributed to the relevant authorities, especially urban planners by enlightening them on the importance of modifying physical design for outdoor spaces and buildings to be more elder-friendly to improve accessibility and walkability [50].

The community support and health services domain is perceived as another significant age-friendly feature. It serves as a proactive intervention in light of increasing healthcare cost resulting from poor health and chronic diseases among aging people. These findings are strongly in line with the need for a reform in the local healthcare system [51]. The main healthcare system in Malaysia concentrates predominantly on acute treatment, which may be inadequate to cater to the growing number of the elderly people, especially those with chronic illness and disabilities [52]. Healthy living can be promoted with the availability of public exercise areas in the communities [18]. This is also in line with the findings from the University of Hong Kong [53], where a practical community support system is included in an age-friendly environment. Given the limited physiotherapy facilities in the current communities in Malaysia and that fact that this service is essential for the recovery of the disabled elderly especially those suffering from stroke [54], we strongly suggest that the Malaysian government provides more public rehabilitation centers or physical exercise centers.

It is worth noting that the other four domains of the age-friendly features are perceived to be not significant in the Malaysian context. They are respect and social inclusion, social participation, civic participation and employment, and communication and information. Possible explanations are discussed below.

First, the lack of reliable and accessible transportation may have created barriers for the middle-aged and above respondents from participating in social, civic, and employment activities within their communities. As a result, they seldom have the opportunities to be included in social activities. It is perceived that limited interaction between the older and younger generations has indirectly led to the lack of respect of the younger generation towards older people.

Second, given that the age-friendly community concept is still very new in Malaysia, not all the outdoor spaces and buildings as well as working environments are elderly friendly. At the same time, modification plans to improve accessibility and walkability are limited. With limited working opportunities for the older people especially after retirement, it may hinder the elderly from being eligible for work and community participation [55].

Last but not least, high Internet connection cost as perceived by the respondents has indirectly discouraged them from accessing information and communication technologies. Some older respondents especially those with a lower education do not have the technical know-how to use advanced technologies, such as personal computers and smart phones. In view of this, we propose that lifelong learning classes should be organized for older adults by nongovernment organizations or local authorities.

Menec et al. [5] state that age-friendly domains related to social environment are easier to address than physical environment; however, this is not the case in the Malaysian environment context. As Malaysia is still a developing nation, many physical environments and infrastructures such as modern public transportation are yet to be fully developed. Hence, the findings strongly suggest that Malaysian policy makers need to prioritize the development of friendly built environments to reduce these structural barriers when building an age-friendly environment.

It should be pointed out that an enabling social environment is just as important as material conditions in determining the well-being for older people. As a whole, an age-friendly community should provide a comprehensive and accessible physical and social environment in which health, social involvement, and security of the elderly can be supported [4, 44].

The findings provide better understandings of an age-friendly environment which supports the well-being of the middle-agers and the elderly by enabling them to continue to be active in society as they age. The findings have potential to reduce social isolation among the aged. Nevertheless, the final model explains 70% of the age-friendly environment, 2% of social connectedness, and 21% of active aging. Hence, certain percentages of variables are yet to be explained especially the variable of social connectedness and active aging which would be of great interest for future studies.

6. Conclusions

Overall, the concept of age-friendly is still very new to Malaysia. Age-friendly transportation, outdoor spaces and buildings, and community and health services emerge as the three most important features in building an age-friendly environment. A structural model with satisfactory goodness-of-fit is built. Improved transportation services as well as modifications to outdoor spaces and buildings such as accessible public toilets and senior buses are essential as short-term solutions to reduce the structural barriers for the aged group to age actively and maintain connectedness to their community. Similarly, wide pavements and traffic signals for crossings as well as recreational activities are age-friendly features that can assist the adult groups in a physical environment. Not only that but also affordable medical care services and physiotherapy centers as well as convenient health services are identified as significant domains in building an age-friendly community. Domains related to social participation, respect and social inclusion, and civic engagement need more emphasis.

The findings provide better understandings for the state and municipal governments to implement age-friendly community initiatives to support the well-being of the residents by enabling them to continue to be active in society when they age. The findings have potential to reduce social isolation among the aged. Future research to examine the applicability and readiness of age-friendly features and outcomes in local communities would be of great interest. Last but not least, an age-friendly community index should be proposed to indicate the degree of age-friendliness.

Competing Interests

The authors declare that there are no competing interests regarding the publication of this paper and the received funding did not lead to any competing interests regarding it.

Acknowledgments

This work was supported by the Ministry of Higher Education, Malaysia, under Exploratory Research Grant Scheme [ERGS/1/2012/SS05/MMU/02/4]. The authors are grateful for the financial support received from the ministry. This work was inspired by Madam Tai Ching Kin's personal health story. The authors would like to thank all those who participated in this survey.

References

[1] International Living, "The world's best places to retire in 2014," 2014, http://internationalliving.com/2014/01/the-best-places-to-retire-2014/.

[2] Population Division of the Department of Economics and Social Affairs of the United Nations Secretariat, *World Population Prospects: The 2008 Revision*, United Nations, New York, NY, USA, 2008.

[3] N. S. Ambrose, "Who will care for our old?" *The Sun Daily*, 2012, http://www.thesundaily.my/news/289751.

[4] World Health Organization (WHO), *Global Age-Friendly Cities: A Guide*, WHO, Geneva, Switzerland, 2007.

[5] V. H. Menec, L. Hutton, N. Newall, S. Nowicki, J. Spina, and D. Veselyuk, "How 'age-friendly' are rural communities and what community characteristics are related to age-friendliness? The case of rural Manitoba, Canada," *Ageing and Society*, vol. 35, no. 1, pp. 203–223, 2015.

[6] R. B. Kline, *Principles and Practice of Structural Equation Modeling*, Guilford Press, New York, NY, USA, 3rd edition, 2011.

[7] M. P. Lawton, "Social ecology and the health of older people," *American Journal of Public Health*, vol. 64, no. 3, pp. 257–260, 1974.

[8] U. Bronfenbrenner, "Toward an experimental ecology of human development," *American Psychologist*, vol. 32, no. 7, pp. 513–531, 1977.

[9] C. A. Emlet and J. T. Moceri, "The importance of social connectedness in building age-friendly communities," *Journal of Aging Research*, vol. 2012, Article ID 173247, 9 pages, 2012.

[10] P. H. Feldman and M. R. Oberlink, "The advantage initiative: developing community indicators to promote the health and well-being of older people," *Family & Community Health*, vol. 26, no. 4, pp. 268–274, 2003.

[11] D. Alley, P. Liebig, J. Pynoos, T. Banerjee, and I. H. Choi, "Creating elder-friendly communities: preparations for an aging society," *Journal of Gerontological Social Work*, vol. 49, no. 1-2, pp. 1–18, 2007.

[12] C.-W. Lui, J.-A. Everingham, J. Warburton, M. Cuthill, and H. Bartlett, "What makes a community age-friendly: a review of international literature," *Australasian Journal on Ageing*, vol. 28, no. 3, pp. 116–121, 2009.

[13] Y. Kadoya, "Toward an age-friendly city: the constraints preventing the elderly's participation in community programs in Akita city," *Working with Older People*, vol. 17, no. 3, pp. 101–108, 2013.

[14] World Health Organization (WHO), *Active Ageing: A Policy Framework*, WHO, Geneva, Switzerland, 2002.

[15] Y. L. Michael, M. K. Green, and S. A. Farquhar, "Neighborhood design and active aging," *Health & Place*, vol. 12, no. 4, pp. 734–740, 2006.

[16] A. Bowling, "Enhancing later life: how older people perceive active ageing?" *Aging and Mental Health*, vol. 12, no. 3, pp. 293–301, 2008.

[17] C. Paúl, O. Ribeiro, and L. Teixeira, "Active ageing: an empirical approach to the WHO model," *Current Gerontology and Geriatrics Research*, vol. 2012, Article ID 382972, 10 pages, 2012.

[18] S. An, Y. Lee, and J. T. Kim, "The effect of the public exercise environment on the physical activity for the active ageing of the elderly," *Indoor and Built Environment*, vol. 22, no. 1, pp. 319–331, 2013.

[19] L. Fratiglioni, S. Paillard-Borg, and B. Winblad, "An active and socially integrated lifestyle in late life might protect against dementia," *The Lancet Neurology*, vol. 3, no. 6, pp. 343–353, 2004.

[20] B. Horner and D. P. Boldy, "The benefit and burden of 'ageing-in-place' in an aged care community," *Australian Health Review*, vol. 32, no. 2, pp. 356–365, 2008.

[21] J. M. Cramm, H. M. van Dijk, and A. P. Nieboer, "The importance of neighborhood social cohesion and social capital for the well being of older adults in the community," *Gerontologist*, vol. 53, no. 1, pp. 142–150, 2013.

[22] T. Franke, C. Tong, M. C. Ashe, H. McKay, and J. Sims-Gould, "The secrets of highly active older adults," *Journal of Aging Studies*, vol. 27, no. 4, pp. 398–409, 2013.

[23] D. O. Cowgill, "The aging of populations and societies," *The Annals of the American Academy of Political and Social Science*, vol. 415, no. 1, pp. 1–18, 1974.

[24] J. J. Dowd, "Aging as exchange: a preface to theory," *Journals of Gerontology*, vol. 30, no. 5, pp. 584–594, 1975.

[25] K. Backman and M. Hentinen, "Model for the self-care of home-dwelling elderly," *Journal of Advanced Nursing*, vol. 30, no. 3, pp. 564–572, 1999.

[26] E. Jaques, "Death and the mid-life crisis," *The International Journal of Psycho-Analysis*, vol. 46, no. 4, pp. 502–514, 1965.

[27] D. Avramov and M. Maskova, *Active Ageing in Europe*, vol. 2, Council of Europe, Strasbourg, France, 2003.

[28] P. J.-H. Poi, D. R. Forsyth, and D. K. Y. Chan, "Services for older people in Malaysia: issues and challenges," *Age and Ageing*, vol. 33, no. 5, pp. 444–446, 2004.

[29] L. K. Brennan Ramirez, C. M. Hoehner, R. C. Brownson et al., "ndicators of activity-friendly communities: an evidence-based consensus process," *American Journal of Preventive Medicine*, vol. 31, no. 6, pp. 515–524, 2006.

[30] World Health Organization (WHO), *Checklist of Essential Features of Age-Friendly Cities*, WHO, Geneva, Switzerland, 2007.

[31] S. R. Cotten, W. A. Anderson, and B. M. McCullough, "Impact of internet use on loneliness and contact with others among older adults: cross-sectional analysis," *Journal of Medical Internet Research*, vol. 15, no. 2, p. e39, 2013.

[32] R. M. Lee and S. B. Robbins, "Measuring belongingness: the social connectedness and the social assurance scales," *Journal of Counseling Psychology*, vol. 42, no. 2, pp. 232–241, 1995.

[33] S. Senapaty, "What is better to use as a first validation attempt: exploratory Factor Analysis or Confirmatory Factor Analysis?" 2014, https://www.researchgate.net/post/What_is_better_to_use_as_a_first_validation_attempt_Exploratory_Factor_Analysis_or_Confirmatory_Factor_Anaylsis.

[34] H. Li, S. M. Edwards, and J.-H. Lee, "Measuring the intrusiveness of advertisements: scale development and validation," *Journal of Advertising*, vol. 31, no. 2, pp. 35–46, 2002.

[35] H. Y. Kim, "Statistical notes for clinical researchers: assessing normal distribution (2) using skewness and kurtosis," *Restorative Dentistry & Endodontics*, vol. 38, no. 1, pp. 52–54, 2013.

[36] J. B. Schreiber, F. K. Stage, J. King, A. Nora, and E. A. Barlow, "Reporting structural equation modeling and confirmatory factor analysis results: a review," *The Journal of Educational Research*, vol. 99, no. 6, pp. 323–337, 2006.

[37] J. F. Hair, W. C. Black, B. J. Babin, and R. E. Anderson, *Multivariate Data Analysis*, Pearson Prentice Hall, New Jersey, NJ, USA, 7th edition, 2010.

[38] C. Fornell and D. F. Larcker, "Evaluating structural equation models with unobservable variables and measurement error," *Journal of Marketing Research*, vol. 18, no. 1, pp. 39–50, 1981.

[39] K. J. Preacher, D. D. Rucker, and A. F. Hayes, "Addressing moderated mediation hypotheses: theory, methods, and prescriptions," *Multivariate Behavioral Research*, vol. 42, no. 1, pp. 185–227, 2007.

[40] D. Y. K. Tong, D. Rasiah, X. F. Tong, and K. P. Lai, "Leadership empowerment behaviour on safety officer and safety teamwork in manufacturing industry," *Safety Science*, vol. 72, pp. 190–198, 2015.

[41] D. D. Rucker, K. J. Preacher, Z. L. Tormala, and R. E. Petty, "Mediation analysis in social psychology: current practices and new recommendations," *Social and Personality Psychology Compass*, vol. 5, no. 6, pp. 359–371, 2011.

[42] K. J. Preacher and G. J. Leonardelli, "Calculation for the Sobel test: an interactive calculation tool for mediation tests," 2001, http://quantpsy.org/sobel/sobel.htm.

[43] L. Nahemow and M. P. Lawton, "Toward an ecological theory of adaptation and aging," in *Environmental Design Research*, vol. 1, pp. 24–32, 1973.

[44] L. A. Plouffe and A. Kalache, "Making communities age friendly: state and municipal initiatives in Canada and other countries," *Gaceta Sanitaria*, vol. 25, no. 2, pp. 131–137, 2011.

[45] A. Zaidi, K. Gasior, M. M. Hofmarcher et al., *Active Ageing Index 2012: Concept, Methodology, and Final Results*, European Centre, Vienna, Austria, 2013.

[46] T. J. Durant Jr. and O. G. Christian, "Caregiving to aging parents," Forum on Public Policy, 2006, http://forumonpublicpolicy.com/archive07/durant.pdf.

[47] A. Nurdden, R. A. O. K. Rahmat, and A. Ismail, "Effect of transportation policies on modal shift from private car to public transport in Malaysia," *Journal of Applied Sciences*, vol. 7, no. 7, pp. 1013–1018, 2007.

[48] A. Sixsmith and J. Sixsmith, "Ageing in place in the United Kingdom," *Ageing International*, vol. 32, no. 3, pp. 219–235, 2008.

[49] A. S. I. Almselati, R. A. O. K. Rahmat, and O. Jaafar, "An overview of urban transport in Malaysia," *The Social Sciences*, vol. 6, no. 1, pp. 24–33, 2011.

[50] G. Miller, G. Harris, and I. Ferguson, "Bracing for the demographic tsunami—can Canada's senior escape unpleasantville?" *Ontario Planning Journal*, vol. 21, no. 6, pp. 1–3, 2006.

[51] K. S. Ambigga, A. S. Ramli, A. Suthahar, N. Tauhid, L. Clearihan, and C. Browning, "Bridging the gap in ageing: translating policies into practice in Malaysian primary care," *Asia Pacific Family Medicine*, vol. 10, no. 2, pp. 1–7, 2011.

[52] M. Mafauzy, "The problems and challenges of the aging population of Malaysia," *Malaysian Journal of Medical Sciences*, vol. 7, no. 1, pp. 1–3, 2000.

[53] University of Hong Kong, *Consultancy Study on Community Care Services for the Elderly*, Sau Po Center on Ageing and Department of Social Work & Social Administration the University of Hong Kong, Hong Kong, 2011.

[54] N. A. Mohd Nordin, N. A. A. Aziz, A. F. Abdul Aziz et al., "Exploring views on long term rehabilitation for people with stroke in a developing country: findings from focus group discussions," *BMC Health Services Research*, vol. 14, no. 1, pp. 118–127, 2014.

[55] K. Lawler, "Age-friendly communities: go big or go home," *Public Policy & Aging Report*, vol. 25, no. 1, pp. 30–33, 2015.

20

Relating Sensory, Cognitive, and Neural Factors to Older Persons' Perceptions about Happiness

Alexandra J. Horne,[1,2] Kimberly S. Chiew,[3] Jie Zhuang,[4] Linda K. George,[5,6] R. Alison Adcock,[3,7] Guy G. Potter,[7] Eleonora M. Lad,[8] Scott W. Cousins,[8] Frank R. Lin,[9] Sara K. Mamo,[10] Nan-Kuei Chen,[4] Abigail J. Maciejewski,[4] Xuan Duong Fernandez,[4] and Heather E. Whitson[6,8,11,12]

[1]*Duke University School of Medicine, Durham, NC, USA*
[2]*Johns Hopkins University, Baltimore, MD, USA*
[3]*Center for Cognitive Neuroscience, Duke University, Durham, NC, USA*
[4]*Brain Imaging and Analysis Center, Duke University, Durham, NC, USA*
[5]*Department of Sociology, Duke University, Durham, NC, USA*
[6]*Center for the Study of Aging and Human Development, Duke University, Durham, NC, USA*
[7]*Department of Psychiatry and Behavioral Sciences, Duke University School of Medicine, Durham, NC, USA*
[8]*Department of Ophthalmology, Duke University School of Medicine, Durham, NC, USA*
[9]*Department of Otolaryngology, Johns Hopkins University School of Medicine, Baltimore, MD, USA*
[10]*Department of Communication Disorders, University of Massachusetts, Amherst, MA, USA*
[11]*Geriatrics Research Education and Clinical Center, Durham VA Medical Center, Durham, NC, USA*
[12]*Department of Medicine, Duke University School of Medicine, Durham, NC, USA*

Correspondence should be addressed to Heather E. Whitson; heather.whitson@duke.edu

Academic Editor: F. R. Ferraro

Despite increased rates of disease, disability, and social losses with aging, seniors consistently report higher levels of subjective well-being (SWB), a construct closely related to happiness, than younger adults. In this exploratory study, we utilized an available dataset to investigate how aspects of health commonly deteriorating with age, including sensory (i.e., vision and hearing) and cognitive status, relate to variability in self-described contributors to happiness. Community-dwelling seniors ($n = 114$) responded to a single-item prompt: "name things that make people happy." 1731 responses were categorized into 13 domains of SWB via structured content analysis. Sensory health and cognition were assessed by Snellen visual acuity, pure-tone audiometry, and in-person administration of the Brief Test of Adult Cognition by Telephone (BTACT) battery. A subset of eligible participants ($n = 57$) underwent functional magnetic resonance imaging (fMRI) to assess resting state functional connectivity (FC) within a previously described dopaminergic network associated with reward processing. SWB response patterns were relatively stable across gender, sensory status, and cognitive performance with few exceptions. For example, hearing-impaired participants listed fewer determinants of SWB (13.59 vs. 17.16; $p < 0.001$) and were less likely to name things in the "special events" category. Participants with a higher proportion of responses in the "accomplishments" domain (e.g., winning, getting good grades) demonstrated increased FC between the ventral tegmental area and nucleus accumbens, regions implicated in reward and motivated behavior. While the framework for determinants of happiness among seniors was largely stable across the factors assessed here, our findings suggest that subtle changes in this construct may be linked to sensory loss. The possibility that perceptions about determinants of happiness might relate to differences in intrinsic connectivity within reward-related brain networks also warrants further investigation.

1. Introduction

Subjective well-being (SWB) refers to a subjective state encompassing people's longer-term levels of pleasant affect, lack of unpleasant affect, and life satisfaction [1]. Although well-being is a complex and multifaceted construct [2, 3], SWB can be generally understood as an index of happiness [4–6]. Research characterizing SWB over the lifespan has identified a paradox: although older adults experience declining physical health and increased personal losses (e.g., the deaths of spouse and friends), they report relatively stable or even increased levels of SWB [7, 8] and an increased ratio of positive to negative emotions relative to younger adults [9–11]. This "positivity effect" has been interpreted as partially reflecting a phenomenon termed *socioemotional selectivity*; that is, as individuals advance towards the end of their lifespan and perceive limitations in time, their goals shift such that they prioritize emotional satisfaction over goals that will pay off in the future (e.g., knowledge or power acquisition), thus promoting positive affect or greater happiness [12]. Furthermore, prior work suggests that the life domains (e.g., social relationships, wealth) that contribute to happiness may change with age; this may be due to changes in life situations, such as retirement or widowhood, or changes in health status [7].

Two aspects of health status that are prone to age-related decline and directly mediate one's lived experience are cognitive and sensory health. Mild cognitive impairment (MCI) is present in 3% to 19% of adults over the age of 65 years, with more than half of these individuals progressing to dementia over 5 years [13]. Compared to older adults with intact cognition, seniors with mild cognitive impairment tend to exhibit higher rates of loneliness and anxiety and increased difficulty in performing daily activities [14]. Likewise, impairments in vision and hearing may affect one's subjective state and become increasingly common in late life. The prevalence of uncorrectable vision impairment among Americans has been estimated as 16.1% among those aged 60–69 years and increases to 50% in Americans over age 80 years [15]. The prevalence of hearing loss among Americans over age 70 years has been estimated as 63.1% [16]. Multiple studies have demonstrated a relationship between vision and hearing impairments and lower quality of life, SWB, and other patient-centered outcomes [17–20].

Understanding how cognitive, vision, and hearing statuses relate to variability in self-described contributors to happiness may add to our understanding of age-related changes in SWB. One challenge to research in this area is that it can be difficult to study determinants of SWB in the setting of cognitive impairment, given inherent issues with measuring patient-reported variables in this population. In this exploratory analysis, we address these gaps with a novel approach to capture self-specified contributors to SWB, or happiness. We made use of data from a group of older adults with well-characterized sensory and cognitive status who had been asked to respond to the prompt, "Name things that make people happy." While this task departs from multi-item scales traditionally used to characterize various dimensions of well-being [1, 7], the simple and open-ended nature of our measure allows feasible data collection among participants with varying degrees of age-related impairment and generates a diversity of responses that may reflect participants' own notions about determinants of happiness.

Next, in order to further explore relationships between self-described determinants of happiness and activity in a functional brain network of interest, we examined intrinsic, resting-state brain activity in a subset of our cohort that was eligible to undergo brain MRI. We were specifically interested in investigating resting-state activity within a functional network associated with reward anticipation and mesolimbic dopamine function [21], given the central role of dopamine in reward processing and motivated behavior [22, 23]. Our interest in relationships between perceived determinants of happiness and activity in this functional neural network was motivated by prior work that has suggested that individual variability in well-being might relate to brain function [24], particularly in regions associated with reward processing, such as the ventral striatum [25]. Although Heller et al. [25] characterized neural correlates of eudaimonic well-being, or one's sense of purpose, fulfillment, or meaning, as opposed to SWB, which is more typically linked to pleasure and happiness, we reasoned that pleasure is an integral component of reward [26]. Thus, we hypothesized that individual variation in perceived determinants of happiness might similarly scale with activity in reward-related brain regions. Exploring this relationship in older adults is novel and of interest, considering that age-related decline in dopaminergic activity has been well documented [27], just as the domains that contribute to SWB are also thought to shift with age [7, 28].

Overall, the present study seeks to advance our understanding of the complex relationships among sensory, cognitive, and neural health status and older adults' perceptions about determinants of SWB, or happiness. In an exploratory approach, we made use of qualitative data generated from a patient-centered and feasible task that asks individuals to "name things that make people happy." A better understanding of how older adults' notions about happiness are linked to common, age-related impairments may shed light on SWB across the lifespan and is a necessary step toward our ultimate goal of designing programs and services to optimize happiness in seniors coping with insults to neural organs.

2. Methods

2.1. Study Population. Data were acquired from an ongoing study that examines cognitive and brain changes associated with age-related macular degeneration (AMD) (National Clinical Trial Registry #: NCT01996215). The parent study has enrolled 81 individuals with AMD as well as an age-balanced control group of 85 individuals with healthy eyes and normal vision. AMD is a condition that may affect one or both eyes and has a variable effect on visual acuity, depending on the stage and severity of the disease. The present analysis includes 114 community-dwelling individuals who had complete data on variables of interest, including neurocognitive assessment, eye examinations, audiology assessments, and health surveys. Participants were recruited from the Duke Eye Center clinics and Duke Aging Center registries. Exclusion criteria for the study were as follows: vision-limiting eye conditions other than AMD, diagnosis of moderate or severe dementia (per chart review or self-report from participant or family) or lack of capacity to provide consent (as assessed by trained study staff), and hearing loss severe enough to preclude participation in study interviews. Of the 114 participants in this analysis, 57 were willing and eligible to undergo functional MRI to characterize resting-state brain activity. Participants were excluded from the MRI portion of the study if they were left-handed, had history of brain surgery or brain pathology (e.g., brain tumor, history of stroke), significant claustrophobia, body weight >300 pounds, or had other contraindications to MRI (e.g., cardiac pacemakers, noncompatible implants).

2.2. Qualitative Data on SWB: Things that Make People Happy. We derived qualitative data about determinants of SWB from a single-item task that required participants to name, in a 60-second period, as many unique responses as possible within the category: "things that make people happy". Neuropsychological assessments were administered by trained study personnel under standardized conditions. The "happy task" was administered as part of the Fuld Object Memory Evaluation [29], in which the task is used to distract participants between memory trials. The assessments were audio-recorded and individual responses were later transcribed into the study database.

The present investigation was conducted on an exploratory basis because, within the data of the parent study, we noted striking heterogeneity in the content of responses generated by the "happy task." We hypothesized that the nature of responses may provide a unique window on individual differences in perceptions about SWB within an older-adult population with varying degrees of sensory and cognitive impairment.

2.3. Vision and Hearing Impairment. Visual acuity was measured in the Duke Eye Center Clinical Research Unit. Vision impairment was defined as Snellen best-corrected visual acuity of 20/40 or less in the better eye. We chose this definition because, in people with central vision loss from AMD, quality of life has been more closely linked to vision in the better seeing eye (as opposed to the worse seeing eye) [30]. Audiometry was assessed with an Interacoustics AD629 Audiometer with ER3A insert earphones in a sound-attenuating booth. Hearing loss was defined as a pur-tone average greater than 25 dB HL in the better ear, averaged over frequencies of 0.5, 1, 2, and 4 kHz, which is a standard definition of function-limiting hearing impairment [16].

2.4. Cognitive Measures. The parent study assessed global cognitive performance with the Brief Test of Adult Cognition by Telephone (BTACT), a validated cognitive battery that evaluates episodic verbal memory, working memory span, verbal fluency, inductive reasoning, and speed of processing [31]. Because it was designed for administration by telephone, the BTACT does not include any items or tasks that rely on vision, which was ideal in this patient population. The BTACT was administered to participants in person by a trained individual in a quiet exam room. In the present study, global cognitive status was quantified via a composite score derived from BTACT performance data via factor analysis. To assign a composite score to each individual, a principal axis factor was performed on the six BTACT measures, which suggested a single-factor solution (one eigenvalue > 1), consistent with the previous literature [31]. The factor matrix showed moderate to strong loadings for all six tests, ranging from 0.37 to 0.70.

One of the six tests in the BTACT is a semantic verbal fluency task: the Animal Naming task, which requires participants to name as many types of animals as they can in 60 seconds [32]. The total number of responses generated by the "happy task" is also a reflection of verbal fluency. Thus, in analyses that considered total number of responses to the "happy task," we used scores on the Animal Naming task as a covariable to adjust for semantic fluency ability.

2.5. Health and Demographic Variables. Participant age was recorded from the medical record. Gender and education level were collected by self-report. Depression screening was performed via verbal administration of the 15-question Geriatric Depression Scale (GDS) [33]. A comorbidity count was created based on the number of affirmative response to a question that asked: "Has a doctor ever told you that you have any of the following health conditions: coronary artery disease, congestive heart failure, heart arrhythmias, arthritis, COPD, stroke/TIAs, diabetes, hypertension, liver disease, kidney disease, cancer, dementia or Alzheimer's disease, Parkinson's disease, osteoporosis, ulcers in the stomach or duodenum, urinary or stool incontinence, and/or insomnia?"

2.6. MRI Data Acquisition. Structural and functional MRI data were collected on a 3T GE MR750 scanner at the Duke/UNC Brain Imaging and Analysis Center (BIAC). An eight-channel head coil was used for radio frequency (RF) reception (General Election, Milwaukee Wisconsin, USA). Sagittal T1-weighted localizer images were acquired and used to define a volume for data collection and high-order shimming. High-resolution structural images were acquired using a 3D fSPGR pulse sequence (TR = 8.156 ms; TE = 3.18 ms; TI = 450 ms; FOV = 25.6 cm^2; flip angle = 12°; voxel size = 1 × 1 × 1 mm; 166 contiguous slices, sense factor = 2). A semiautomated high-order shimming program was used to ensure global field homogeneity. T2*-weighted functional images were acquired during resting state, using a gradient echo-planar sequence sensitive to BOLD contrast (TR = 2 s; TE = 27 ms; flip angle 77°; FOV = 24 cm^2; SENSE factor = 1; voxel size = 3.75 × 3.75 × 4 mm; 34 contiguous oblique axial slices, parallel to the anterior commissure-posterior commissure line, interleaved acquisition) in two 180-volume (~6 minute) runs. In each of these two runs, four initial radio-frequency (RF) excitations were performed to achieve steady-state equilibrium and were subsequently discarded.

During these resting state runs, participants were instructed to "stay awake and think about nothing in particular". Due to the varying visual abilities in this cohort, all participants were instructed to close their eyes during imaging acquisition. Participants remained awake for the duration of MRI data acquisition, which was confirmed by verbal communication between runs.

2.7. MRI Preprocessing. Preprocessing was conducted through Duke/UNC BIAC processing daemons based on the tools from the Oxford Centre for Functional MRI of the Brain's Software Library (FSL version 4.0, https://www.fmrib.ox.ac.uk/fsl). The first four images were removed from each resting state run to achieve steady-state equilibrium. All remaining functional images were aligned with respect to the first image within each run to correct for head movements during data acquisition. A bandpass filter was applied to filter the functional data in the time dimension so that frequencies were retained between 0.001 Hz and 0.08 Hz. The aligned and filtered images were spatially normalized to Montreal Neurological Institute (MNI) space during a 12-degree-of-freedom affine transformation implemented in FSL's Linear Image Registration Tool (FLIRT). We further removed constant offsets and linear drift over each run and regressed out the six rigid body head motion parameters, the signal averaged over the white matter, and the signal averaged over the cerebrospinal fluid regions to reduce nonneuronal influence to BOLD corrections. The normalized images were smoothed using an isotropic Gaussian kernel of 5 mm full-width-half-maximum. The resulting voxel size was $3.75 \times 3.75 \times 4$ mm.

2.8. Data Analysis

2.8.1. Qualitative Analysis of SWB Data. A qualitative content analysis [34] was performed to characterize differences in responses to the "happy task." As a first step, two independent reviewers categorized the responses into 10 mutually exclusive domains. The original framework of 10 domains was based on seven determinants of SWB that have been well described in the literature (social relationships, financial/material wealth, health factors, religious involvement, volunteerism/altruism, exercise and physical activity, and accomplishments) [35], plus three domains that were observed to be recurring categories in our data: avocation (e.g., hobbies), ingestibles (e.g., food and beverages), and special events (birthdays and weddings). Next, the two reviewers met to compare categorizations and revise the framework. An eleventh domain ("nature") was created to capture nature-related responses as an emergent theme identified independently by both reviewers, for which responses did not neatly fit into the initial categories. The nature domain included responses such as "mountains" and "sunsets." Some decision rules were established to guide categorization (e.g., include pets in the social relationship category). Responses were recategorized as needed based on the revised framework and decision rules. Finally, a committee of three coauthors met to adjudicate any remaining disparate categorizations and discuss all responses that had not been assigned to a category. At this meeting, a twelfth domain ("positive emotion") was added to our framework to capture responses such as "smiles" and "laughter" that were felt to represent a small but recurrent theme. Additional decision rules were agreed upon to resolve discordant categorizations (e.g., if the response used active voice for a sporting activity (e.g., "playing basketball"), it was categorized as "exercise/physical activity", whereas passive references to sports (e.g., "basketball"), for which it could not be determined whether the enjoyment was derived from playing or spectating, were categorized as avocation/hobby). This iterative process produced almost complete theme saturation, with 99.08% of responses (1715/1731) categorized into one of 12 mutually exclusive domains (as noted above: social relationships, financial/material wealth, health factors, religious involvement, volunteerism/altruism, exercise and physical activity, accomplishments, avocation/hobbies, ingestibles, special events, nature, and positive emotion).

Next, to explore potential contributions of sensory health to individual variability in perceived determinants of happiness in this sample, we created a secondary category of "vision-dependent" responses. All responses that were determined by reviewer consensus to rely heavily on visual ability (e.g., working crossword puzzles, watching television, driving a vehicle, and reading) were assigned to this category, regardless of their primary assignment in one of the 12 mutually exclusive categories.

2.8.2. MRI Data Analysis. The BOLD signal, measured via fMRI, is used as a marker of region-specific metabolic activity within the brain. Regions whose BOLD signal fluctuations show a high degree of temporal correlation are presumed to constitute a tightly coupled neural network and are said to be functionally connected [36]. Here, we estimated the functional connectivity (FC) within selected regions associated with reward anticipation within the dopaminergic mesolimbic system (reward network; i.e., ventral tegmental area, nucleus accumbens, and dorsolateral prefrontal cortex) [21]. Regions of interest (ROIs) were drawn as 8 mm spheres centered on peak coordinates identified via prior work [21] and were converted to MNI space. These ROIs are displayed in Figure 1. To quantify FC, participants' BOLD time series data were averaged within each selected ROI and Pearson correlation coefficients were calculated to examine relationships between average levels of BOLD activity in pairs of regions within the network.

2.9. Statistical Analyses. Descriptive statistics were used to characterize the sample. For each participant, we calculated the total number of responses to the "happy task" as well as the proportion of responses belonging to each of the 12 mutually exclusive domains as well as the "vision-dependent" task domain. Additionally, we created a dichotomous variable for each of the 12 SWB domains that indicated whether or not the participant gave any response within that domain.

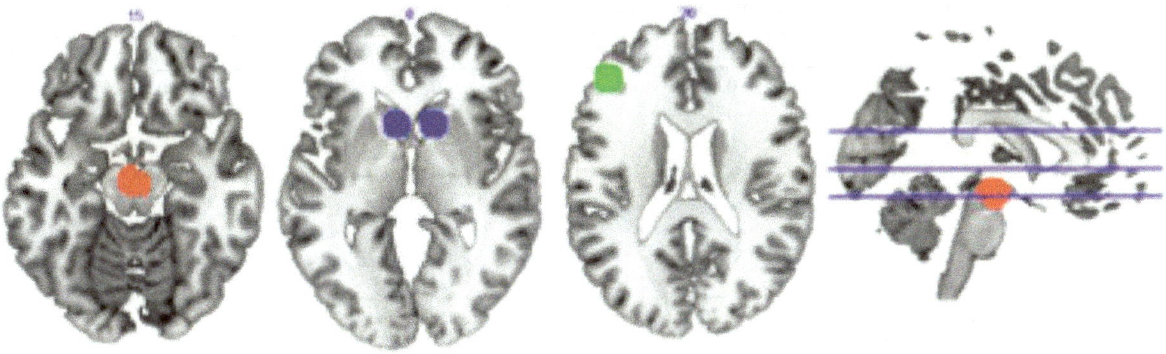

Figure 1: Map demonstrating the selected mesocorticolimbic structures in the dopaminergic reward network, using peak coordinates described by Ballard et al. [21]. Note: red = ventral tegmental area (VTA), blue = nucleus accumbens (NAcc), green = dorsolateral prefrontal cortex (dlPFC).

2.9.1. SWB/Happiness Responses and Gender, Vision, and Hearing Status. Two-tailed *t*-tests were used to compare the mean proportion of responses in each domain category, across three dichotomous groups: gender (male vs female), hearing status (unimpaired vs impaired), and vision status (unimpaired vs impaired). We used Pearson's chi-squared tests to compare the proportions of individuals in each of these dichotomous groupings who listed at least one response in each domain.

2.9.2. SWB/Happiness Responses and Cognitive Performance. Global cognitive performance, indexed via BTACT composite score (derived via factor analysis on our sample of data), exhibited a Gaussian distribution and was analyzed as a continuous variable. We do not dichotomize the cognitive variable because we lack the data to determine a valid cut-point to delineate normal cognition based on this composite score. Pearson correlations assessed the relationship between cognitive performance and total number of "happy task" responses, as well as the proportion of responses in each of the 13 domains.

2.9.3. Adjusted Models. After examining the bivariate relationships between SWB response patterns and gender, vision status, and hearing status, fully adjusted regression models were built. All models included the following independent variables included as predictors: age, gender, education level, GDS score, number of comorbid medical conditions, hearing status (unimpaired or impaired), and vision status (unimpaired or impaired). We constructed adjusted models with the following dependent variables: total number of SWB responses, proportion of responses in any domain with a mean proportion ≥20%. We did not examine adjusted models of proportions if the mean proportion was <20% because in such cases, the distribution of proportions is highly skewed, with many participants having zero responses in that domain. In models where the dependent variable was the total number of SWB responses, Animal Naming score was also included as an independent variable, to control for verbal fluency ability. In models where the dependent variable was proportion of responses in a given domain, BTACT composite score was included as an independent variable to adjust for global cognitive status. We did not include both Animal Naming score and BTACT composite score in the same models, as these two cognitive test scores were highly collinear. Collinearity of the other variables in the models was evaluated, and no two variables exceeded our threshold for unacceptable collinearity, which was a Pearson's correlation coefficient (CC) >0.7 (the highest CC was 0.49 for hearing impairment and age) (Table 1).

2.9.4. SWB/Happiness Responses and Brain Connectivity. To examine relationships between the SWB data and reward network activity, average FC between pairs of selected regions in this network, as previously described [21], was calculated. The regions in the previously described network included the ventral tegmental area (VTA) (left and right VTA averaged together), nucleus accumbens (NAcc) (left and right NAcc averaged together), and left dorsolateral prefrontal cortex (DLPFC). We examined connectivity between each pairwise combination of nodes (VTA-NAcc; VTA-DLPFC; NAcc-DLPFC). FC between each pair of regions was subsequently correlated to the proportion of responses belonging to each of the 12 domains. Fully adjusted regression models were built with FC (of each region pairing) as the dependent variable and the following independent variables: proportion of responses in a domain, age, gender, education, GDS score, number of comorbidities, vision status (impaired/not impaired), hearing status (impaired/not impaired), and BTACT composite score.

Statistical analyses were performed using JMP software from SAS (Cary, NC). Due to multiple comparisons performed in this exploratory analysis, to reduce the risk of alpha error accounting for spurious conclusions, we set our *p* value threshold for significance at 0.01, which is more conservative than the traditional level of 0.05.

3. Results

3.1. Participant Characteristics. Participant demographics and clinical characteristics are summarized in Table 2. Mean

Table 1: Correlation coefficient matrix of variables included in adjusted models.

	Age	Gender	Education	GDS	CC	VI	HI	BTACT
Age	1.0	−0.07	−0.01	−0.04	0.14	0.13	0.49***	−0.29**
Gender		1.0	−0.07	0.03	−0.15	0.10	−0.19*	0.08
Education			1.0	−0.14	−0.30**	0.10	−0.19*	0.36***
GDS				1.0	0.48***	0.07	0.08	−0.10
CC					1.0	−0.07	0.20*	−0.26**
VI						1.0	0.14	−0.16
HI							1.0	−0.27**
BTACT								1.0

GDS, geriatric depression screen score; CC, chronic condition count; VI, vision impairment; HI, hearing impairment; BTACT, Brief Test of Adult Cognition by Telephone. * $p < 0.05$, ** $p < 0.01$, *** $p < 0.001$.

Table 2: Participant demographics and clinical characteristics.

Characteristics	All participants (n = 114)	Subset with fMRI (n = 57)
Age, mean (SD), y	74.6 (7.8)	73.4 (8.1)
Women, %	54.4	64.9
College degree or higher, %	57.9	61.4
Chronic medical conditions, mean (SD)	2.9 (2.1)	2.2 (1.5)[d]
Geriatric depression scale (GDS), mean (SD)[a]	1.4 (1.9)	1.2 (1.6)
Vision-impaired, %[b]	21.9	24.6
Hearing impaired, %[c]	55.3	49.1

[a]Geriatric depression scale (GDS) short-form: 15-item screening tool used to identify depression in older adults. [b]Defined as visual acuity 20/40 or less in the better eye. [c]Defined as pure-tone average >25 dB HL in the better ear averaged over frequencies of 0.5, 1, 2, and 4 kHz. [d]fMRI subset significantly differs from participants without fMRI (at $p < 0.05$ level).

age of participants was 74.6 years with 54.4% females. Mean short-form GDS score was 1.4 (out of 15) and only three of 114 participants scored within ranges suggestive of depression (i.e., GDS score > 5). While 52.6% of our study samples are diagnosed with AMD in at least one eye, only 21.9% meet our definition of function-limiting vision impairment, which is based on visual acuity in the better-seeing eye. Some AMD participants had unilateral AMD and/or relatively preserved visual acuity despite AMD. Participants with bilateral hearing impairment represented 55.3% of the cohort. Seventeen participants had both vision and hearing impairments, meaning that dual sensory impairment affected 14.9% of the cohort.

With respect to most characteristics, the 57 participants who received an fMRI were similar to those who did not, although those who were eligible and willing to under fMRI tended to report fewer chronic conditions (fMRI subset M = 2.2, SD = 1.5; all participants M = 2.9, SD = 2.1).

3.2. Determinants of SWB: "Happy Task" Response Patterns. The mean number of responses to the "happy task" was 15.2 (SD: 5.5, range 4–38). Of the 1731 responses across all participants, 1715 (99.08%) were categorized into one of 12 mutually exclusive domains of SWB, as described in the Methods section. 237 (13.7%) of the 1731 total responses to the SWB task were additionally categorized in the "vision-dependent" category. The results of the qualitative content analysis are summarized in Table 3. Responses most frequently belonged to the domains of social relationships and avocation/hobbies. Other highly prevalent domains included financial/material wealth, ingestibles (i.e., food, beverage), and nature-themed responses.

3.3. Response Patterns According to Gender, Vision Status, and Hearing Status. There was no significant difference in the number of responses to the "happy task" by gender (male: M = 14.27, SD = 4.79; female: M = 15.95, SD = 5.99; $t(112)$ = 1.67, p = 0.11). As shown in Table 4, no gender-based differences in response patterns met our criteria for statistical significance ($p < 0.01$), although males were somewhat more likely to list responses in categories of ingestibles (73.08% vs. 54.84%, p = 0.04) and financial wealth (65.38% vs. 48.39%, p = 0.07), while females were more likely to list social relationship responses (96.77% vs. 86.54%, p = 0.04). Individuals with and without vision impairment listed similar numbers of responses to the SWB prompt (vision-impaired: M = 14.52, SD = 4.82; non-vision-impaired: M = 15.37, SD = 5.71; $t(45)$ = 0.75, p = 0.50). Visually impaired participants were more likely to express avocation (100% vs. 84.27%, p = 0.03) and vision-dependent (92.00% vs. 69.66%, p = 0.02) responses (e.g., completing a crossword puzzle), compared to nonvisually impaired peers, although these differences do not meet our threshold for significance. Participants with hearing impairment listed significantly fewer responses overall (hearing-impaired: M = 13.59, SD = 4.72; non-hearing-impaired: M = 17.16, SD = 5.83; $t(96)$ = 3.53, p = 0.001), although this result did not retain significance after adjustment for age, gender, education, GDS score, Animal Naming score, number of comorbid medical conditions, and vision impairment status (p = 0.06; see Table 5). Also, adjusted analyses (Table 5) revealed that hearing-impaired participants listed higher proportions of social relationship responses ($t(111)$ = 3.22, p = 0.01) and in unadjusted analyses (Table 4), lower proportions of special events responses (e.g., holidays and parties, $t(85)$ = 2.51, p = 0.01), compared to non-hearing-impaired peers.

Table 3: Qualitative content analysis of responses to the task "name things that make people happy" (n = 114 participants, n = 1731 responses).

Domains	% participants with at least one response in the corresponding domain (%)	Mean proportion of responses per participant
Social relationships[a]	92.11	0.23
Material wealth[b]	56.14	0.08
Physical activity[c]	47.37	0.06
Accomplishments[d]	33.33	0.04
Religious involvement[e]	19.30	0.01
Health factors[f]	15.79	0.02
Volunteerism/altruism[g]	12.28	0.02
Avocation/hobbies[h]	87.72	0.28
Ingestibles[i]	63.16	0.09
Special events[j]	37.72	0.06
Nature[k]	50.88	0.08
Positive emotion[l]	31.58	0.03
Vision-dependent tasks[m]	74.56	0.14

[a]Examples include marriage, love, spouse, family, children, companionship, and friends. [b]Examples include money, new house, nice clothes, and jewelry. [c]Examples include going to the gym, exercise, running, swimming, and playing sports. [d]Examples include getting a promotion, earning a good grade, succeeding, and winning a prize. [e]Examples include prayer, fellowship, attending church, and faith. [f]Examples include good health, sight, dressing oneself, and hearing. [g]Examples include volunteer work, being helpful, visiting the sick, and doing favors for others. [h]Examples include watching sports, playing cards, reading, gardening, and fishing. [i]Examples include eating, specific food items, wine, and beer. [j]Examples include holidays, birthdays, parties, graduations, and weddings. [k]Examples include scenery, sunshine, ocean, mountains, and nice weather. [l]Examples include laughter, smiles, fun, jokes, and happiness. [m]Examples include completing a crossword puzzle, watching television, and driving a vehicle.

Table 4: Name things that make people happy: comparison of response patterns by gender, vision, and hearing status.

Domains of SWB	Gender			Vision			Hearing		
	Male	Female	p^a	Nml	Abn	p^a	Nml	Abn	p^a
Social relationships	86.54	96.77	0.04	89.89	100.0	0.10	86.27	96.83	0.04
Material wealth	65.38	48.39	0.07	59.55	44.00	0.17	56.86	55.56	0.89
Physical activity	40.38	53.23	0.17	44.94	56.00	0.33	54.90	41.27	0.15
Accomplishments	32.69	33.87	0.89	37.08	20.00	0.11	31.37	34.92	0.69
Religion	21.15	17.74	0.21	19.10	20.00	0.92	15.69	22.22	0.38
Health factors	15.38	16.13	0.91	15.73	16.00	0.97	15.69	15.87	0.98
Volunteerism/altruism	7.69	16.13	0.17	11.24	16.00	0.52	7.84	15.87	0.19
Avocation/hobbies	84.62	90.32	0.36	84.27	100.0	0.03	92.16	84.13	0.19
Ingestibles	73.08	54.84	0.04	64.04	60.00	0.71	66.67	60.32	0.48
Special events	32.69	41.94	0.31	40.45	28.00	0.26	50.98	26.98	<0.01
Nature	44.23	56.45	0.19	52.81	44.00	0.44	58.82	44.44	0.13
Positive emotion	34.62	29.03	0.52	28.09	44.00	0.13	35.29	28.57	0.44
Vision-dependent tasks	69.23	79.03	0.23	69.66	92.00	0.02	80.39	69.84	0.20

SWB, subjective well-being; Nml, normal; Abn, abnormal. [a]p values for the comparison of the proportion of individuals in each group who listed any response in that domain (by two-tailed t-test). Due to multiple comparisons in this exploratory analysis, our alpha error threshold for statistical significance was set at $p \leq 0.01$.

3.4. Response Patterns and Cognitive Status. As expected, number of responses to the "happy task" was associated with both Animal Naming task verbal fluency scores (R^2 (112) = 0.28, p = 0.001) and BTACT composite scores (R^2 (112) = 0.23, p = 0.001). As BTACT composite score declined, the proportion of responses belonging to the social relationships category increased (R^2 (112) = 0.06, p = 0.01). No significant relationships were observed between cognitive status and proportion of responses in other SWB domains.

3.5. Response Patterns and Brain Connectivity in the Mesolimbic Dopaminergic Reward Network. As summarized in Table 6, participants who listed an accomplishment-themed response (e.g., getting a promotion, earning an "A" on an exam, winning a prize) had significantly higher mean resting FC between VTA and NAcc, compared to those who did not list an accomplishment-themed response (M = 0.624, SD = 0.182 vs. M = 0.477, SD = 0.200; t(55) = 2.58, p = 0.01). In addition, as the proportion of responses belonging to the accomplishment domain increased, mean connectivity between VTA and NAcc increased (R^2 (55) = 0.104, p = 0.01) and remained significant in fully adjusted multivariate regression models. Participants with higher GDS scores tended to have lower mean functional connectivity between VTA and NAcc (R^2 (55) = 0.09, p = 0.02); however, this relationship was attenuated in the fully adjusted model.

4. Discussion

This exploratory study investigates how interperson variability in self-expressed determinants of happiness,

TABLE 5: Predictors of response patterns: results of multivariate regression models.

Model variables	"Happy" task score[a]		Proportion of responses belonging to the "social relationship" domain		Proportion of responses belonging to the "avocation/ hobbies" domain	
	β	P	β	p	β	p
Age	−0.01	0.93	−0.20	0.05	0.00	0.08
Gender	0.97	0.29	0.10	0.28	0.06	0.12
Education level	0.38	0.37	0.08			0.89
< High school	—	—	0.18	—	−0.02	—
High school	—	—	0.17	—	−0.04	—
College	—	—	−0.35	—	−0.14	—
Graduate	—	—	0.08	—	−0.01	—
GDS-SF score	−0.13	0.61	0.05	0.63	0.00	0.69
Comorbid medical conditions	−0.26	0.27	−0.05	0.65	0.01	0.26
BTACT composite score	N/A	N/A	−0.17	0.09	0.03	0.23
Animal Naming score	0.45	<0.001	N/A	N/A	N/A	N/A
Hearing status	−2.00	0.06	−0.39	<0.001	−0.01	0.76
Vision status	−0.65	0.55	−0.03	0.71	0.09	0.04

Note. In the model that predicted SWB "happy" task score, Animal Naming score was included to control for intrinsic semantic fluency ability; in the model that predicted the proportion of responses (not total number of responses), we adjusted instead for global cognitive BTACT score. GDS-SF, geriatric depression scale short-form; BTACT, Brief Test of Adult Cognition by Telephone. [a]Total number of responses to the 60-second "name things that make people happy" task.

TABLE 6: Resting-state functional connectivity of meso-corticolimbic regions in a reward network, among participants with and without "Happy task" responses in the accomplishment domain (n = 57).

Regions of interest	Function connectivity, mean		p^a
	+ Accomplishment	− Accomplishment	
VTA - NAcc	0.63	0.48	0.01
VTA - dlPFC	−0.07	−0.03	0.61
NAcc - dlPFC	−0.15	−0.04	0.20

VTA, ventral tegmental area; NAcc, nucleus accumbens; dlPFC, dorsolateral prefrontal cortex. [a]p values derived from regression models in which dependent variable is functional connectivity (FC). Adjusted models included the following independent variables: proportion of responses in accomplishment domain, age, gender, education level, depression score, comorbidity count, BTACT cognitive score, vision status (impaired/unimpaired), hearing status (impaired/unimpaired). The p value indicates whether there was a significant association between FC and proportion of responses in the accomplishment domain.

generated by the simple task "name things that make people happy," relates to sensory and cognitive health in a group of older adults. We additionally investigated relationships between response patterns and neural activity in a prespecified brain network. To our knowledge, this is the first study to examine potential neural underpinnings of SWB determinants among older adults with varying levels of age-related sensory and cognitive function.

Qualitative content analysis and subsequent statistical analyses revealed few significant differences in response patterns based on participants' gender, vision, hearing, or cognitive status. Hearing-impaired individuals listed fewer responses overall, but this difference did not remain statistically significant after adjusting for demographic variables, depressive symptoms, comorbidity, vision status, and semantic fluency score (Animal Naming). The proportion of responses categorized into 13 different "domains" of SWB was also fairly consistent across the participant groups. The fact that a relatively stable pattern of responses was elicited in this cohort, in men and women and across varying degrees of sensory and cognitive function, supports the validity of existing SWB frameworks and important commonalities in perceptions of happiness.

A few group differences in response patterns did exceed our conservative threshold for statistical significance and are notable. Worse global cognitive scores were significantly associated with higher proportions of responses in the social relationship domain, which was also the most common domain overall. Hearing-impaired individuals also listed higher proportions of social relationship responses and lower proportions of special event responses, compared to individuals with unimpaired hearing. The reasons for these patterns cannot be determined from available data, and there is a paucity of literature on how changes in cognition and sensory function may influence the drivers of one's happiness. One possibility is that impaired individuals are more dependent on friends and family, and thus the role of social relationships in determining happiness becomes especially salient in the setting of cognitive and sensory impairment. An alternative possibility is that hearing or cognitive impairments may challenge social relationships, creating a tendency for impaired individuals to be more aware of them. This rationale may be consistent with the separate (but not statistically significant) finding that vision-impaired individuals were more likely to list responses in the category of vision-dependent activities (e.g., painting and working crossword puzzles). A tendency to list more of these activities as "things that make people happy" may reflect nostalgic thoughts, or greater appreciation for activities that have been rendered more difficult (or impossible) by one's sensory loss. On the contrary, the tendency for hearing-impaired individuals to exhibit a lower proportion of responses about special events (e.g., weddings, Christmas parties) may reflect reduced enjoyment of such events due to hearing impairment.

In light of the high prevalence of sensory and cognitive impairment in the aging population, further research to understand how these aspects of function shape one's happiness is merited. Our study was motivated by previous work which has shown that individuals with sensory and cognitive deficits tend to report diminished quality of life and life satisfaction [37–40]. By identifying differences in perceived contributors to happiness, we hoped the present study would hint at which domains of SBW are most threatened by age-related impairments, or may suggest opportunities to preserve quality of life for impaired individuals. Overall, our findings point toward a relatively stable framework of determinants of happiness, but suggest that interventions that bolster social relationships may be especially valuable for people with cognitive and hearing impairments.

We also examined relationships between self-described determinants of happiness and average connectivity levels within a functional brain network. We observed that functional connectivity between the VTA and NAcc was higher in those who listed accomplishment-themed responses, versus those who listed fewer or no responses in that domain. Responses in the accomplishment domain included items such as "winning" or "getting promoted", and it is possible that individuals who listed responses in that domain were primed, at a neural level, to associate feelings of happiness or pleasure with reward pursuit.

Primate studies have identified structural connectivity between the VTA and both the NAcc and PFC [41]. Importantly, the network we examined was identified in the context of a reward anticipation task [21]. A more recent human study examined resting-state connectivity of dopaminergic midbrain regions and observed intrinsic coupling between the VTA and NAcc, but not the VTA and PFC, at rest [42]. The authors suggest that VTA-PFC coupling might be observed specifically during task engagement or initiation of motivated behavior (hence observation of VTA-PFC connectivity during task performance in Ballard et al. [21]), but not during rest. Additionally, animal studies have shown that the VTA sends dopaminergic projections to the NAcc [43, 44] and the NAcc sends back modulatory input to VTA [45]. In general, these reciprocal communications are thought to be an integral component of the mesolimbic dopamine circuit mediating reward and motivation—a circuit which might include PFC during task engagement, but potentially not while in the resting state. If this is the case, our observation that participants with more reward-themed responses did not exhibit higher connectivity between VTA-PFC or NAcc-PFC at rest is not unexpected, although these individuals might exhibit stronger connections between these regions during task performance. Testing this prediction remains a direction for future research.

Another novel aspect of our analysis was the use of qualitative data from the patient-centered SWB task, which is based on unique lists generated by our participants. The tool is feasible, even in people with some degree of cognitive and hearing impairments, and it provides a rich diversity in the types of responses generated. In addition, the open-ended nature of the prompt allows for spontaneous insights about perceived contributors to happiness, rather than eliciting SWB data through any particular theoretical lens. In addition, because participants are asked to name things that make people happy (rather than "make *you* happy"), the tool may reveal perceptions about societal expectations of happiness, as opposed to more personal determinants of happiness. The pattern of responses elicited is consistent with prior literature which suggests that global life satisfaction, or personal happiness, might be characterized as a multidimensional construct with many domain-specific determinants [7].

Our study has important limitations. The "happy task" we used to gain insights about determinants of SWB has not been validated for this purpose, and this approach should be considered exploratory. If participants were asked about determinants of their own happiness (rather than "name things that make people happy"), we may have observed greater differences in response patterns as a function of sensory and cognitive status. Additionally, we cannot infer from the data how the specific SWB categories we identified relate to the respondents' concept of happiness (e.g., did respondents perceive happiness as a multidimensional construct, or a unidimensional construct with multiple potential predictors?). Another limitation is that although the task is feasible in people with some cognitive impairment, certain cognitive deficits likely influence performance on the task. The parent study excluded individuals with a known diagnosis of dementia or who lacked capacity to give consent, but we did observe variations in cognitive test performance within the study population. Although we attempted to adjust for cognitive ability statistically, formal testing for dementia-related diagnoses was not performed. Despite these limitations, we believe the tool has face validity as a means to reveal individual perspectives about factors that contribute to subjective sense of happiness.

Additional limitations of the study include its cross-sectional design, which prohibits us from inferring causal attributions from the observed correlations. Despite attempts to control for a number of confounders, including demographics and health factors, it remains possible that additional confounding factors influenced the relationships and group differences described here. Further, this study examined the effect of visual, hearing, and cognitive impairment separately, but future studies should investigate how multiple, coexisting impairments might interact to impact well-being. Lastly, given the exploratory nature of our investigation, analysis was conducted without correction for multiple comparisons, although we applied a conservative statistical significance threshold. Given that this particular single-item measure is unique to the present study, we felt that the use of an exploratory approach was justified in characterizing the types of response patterns generated in different populations; however, these findings require confirmation, as well as characterization of test-retest reliability, in a follow-up sample.

In conclusion, in an older adult sample, we found that sensory and cognitive statuses were associated with relatively few differences in the types and patterns of responses elicited by a simple prompt: "name things that make people happy". The most notable exception was that individuals with hearing impairment produced a higher proportion of responses related to "social relationships" and a lower proportion of responses related to "special events". Although it is perhaps intuitive that subjective perceptions about determinants of happiness and well-being might be influenced by our ability to perceive the environment, interact with people around us, and make sense of those inputs and experiences, this study identified a specific relationship between an age-related sensory deficit and determinants of SWB. In addition, we found that individual differences in intrinsic functional connectivity within a brain network associated with reward processing may be associated with differences in perceived contributors to happiness. These results are exploratory, but were motivated by prior work indicating relationships between neural function and individual variability in well-being [24, 25]. Future longitudinal studies, qualitative research, and task-based MRI research will help elucidate further how age-related health changes may affect SWB, and how differences in our notions about happiness may be supported by neural function, with the ultimate goal of optimizing programs and services that promote SWB in seniors coping with sensory and cognitive loss.

Conflicts of Interest

The authors declare that they have no conflicts of interest.

Acknowledgments

This work was supported by grants from the National Institute on Aging (R01AG043438 and P30 AG028716). The funding agencies had no role in the conduct of the study or interpretation of results.

References

[1] E. Diener, "Assessing subjective well-being: progress and opportunities," *Social Indicators Research*, vol. 31, no. 2, pp. 103–157, 1994.

[2] D. J. Disabato, F. R. Goodman, T. B. Kashdan, J. L. Short, and A. Jarden, "Different types of well-being? A cross-cultural examination of hedonic and eudaimonic well-being," *Psychological Assessment*, vol. 28, no. 5, pp. 471–482, 2016.

[3] A. S. Waterman, "Two conceptions of happiness: contrasts of personal expressiveness (eudaimonia) and hedonic enjoyment," *Journal of personality and social psychology*, vol. 64, no. 4, pp. 678–691, 1993.

[4] L. Lu and J. B. Shih, "Sources of happiness: a qualitative approach," *Journal of Social Psychology*, vol. 137, no. 2, pp. 181–187, 1997.

[5] R. Layard, "Measuring subjective well-being," *Science*, vol. 327, no. 5965, pp. 534-535, 2010.

[6] B. Vanhoutte, "The multidimensional structure of subjective well-being in later life," *Journal of Population Ageing*, vol. 7, no. 1, pp. 1–20, 2014.

[7] L. K. George, "Still happy after all these years: research frontiers on subjective well-being in later life," *Journals of Gerontology Series B: Psychological Sciences and Social Sciences*, vol. 65B, no. 3, pp. 331–339, 2010.

[8] U. Kunzmann, T. D. Little, and J. Smith, "Is age-related stability of subjective well-being a paradox? Cross-sectional and longitudinal evidence from the Berlin Aging Study," *Psychology and aging*, vol. 15, no. 3, pp. 511–526, 2000.

[9] L. L. Carstensen, M. Pasupathi, U. Mayr, and J. R. Nesselroade, "Emotional experience in everyday life across the adult life span," *Journal of Personality and Social Psychology*, vol. 79, no. 4, pp. 644–655, 2000.

[10] D. K. Mroczek and C. M. Kolarz, "The effect of age on positive and negative affect: a developmental perspective on happiness," *Journal of Personality and Social Psychology*, vol. 75, no. 5, pp. 1333–1349, 1998.

[11] M. Mather and L. L. Carstensen, "Aging and motivated cognition: the positivity effect in attention and memory," *Trends in Cognitive Sciences*, vol. 9, no. 10, pp. 496–502, 2005.

[12] L. L. Carstensen, D. M. Isaacowitz, and S. T. Charles, "Taking time seriously: a theory of socioemotional selectivity," *American Psychologist*, vol. 54, no. 3, pp. 165–181, 1999.

[13] S. Gauthier, B. Reisberg, M. Zaudig et al., "Mild cognitive impairment," *The Lancet*, vol. 367, no. 9518, pp. 1262–1270, 2006.

[14] H. C. Comijs, M. G. Dik, M. J. Aartsen, D. J. H. Deeg, and C. Jonker, "The impact of change in cognitive functioning and cognitive decline on disability, well-being, and the use of healthcare services in older persons," *Dementia and geriatric cognitive disorders*, vol. 19, no. 5-6, pp. 316–323, 2005.

[15] R. Varma, T. S. Vajaranant, B. Burkemper et al., "Visual impairment and blindness in adults in the United States," *JAMA Ophthalmology*, vol. 134, no. 7, pp. 802–809, 2016.

[16] F. R. Lin, R. Thorpe, S. Gordon-Salant, and L. Ferrucci, "Hearing loss prevalence and risk factors among older adults in the United States," *Journals of Gerontology Series A: Biological Sciences and Medical Sciences*, vol. 66A, no. 5, pp. 582–590, 2011.

[17] E.-M. Chia, P. Mitchell, E. Rochtchina, S. Foran, M. Golding, and J. J. Wang, "Association between vision and hearing impairments and their combined effects on quality of life," *Archives of Ophthalmology*, vol. 124, no. 10, pp. 1465–1470, 2006.

[18] C. D. Mulrow, C. Aguilar, J. E. Endicott et al., "Association between hearing impairment and the quality of life of elderly individuals," *Journal of the American Geriatrics Society*, vol. 38, no. 1, pp. 45–50, 2015.

[19] M. Bazargan, R. S. Baker, and S. H. Bazargan, "Sensory impairments and subjective well-being among aged African American persons," *Journals of Gerontology Series B: Psychological Sciences and Social Sciences*, vol. 56, no. 5, pp. P268–P278, 2001.

[20] H.-W. Wahl, P. M. Drapaniotis, and V. Heyl, "Functional ability loss in sensory impaired and sensory unimpaired very old adults: analyzing causal relations with positive affect

across four years," *Experimental Gerontology*, vol. 59, pp. 65–73, 2014.

[21] I. C. Ballard, V. P. Murty, R. M. Carter, J. J. MacInnes, S. A. Huettel, and R. A. Adcock, "Dorsolateral prefrontal cortex drives mesolimbic dopaminergic regions to initiate motivated behavior," *Journal of Neuroscience*, vol. 31, no. 28, pp. 10340–10346, 2011.

[22] R. A. Bressan and J. A. Crippa, "The role of dopamine in reward and pleasure behaviour—review of data from preclinical research," *Acta Psychiatrica Scandinavica*, vol. 111, no. 427, pp. 14–21, 2005.

[23] J. D. Salamone, M. Correa, A. Farrar, and S. M. Mingote, "Effort-related functions of nucleus accumbens dopamine and associated forebrain circuits," *Psychopharmacology*, vol. 191, no. 3, pp. 461–482, 2007.

[24] H. L. Urry, J. B. Nitschke, I. Dolski et al., "Making a life worth living," *Psychological Science*, vol. 15, no. 6, pp. 367–372, 2016.

[25] A. S. Heller, C. M. van Reekum, S. M. Schaefer et al., "Sustained striatal activity predicts eudaimonic well-being and cortisol output," *Psychological Science*, vol. 24, no. 11, pp. 2191–2200, 2013.

[26] M. L. Kringelbach and K. C. Berridge, "Towards a functional neuroanatomy of pleasure and happiness," *Trends in cognitive sciences*, vol. 13, no. 11, pp. 479–487, 2009.

[27] L. Bäckman, L. Nyberg, U. Lindenberger, S.-C. Li, and L. Farde, "The correlative triad among aging, dopamine, and cognition: current status and future prospects," *Neuroscience & Biobehavioral Reviews*, vol. 30, no. 6, pp. 791–807, 2006.

[28] M. M. Baltes and L. L. Carstensen, "The process of successful aging: selection, optimization, and compensation," in *Understanding Human Development*, pp. 81–104, Springer, Berlin, Germany, 2003.

[29] P. A. Fuld, "The fuld object-memory evaluation," in *Company SI*, Stoelting Company, Chicago, IL, USA, 1981.

[30] C. Hirneiss, "The impact of a better-seeing eye and a worse-seeing eye on vision-related quality of life," *Clinical Ophthalmology*, vol. 8, pp. 1703–1709, 2014.

[31] P. A. Tun and M. E. Lachman, "Telephone assessment of cognitive function in adulthood: the brief test of adult cognition by telephone," *Age and Ageing*, vol. 35, no. 6, pp. 629–632, 2006.

[32] A. U. Monsch, M. W. Bondi, N. Butters, D. P. Salmon, R. Katzman, and L. J. Thal, "Comparisons of verbal fluency tasks in the detection of dementia of the Alzheimer type," *Archives of Neurology*, vol. 49, no. 12, pp. 1253–1258, 1992.

[33] J. I. Sheikh and J. A. Yesavage, "Geriatric Depression Scale (GDS): recent evidence and development of a shorter version," *Clinical Gerontologist*, vol. 5, pp. 165–173, 1986.

[34] S. Elo and H. Kyngäs, "The qualitative content analysis process," *Journal of Advanced Nursing*, vol. 62, no. 1, pp. 107–115, 2008.

[35] P. Dolan, T. Peasgood, and M. White, "Do we really know what makes us happy? A review of the economic literature on the factors associated with subjective well-being," *Journal of Economic Psychology*, vol. 29, no. 1, pp. 94–122, 2008.

[36] M. D. Greicius, B. Krasnow, A. L. Reiss, and V. Menon, "Functional connectivity in the resting brain: a network analysis of the default mode hypothesis," *Proceedings of the National Academy of Sciences*, vol. 100, no. 1, pp. 253–258, 2002.

[37] C. Carabellese, I. Appollonio, R. Rozzini et al., "Sensory impairment and quality of life in a community elderly population," *Journal of the American Geriatrics Society*, vol. 41, no. 4, pp. 401–407, 2015.

[38] F. Cacciatore, C. Napoli, P. Abete, E. Marciano, M. Triassi, and F. Rengo, "Quality of life determinants and hearing function in an elderly population: Osservatorio Geriatrico Campano Study Group," *Gerontology*, vol. 45, no. 6, pp. 323–328, 1999.

[39] W. J. Strawbridge, M. I. Wallhagen, S. J. Shema, and G. A. Kaplan, "Negative consequences of hearing impairment in old age," *Gerontologist*, vol. 40, no. 3, pp. 320–326, 2000.

[40] N. L. Hill, C. McDermott, J. Mogle et al., "Subjective cognitive impairment and quality of life: a systematic review," *International Psychogeriatrics*, vol. 29, no. 12, pp. 1965–1977, 2017.

[41] S. N. Haber and J. L. Fudge, "The primate substantia nigra and VTA: integrative circuitry and function," *Critical Reviews in Neurobiology*, vol. 11, no. 4, pp. 323–342, 1997.

[42] V. P. Murty, M. Shermohammed, D. V. Smith, R. M. Carter, S. A. Huettel, and R. A. Adcock, "Resting state networks distinguish human ventral tegmental area from substantia nigra," *Neuroimage*, vol. 100, pp. 580–589, 2014.

[43] H. L. Fields, G. O. Hjelmstad, E. B. Margolis, and S. M. Nicola, "Ventral tegmental area neurons in learned appetitive behavior and positive reinforcement," *Annual Review of Neuroscience*, vol. 30, no. 1, pp. 289–316, 2007.

[44] M. F. Roitman, R. A. Wheeler, R. M. Wightman, and R. M. Carelli, "Real-time chemical responses in the nucleus accumbens differentiate rewarding and aversive stimuli," *Nature Neuroscience*, vol. 11, no. 12, pp. 1376-1377, 2008.

[45] A. A. Grace, S. B. Floresco, Y. Goto, and D. J. Lodge, "Regulation of firing of dopaminergic neurons and control of goal-directed behaviors," *Trends in Neurosciences*, vol. 30, no. 5, pp. 220–227, 2007.

21

Perspectives on the Role and Synergies of Architecture and Social and Built Environment in Enabling Active Healthy Aging

Evangelia Chrysikou,[1] Richard Rabnett,[2] and Chariklia Tziraki[3]

[1]*Faculty of the Built Environment, UCL Bartlett School of Architecture, 140 Hampstead Rd., London NW1 2BX, UK*
[2]*AM-GAR, Hashdera Hamerkazit 15, Ligad 1, 7173003 Modi'in, Israel*
[3]*MELABEV-Community Elders Club, Research and Evaluation Department and Hebrew University of Jerusalem, Israel Gerontological Data Center, 9190501 Mount Scopus, Israel*

Correspondence should be addressed to Evangelia Chrysikou; e.chrysikou@ucl.ac.uk

Academic Editor: Illario Maddalena

Research has demonstrated that enabling societal and physical infrastructure and personal accommodations enhance healthy and active aging throughout the lifespan. Yet, there is a paucity of research on how to bring together the various disciplines involved in a multidomain synergistic collaboration to create new living environments for aging. This paper aims to explore the key domains of skills and knowledge that need to be considered for a conceptual prototype of an enabling educational process and environments where healthcare professionals, architects, planners, and entrepreneurs may establish a shared theoretical and experiential knowledge base, vocabulary, and implementation strategies, for the creation of the next generation of living communities of active healthy adults, for persons with disabilities and chronic disease conditions. We focus on synergistic, paradigmatic, simple, and practical issues that can be easily upscaled through market mechanisms. This practical and physically concrete approach may also become linked with more elaborate neuroscientific and technologically sophisticated interventions. We examine the domains of knowledge to be included in establishing a learning model that focuses on the still-understudied impact of the benefits toward active and healthy aging, where architects, urban planners, clinicians, and healthcare facility managers are educated toward a synergistic approach at the operational level.

1. Introduction

According to the World Health Organization (WHO), physical and social environments are key determinants in maintaining an autonomous, meaningful life along the aging process [1]. Research from epidemiological studies and social sciences has provided sufficient evidence that maintaining health, independency, and autonomy would imbue longevity with wellbeing, a more meaningful life span, and lower healthcare costs. Urban planning, architecture of healthcare facilities that promote healing, and domestic buildings supporting autonomy are important elements in enabling a more active and healthy aging process throughout the life span. Yet, in practice, the fields of traditional healthcare and architecture or urban planning seldom cross paths in either the academic curricula, the research arena, or the actual execution of theory and evidence-based research and planning of these physical spaces within which individuals and societies age [2]. This paper aims to outline the domains of a new model of multidisciplinary learning which takes place in face-to-face interactions with all the interested parties: architects, healthcare providers and managers, and planners. Aging is not a disease, but rather a normal and valued part of the life course, as defined by the WHO [1, p. 103]. In this paper, we briefly present the theoretical complexity and the multidisciplinary nature involved in the planning of the healthcare facilities and domestic living spaces. The three elements comprising this planning: the healthcare framework, the social context and the physical milieu, and their interrelationships. We then present the argument that by examining how to intergrade these three elements in a potentially synergistic enabling educational process would lead the participants to ponder on the integration of these elements in real market scenarios. Our approach is informed by the synergies groups generated by the EIP AHA [3] and planned activities of our commitment to A2 group of the EIP AHA [4].

2. Theoretical Framework

2.1. Health and Society and Space: An Integrated Perspective. Epidemiological studies have identified a strong link between health status and societal domains [5]. The healthcare system and its practitioners are aiming to use this evidence-based knowledge in supporting and advocating policy at the local level for improvement of the social determinants of health including the built environment [6]. Hillier and Hanson's [7] work has contributed significantly to the interconnection and synergies of the built environment, society, and space, arguing that there is a social logic of space and that the linkage is cross-cultural and not age specific [8]. Thus, the link between health and society has been established through public health, and the link between society and space has been established through space syntax [9]. The theory of salutogenesis [10] joints all three domains bridging health and physical space. Salutogenesis, derived from medical sociology, was conceived by Antonovsky [11] who looked at the relationship between stress and wellbeing, through the "Sense of Coherence." Antonovsky's salutogenesis theory focuses on the factors and mechanisms that promote health, not on illness [12]. The multidisciplinary and the intercultural application of the "Sense of Coherence," an essential element of the salutogenic theory [13], has influenced a growing body of research based design framework of the built environment, creating a platform for a creative dialogue between healthcare and architecture [14–16]. Although Antonovsky did not aim directly at the spatial elements, which are considered part of the physical pillar [17] that lead to increase somebody's "Sense of Coherence" [18], his theories has prompted the generation of a variety of fields, including practitioners of medical architecture, salutogenic design or design and health field [19–21], and Healing Gardens [22].

The work of Zeisel on Alzheimer's [23] is a paradigmatic example of the three pillars of Salutogenesis connecting health, space, and society and stresses the benefits deriving from their synergy, as depicted in Figure 1.

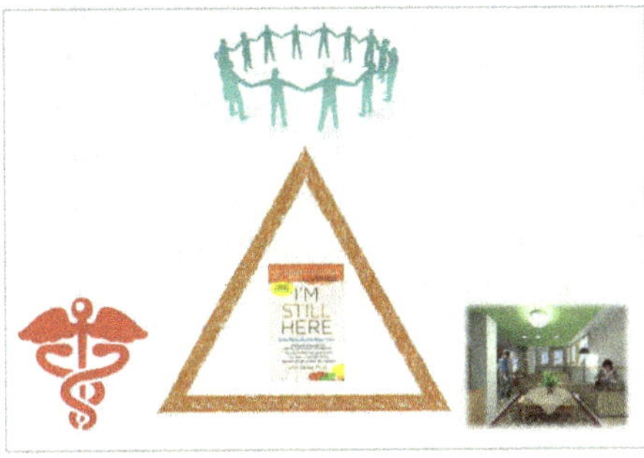

Figure 1: Visual interpretation of Zeisel's three key elements in the treatment and care of people with dementia—the medication, the human interaction, and the physical environment.

Zeisel advocates that although there are three key elements in the treatment and care of people with Alzheimer's, that is, the medication, the human interaction, and the physical environment, funding and research concentrate on the first, reducing considerably the resources allocated to the other two. This disproportionate allocation of resources happens despite the fact that space and human care may have significant, sustained, and immediate impact on health status of dementia person, when compared to pharmaceuticals where progress still needs to be made [23].

In this paper, we aim to highlight the need for synergy between healthcare systems, the built environment, as well as their social context including public and private domains and urban setting as well as the smallest scale of domestic objects and artefacts that can enhance life during the life span.

Despite the evidence suggesting that space is a key component of any healthcare plan, the design of individual dwellings for encouraging active and healthy aging is a truly underdeveloped area of research, compared, for example, to assistive technologies. Yet, the living space and its impact on quality of life are indeed a very ancient concept [24]. The literature regarding active and healthy aging has in general concluded that healthy life styles through the life span contribute to better quality of life including physical, mental, and cognitive capacity. In general, building and urban design lag behind knowledge from relevant fields such as neuroscience, mental health, rehabilitation, and active healthy aging research. Our aim is to help bridge this gap by creating a learning platform for the relevant disciplines that is experiential and theory driven, while at the same time targeted to generating marketable solutions of the built environment. One area where this leaning platform may be considered of urgent importance is the emerging field of adoption of healthier life style patterns and the need for environmental factors to support these changes.

2.2. Life Style Patterns and Environmental Factors to Support Active Healthy Aging (AHA). "More of the Same Is Not Enough" [25] reviews the most recent research efforts to increase physical activity and thus decrease sedentary life styles, especially among older adults, thus contributing to the top ten chronic diseases worldwide [26]. Understanding how to do more to change this "pandemic" pair of sedentary lifestyles and chronic diseases burden requires new approaches to our theoretical understandings of the causes, as well as the design of innovative interventions to change them at the individual level, since the "one-model-fits-all" approach does not take into account the ecological perspective at the root of the problem. The ecological model for changing toward healthier life styles take into account multiple predisposing factors and barriers such as intrapersonal variables (e.g., personality, health beliefs, knowledge, attitudes, and skills), interpersonal processes, and their likely interactions with genetics as well as community and macro/public policy levels factors [27]. Furthermore, research has shown that interventions for change are likely to take place, not in the conventional healthcare system, but rather in what sociologists have labelled "enabling spaces." Virtual or physical enabling spaces provide the opportunity for peer learning and teaching that could be actualized within a community. Copresence and observation could provide the mechanism that would generate this learning [28, 29].

The diversity of noncommunicable chronic diseases (NCDs), which hamper healthy and active aging, also shares key modifiable life style factors: sedentary lifestyles with lack of physical activity, poor nutritional habits, high stress levels, and lack of social connectivity [30]. Each one of these modifiable lifestyle factors can be improved with appropriate attention to how neighborhoods/workspaces are designed, how architectural design enhances the creation of enabling spaces for mingling and connecting physically, and how green spaces and walkable communities create more active aging environments. The regional authorities, planning agencies, and healthcare systems working in synergies may be able to create an ecosystem that supports active and healthy lifestyles throughout the life span. This includes industries of food production and distribution as well as boutique culinary facilities catering to aging populations and their physical needs.

A crucial component of this ecosystem is the enabling of movement. This is primarily viewed through the concept of universal design. It is the main concept that has provided solutions for the mobility of the general population, yet so far it presents limitations when neurological or mental disorders are concerned [31]. User involvement from the planning stage of these facilities was one of the key elements of fit for purpose. Similarly, when designing for extra care homes accessibility, user involvement at the planning and remodelling stages was a crucial element of success as it was the involvement of all professionals involved including architects and builders that were aware of universal design and assistive technologies [32]. The next domain that our theoretical model for a multidisciplinary teaching program focuses on is the role of what is now a serious priority for the EIP AHA and WHO and generally falls under the title of age-friendly environment [33, 34].

3. Age-Friendly Liveable Environment

3.1. Living Styles Supported by Built Environment. The built environment is commonly used in connection with technology supported aging [35]. However, here we would suggest that the WHO definition of environments is more useful in considering healthy and active aging. This definition is broad: "*all the factors in the extrinsic world that form the context of an individual's life; these include home, communities and the broader society; within these environments are a range of factors, including the built environment, people and their relationships, attitudes and values, health and social policies, systems and services*" [1, p. 240]. As it is important for older people to stay at their homes as long as possible [36] some home adaptations might prolong aging in place, the preferred alternative by persons and also a more cost-effective way from a societal perspective [37]. Yet, even if for supported accommodation, research involves physical environment as a determinant of active aging [38] and links QoL with homelike design traits [39, 40] and the fine balance between requirements for safety and homelike environments [41].

In addition to the homelike age-friendly environment, there is an emerging literature of the important connection to nature and its restorative and therapeutic value, along with space for physical and recreative activities in mental health and healthy aging. We discuss these topics next.

3.2. Mental Wellbeing and Nature. Research has long established the beneficial elements of nature to mental and physical wellbeing [42, 43], and there is a strong link between perceived sense of health and availability of green areas especially for the elderly and even more so for those living in urban environments [44]. Its integration in the architectural environment of home can have multiple benefits for the resident, from a window view, to the beneficial feel of a breeze and sunshine, which can be appreciated even by patients with Alzheimer's disease [23], to mild form of exercise or gardening, especially if combined with raised accessible flower beds. Yet, gardening does not cover all potential benefits of incorporating nature into design. For instance, in more complex healthcare environments, views to gardens can act as orientation elements [14].

3.3. Physical Activity Space. As far as physical activity space is concerned, ergonomic design of healthcare facilities, mainly concentrating on nurses' movement, ignored the complications of confined space for patients without access to the outdoors. Single-loaded corridors for instance could increase the opportunity for walks indoors as well as allow better orientation [21]. At a residential environment, however, there could be other solutions for physical exercise that could be creatively codesigned with appropriately trained architect and the input of the carer and the resident.

3.4. Creativity and Social Interaction Spaces. In healthcare environments creativity could be enhanced through a variety of spaces designed for different uses, such as dancing or exercise and space for horticulture, to give to examples out of the numerous possibilities, rather than the one-type-of-common-room-fits-all approach. Research on long-term care connected architecture and the implementation of therapeutic regime through the availability/lack of such areas [45].

3.5. Adjusting an Older Residential Care Facility to Contemporary Dementia Care Visions. In residential settings suitable comfortable sitting, presenting a variety of types in accordance with individual preferences and functional elements such as task lighting, worktops, and variety of storage could provide opportunity that a variation of the "student bedsit" that is often applied in care environments, that is, one desk, one bed with a side table, and a wardrobe, or hopefully if it is like a 4- or a 5-star hotel room an additional armchair and a coffee table, could not possibly cover.

3.6. Visiospatial Orientation. External views, art, and positive or negative distraction methods [23], such as concealing the external door or using clearly visible clues and colour for bathroom doors, might prove invaluable tools for the orientation and the cognitive function of older people and especially those suffering from dementia.

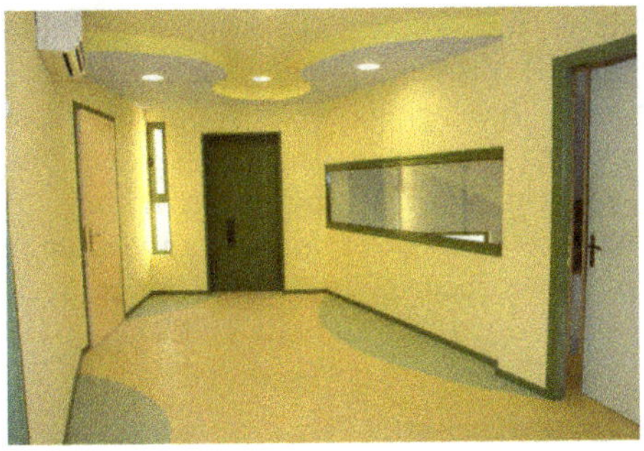

Figure 2: Day Centre for children and adolescents with autism in Paleo Faliro, Greece. Designed by SynThesis Architects.

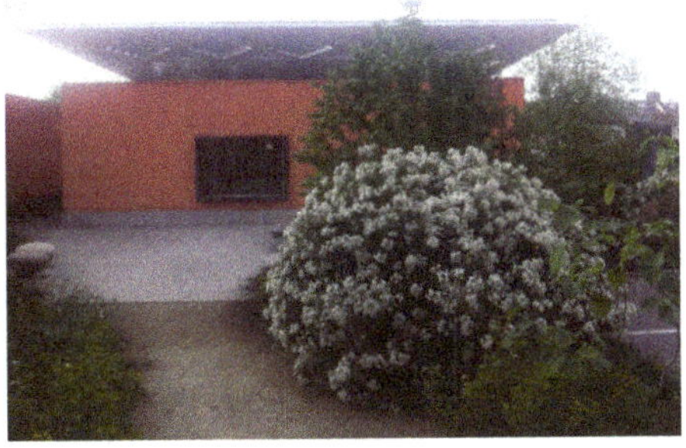

Figure 3: Maggie's West London, located at Charing Cross Hospital. Designed by Rogers Stirk Harbour + Partners.

3.7. Autonomy and Independence. Control is a factor that tends to appear lower in the pyramid of needs, when compared to more basic needs of sustaining life. However, it is linked with improved health [6], mental healthcare [21], and noninstitutional design frameworks that cater for heterogeneity [40, 46]. At a strategic level, control might be expressed through user involvement and through accessibility means that might enter the core of day-to-day life, such as the case of accessible kitchens or fixtures and fittings at a suitable height. In general, the healthcare environments granted significant control to healthcare professionals as opposed to patients [22]. Yet, lately through increasing patient involvement in the design process we have seen projects that grant significant spatial control to the patients (Figure 2). A very interesting example from the area of cancer care provision is the Maggie's Centre initiative (Figure 3), an innovative, holistic type of facility for cancer patients that has been developed from Maggie Jenks, an architect, when she had been diagnosed with terminal cancer [47].

3.8. Fall Prevention Architectural Elements. Lighting, carefully designed circulation spaces, especially in turning points, comfortable and strong grab-rails, preferably cleverly integrated in the decoration rather than the sad and possibly dangerous accessibility devices, opportunities for mind and body exercise for the brain through salutogenic design, and solid and strong furniture at an adequate height for people lifting themselves comfortably are only some of the possibilities that architects can consider as their tools in their aim to design an environment that allows older people to use their body in a safer manner. Yet, the lack of research and the lack of a communication channel between the disciplines have not provided the data that would allow these solutions to be approached systematically and eventually enter the design guidelines documentation allowing their broader implementation.

4. Results and Discussion

Based on the theoretical models and research utilizing these models as cited above, we suggest that the creation of an experiential curriculum for all relevant players in designing and building facilities to meet the needs of an aging society is a goal we should be aspiring to. The planning of this type of curriculum should involve all sectors of the economy, that is, governmental, private, and the third sector, as well as cross-industry from the very beginning. This would utilize the experience of the stakeholders, from policy to user level, and enable the burning issues that are well known to those that deal with the subject on an everyday basis to be addressed in a more systematic way. We are aware, for example, of participatory design initiatives such as the Collectively Commissioned Housing in Casteren, Netherlands, where the architects worked mainly as facilitators and residents were the main decision-makers, which proved a cost-effective solution [48]. Such an approach is important for highlighting the importance of the involvement of the users and the financial gains of similar approaches. Yet for more elaborate dwellings, such as residences for vulnerable populations, this crucial amount of user involvement should be complemented by substantial know-how from the architects on special design aspects and implications. For instance, an excellent case of a synergy between informed architectural intervention and the active involvement of users and carers at all levels of decision-making has been the Foyer Élan Retrouvé in Paris, an accommodation facility for the social reintegration of adult mentally ill patients that generated innovation and at the same time presented high user satisfaction results [21, 49]. Similarly, the close collaboration between staff working on a day centre for children with developmental disabilities and a team including a medical architect and a neuroscientist in Faliro, Athens, presented significant reduction of the autistic behaviour of the children during the time they used the facility. In that case, staff would enable a design that was fully compatible with the care regime and the experts introduced to the design elements such as the evidence-based use of positive and negative distraction through colours, shapes, and patterns [50, 51]. Central to these initiatives has been the task to work on an interdisciplinary language and understanding in order to deliver a more evidence based, inclusive practice.

Medical sciences have a clear knowledge that the perception and the physiology of an older frail person differs from a normative one. Yet, that message has not entered the conscious design process of the built environment professionals, as the perception and visual distraction in architectural literature [52] concentrates on architectural-focused instead of person-focused aims, unrelated to the distortions of perception due to ill health. Moreover, research suggests that architects might have a combination of lack of knowledge and misconceptions on the actual needs and preferences of the elderly and research by design projects, such as the example of a Dementia ward at Flanders [45, 53]. This gap of architectural knowledge and education on the perception and users' needs should make us reflect on the way architectural education is delivered as well as potential for further research.

It would be important, among others, for practitioners, designers, and stakeholders, to understand to what extent the built environment is adequate for its residents. It would be important, for instance, to research the safety of universal design features in an older person's bathroom and ways for improvement. Through learning we could encourage designers to broaden their perspective of what constitutes innovative architecture, in a way more human-focused than the glass and steel iconic landmarks. It would be important to help them understand user needs across the lifespan when designing public outdoor areas. That would be the way to create a series of public space improvements that might encourage people to be confident enough and go out of their home in a not so cold day and engage in social activities. A module should provide students the know-how of facility planning in order to create facilities that could act as a magnet for older and frail people and how these could be intergraded in the urban grid. Through case study learning and fieldtrips they could familiarise themselves with existing examples of good practice that need to be explored and lessons to be learned. They should be able to understand the limitations of the existing definition of accessibility in covering the needs of the largest ever generation approaching old age. It would be also important for all stakeholders to build the skills to comprehend the value of more elaborate and neuroscientific and technologically sophisticated interventions that could generate significant health benefits with relatively low costs. The list is indicative and the authors could by no means cover the whole spectrum of research possibilities and the learning potential in a single paragraph.

4.1. Conclusions. Part of the gap between human science and architecture relates to the educational process of architects, the lack of evidence-based guidelines or best practices that architects could refer to, and the lack of translational research across fields. The article presented a theoretical framework for incorporating into architecture the vision of design for active and healthy living; features medical research suggest would add value toward active and healthy aging.

The challenges aging presents to individuals and society as a whole are complex and multilevel. For example, aging person functionality is impacted by not only one's intrinsic personality but also by ecopsychosocial elements. These multilevel and complex societal domains can be modified through the creation of multidisciplinary knowledge and educational opportunities along with design for wellbeing research to explore the benefits of interlinking space, architecture of living environments, and their impact on physical and cognitive functionality. It is important for medical practitioners to be aware of the developments and opportunities in the built environment and vice versa and at the same time to see the social impact and the extent in terms of social scale of the problem. Creating a multidisciplinary program for the various professionals (architects, doctors, and planners) and aging persons can be accomplished through blended learning curriculum (see, e.g., http://www.eitdigital.eu/eit-digital-academy/master-school/). The EIP AHA through its synergies initiative can play an important leadership role for securing funding to initiate such blended learning environments throughout the EU.

Competing Interests

The authors declare that there is no conflict of interests regarding the publication of this paper.

Acknowledgments

Dr. Evangelia Chrysikou is Chief Investigator of the Planning and Evaluation Methodologies for Mental Healthcare Buildings (PEMETH) project. Dr. Chrysikou's research is funded by the European Union's Horizon 2020 Research and Innovation Programme under the Marie Skłodowska-Curie Grant Agreement no. 658244.

References

[1] WHO, *World Report on Ageing and Health*, World Health Organization, Luxembourg, Luxembourg, 2015.

[2] R. S. Ulrich, L. L. Berry, X. Quan, and J. T. Parish, "A conceptual framework for the domain of evidence-based design," *HERD: Health Environments Research & Design Journal*, vol. 4, no. 1, pp. 95–114, 2010.

[3] European Innovation Partnership on Active and Healthy Ageing, A2 and A3, https://ec.europa.eu/eip/ageing/commitments-tracker/a2/a2-and-a3_en.

[4] European Innovation Partnership on Active and Healthy Ageing, Inclusive Urban and Rural Communities (Commitment), https://ec.europa.eu/eip/ageing/commitments-tracker/d4/inclusive-urban-and-rural-communities_en.

[5] G. P. Westert, F. G. Schellevis, D. H. De Bakker, P. P. Groenewegen, J. M. Bensing, and J. Van Der Zee, "Monitoring health inequalities through general practice: the Second Dutch National Survey of General Practice," *European Journal of Public Health*, vol. 15, no. 1, pp. 59–65, 2005.

[6] M. Marmot, *The Health Gap: The Challenge of an Unequal World*, Bloomsbury Publishing, London, UK, 2015.

[7] B. Hillier and J. Hanson, *Social Logic of Space*, Cambridge University Press, New York, NY, USA, 1988.

[8] C. Alexander, *The Nature of Order, Book Three, Part Two Chapter 3*, Centre for Environmental Structure, Berkeley, Calif, USA, 2003.

[9] A. Penn, "Space syntax and spatial cognition: or why the axial line?" *Environment and Behavior*, vol. 35, no. 1, pp. 30–65, 2003.

[10] A. Antonovsky, "The salutogenic model as a theory to guide health promotion," *Health Promotion International*, vol. 11, no. 1, pp. 11–18, 1996.

[11] A. Antonovsky, *Health, Stress and Coping*, Jossey-Bass, San Francisco, Calif, USA, 1979.

[12] A. Antonovsky, *Unraveling the Mystery of Health: How People Manage Stress and Stay Well*, Jossey Bass Social and Behavioral Science Series, Jossey Bass, San Francisco, Calif, USA, 1987.

[13] M. Eriksson and B. Lindström, "Validity of Antonovsky's sense of coherence scale: a systematic review," *Journal of Epidemiology & Community Health*, vol. 59, no. 6, pp. 460–466, 2005.

[14] I. M. Assali, "Enhance indoor environment in buildings and its effect on improving occupant's health," *International Journal of Civil, Environmental, Structural, Construction and Architectural Engineering*, vol. 10, no. 2, pp. 90–96, 2016.

[15] A. A. Behbehani, *Design for Wellbeing: Investigating the Relationship Between Built Environments and Art Therapy Experiences*, Florida State University, Tallahassee, Fla, USA, 2013.

[16] A. Dilani, "Psychosocially supportive design: a salutogenic approach to the design of the physical environment," *Design and Health Scientific Review*, vol. 1, no. 2, pp. 47–55, 2008.

[17] K. Hudson, "Salutogenesis: the origin of health," *Nursing Management*, vol. 44, no. 11, pp. 12–13, 2013.

[18] European Communities, "Salutogenesis and the promotion of positive mental health in older people," in *Proceedings of the EU Thematic Conference "Mental Health and Well-Being in Older People—Making It Happen"*, Madrid, Spain, April 2010.

[19] A. Dilani, *Healthcare Building as Supportive Environments*, KTH, Landstinget Härnösand, Sweden, 1998.

[20] J. A. Golembiewski, "Start making sense: applying a salutogenic model to architectural design for psychiatric care," *Facilities*, vol. 28, no. 3-4, pp. 100–117, 2010.

[21] E. Chrysikou, *Architecture for Psychiatric Environments: Environments and Therapeutic Spaces*, IOS Press, Amsterdam, Netherlands, 2014.

[22] C. Marcus and M. Barnes, "Introduction: historical and cultural perspective on healing gardens," in *Healing Gardens: Therapeutic Benefits and Design Recommendations*, pp. 1–26, John Wiley & Sons, New York, NY, USA, 1999.

[23] J. Zeisel, *I'm Still Here-A Breakthrough Approach to Understanding Someone Living with Alzheimer's*, Piatkus, London, UK, 2010.

[24] E. M. Sternberg, *Healing Space: The Science of Place and Well-Being*, Harvard University Press, Cambridge, Mass, USA, 2009.

[25] P. C. Hallal, A. E. Bauman, G. W. Heath, H. Kohl III, I. Min Lee, and M. Pratt, *Physical Activity: More of the Same Is Not Enough*, Federal University of Pelotas, Pelotas, Brazil, 2012.

[26] University of Turku, http://www.utu.fi/fi/Sivut/home.aspx.

[27] N. Fitzgerald and K. Spaccarotella, "Barriers to a healthy lifestyle: from individuals to public policy—an ecological perspective," *Journal of Extension*, vol. 47, no. 1, pp. 1–8, 2009.

[28] C. Duff, "Networks, resources and agencies: on the character and production of enabling places," *Health & Place*, vol. 17, no. 1, pp. 149–156, 2011.

[29] A. M. McMurray, "The enabling community for child and family health," *Contemporary Nurse*, vol. 40, no. 1, pp. 2–4, 2011.

[30] S. Ballesteros, E. Kraft, S. Santana, and C. Tziraki, "Maintaining older brain functionality: a targeted review," *Neuroscience & Biobehavioral Reviews*, vol. 55, pp. 453–477, 2015.

[31] E. Chrysikou, "Accessibility for mental healthcare," *Facilities*, vol. 31, no. 9-10, pp. 418–426, 2013.

[32] R. Mayagoitia, E. Van Boxstael, H. Wojgani, F. Wright, J. Hanson, and A. Tinker, "Is extra care housing in England care-neutral?" *Journal of Assistive Technologies*, vol. 9, no. 1, pp. 3–20, 2015.

[33] World Health Organisation, 2016, http://www.who.int/ageing/age-friendly-world/en/.

[34] L. Plouffe and A. Kalache, "Towards global age-friendly cities: determining urban features that promote active aging," *Journal of Urban Health*, vol. 87, no. 5, pp. 733–739, 2010.

[35] Centres for Disease Control and Prevention, *Healthy Aging & The Built Environment*, Centres for Disease Control and Prevention, 2015, http://www.cdc.gov/healthyplaces/healthtopics/healthyaging.htm.

[36] K. Croucher, *Housing Choices and Aspirations of Older People. Research from the New Horizons Programme*, Communities and Local Government, London, UK, 2008.

[37] J. L. Wiles, A. Leibing, N. Guberman, J. Reeve, and R. E. S. Allen, "The meaning of 'aging in place' to older people," *The Gerontologist*, vol. 52, no. 3, pp. 357–366, 2012.

[38] L. Van Malderen, T. Mets, P. De Vriendt, and E. Gorus, "The Active Ageing-concept translated to the residential long-term care," *Quality of Life Research*, vol. 22, no. 5, pp. 929–937, 2013.

[39] S. A. Bradshaw, E. D. Playford, and A. Riazi, "Living well in care homes: a systematic review of qualitative studies," *Age and Ageing*, vol. 41, no. 4, pp. 429–440, 2012.

[40] L. Van Malderen, P. De Vriendt, T. Mets, and E. Gorus, "Active ageing within the nursing home: a study in Flanders, Belgium," *European Journal of Ageing*, vol. 13, no. 3, pp. 219–230, 2016.

[41] I. Van Steenwinkel, S. Baumers, and A. Heylighen, "Home in later life: a framework for the architecture of home environments," *Home Cultures*, vol. 9, no. 2, pp. 195–217, 2012.

[42] C. Maller, M. Townsend, A. Pryor, P. Brown, and L. St Leger, "Healthy nature healthy people: 'contact with nature' as an upstream health promotion intervention for populations," *Health Promotion International*, vol. 21, no. 1, pp. 45–54, 2006.

[43] R. Ulrich, "View through a window may influence recovery from surgery," *Science*, vol. 224, no. 4647, pp. 420–421, 1984.

[44] J. Maas, R. A. Verheij, P. P. Groenewegen, S. de Vries, and P. Spreeuwenberg, "Green space, urbanity, and health: how strong is the relation?" *Journal of Epidemiology and Community Health*, vol. 60, no. 7, pp. 587–592, 2006.

[45] I. Van Steenwinkel, E. Verstraeten, and A. Heylighen, "Adjusting an older residential care facility to contemporary dementia care visions," in *Designing Around People*, P. Langdon, J. Lazar, A. Heylighen, and H. Dong, Eds., Springer, Berlin, Germany, 2016.

[46] T. Marcus, *Buildings and Power: Freedom and Control in the Origin of Modern Building Types*, Routledge, London, UK, 1993.

[47] Maggie's, 2016, https://www.maggiescentres.org.

[48] T. T. Veeger and S. J. E. Maussen, *Dutch Experiment in Co-Creation in a Collectively Commissioned Housing Project*, Architectural Research Addressing Societal Challenges, Taylor & Francis, New York, NY, USA, 2016.

[49] E. Diebolt, *De la Quarantaine au Quarantaine: Histoire dy Foyer de Postcure Psychiatrique de l'Elan*, L' lan Retrouve, Paris, France, 1997.

[50] C. Lustig, K. Giannakopoylou, and E. Chrysikou, "Quality architecture as a means of reducing the functional expenses in health facilities: cooperation of architect, physician and neurologist at a project in Faliro," in *Proceedings of the 4th Panhellenic Congress on Management, Economics and Health Policy*, Athens, Greece, December 2008.

[51] E. Chrysikou and C. Lustig, "Accessibility for fully mobile patients: the case of children with intellectual disabilities and autism spectrum disorder," in *Proceedings of the 7th Cambridge Workshop on Universal Access and Assistive Technology*, P. Langdon, J. Lazar, A. Heylighen, and H. Dong, Eds., chapter 5, pp. 33–38, University of Cambridge, Cambridge, UK, 2014.

[52] A. P. Bader, "A model for everyday experience of the built environment: the embodied perception of architecture," *The Journal of Architecture*, vol. 20, no. 2, pp. 244–267, 2015.

[53] K. Coomans, P.-W. Vermeersch, and A. Heylighen, "How do older residents experience a recently built innovative housing and care facility?" in *Designing Around People*, P. Langdon, J. Lazar, A. Heylighen, and H. Dong, Eds., pp. 209–218, Springer, London, UK, 2016.

22

Do Depressive Traits and Hostility Predict Age-Related Decline in General Intelligence?

Erik Lykke Mortensen,[1,2,3] John Calvin Barefoot,[3,4] and Kirsten Avlund[2,5,6]

[1] *Department of Public Health, Section of Environmental Health, Medical Psychology Unit, University of Copenhagen, Øster Farimagsgade 5 A, 1353 Copenhagen K, Denmark*
[2] *Center for Healthy Aging, Faculty of Health Science, University of Copenhagen, 2200 Copenhagen N, Denmark*
[3] *Institute of Preventive Medicine, Copenhagen University Hospital, Copenhagen, 1353 Copenhagen K, Denmark*
[4] *Department of Psychiatry and Behavioral Sciences, Duke University, Medical Center, Durham, NC 27710, USA*
[5] *Department of Public Health, Section of Social Medicine, University of Copenhagen, 1353 Copenhagen K, Denmark*
[6] *Danish Aging Research Center, Universities of Aarhus, Copenhagen and Southern Denmark, Denmark*

Correspondence should be addressed to Erik Lykke Mortensen, elme@sund.ku.dk

Academic Editor: Denis Gerstorf

Certain personality traits are likely to be associated with stress and distress through the lifespan, and as a consequence these traits may influence the rate of age-related cognitive decline. The present study uses data from the Glostrup 1914 cohort to analyze potential effects of personality on decline in general intelligence over a 30-year period. The Minnesota Multiphasic Personality Inventory was administered at a 50-year baseline exam, and from this inventory the Obvious Depression Scale and an abbreviated version of the Cook-Medley Hostility Scale were derived. At the 50-year baseline and at the 60-, 70-, and 80-year followups the full version of Wechsler's Adult Intelligence Scale (WAIS) was administered to 673, 513, 136, and 184 participants. Mixed effects statistical models were used to evaluate both the effect of the personality scores on level of intelligence and the interaction between the personality scores and the time since followup. Analyses were adjusted for demographic background and a wide range of lifestyle factors. Both obvious depression and hostility were negatively associated with level of intelligence, but personality scores did not influence rate of decline in general intelligence.

1. Introduction

Recent decades have seen a widespread interest in personality and health [1]. This interest partly reflects an increasing focus on personality in a lifespan perspective and on personality and aging. Although personality, aging, and well-being have been investigated in several studies [2], there is very little research on the associations between personality and age-related changes in cognition. This is remarkable because much evidence suggests that stress may impact brain structures involved in cognition [3], and that personality traits associated with increased vulnerability to stress may influence cognition over the lifespan [4]. Thus, Crowe et al. [4] suggested that personality traits associated with stress, depression, and anxiety may be associated with age-related cognitive decline and risk of Alzheimer's disease and demonstrated that the broad personality dimension of neuroticism was in fact associated with higher risk of cognitive impairment. The study was limited by lack of early-life assessment of cognition and by the use of a relatively rough binary measure of cognition based on a telephone interview. However, neuroticism is known to be associated with increased reactivity to environmental stress [5] and has been found to be associated with psychopathology [6], including depression, which is a relatively well-documented risk factor for dementia [7]. If associations between neuroticism and normal age-related cognitive decline could be demonstrated over a wide range of the lifespan, the public health implications would be substantial since normal cognitive decline as a consequence of personality-related vulnerability to stress would affect a much larger part of the general population and presumably would affect individuals over a larger part of their life-span.

Obviously, risk factors for Alzheimer's disease or other forms of dementia are not necessarily risk factors for normal age-related decline. However, studies of personality and normal age-related cognitive decline involve a number of methodological challenges. Thus, cross-sectional studies of old age samples are unable to separate effects of personality on age-related cognitive decline from the associations between personality and cognitive performance which can be demonstrated in younger adults [8]. Studies with short followup intervals will usually observe relatively small age-related changes and may consequently not have sufficient power to detect associations between personality and cognitive decline.

In this perspective, the Glostrup 1914 cohort offers an unusual opportunity to analyze potential associations between personality and cognitive decline as the Minnesota Multiphasic Personality Inventory (MMPI) was administered at age 50 and the cohort was repeatedly assessed with the same cognitive tests for up to 45 years [9]. Among the many scales which can be derived from the MMPI, the Obvious Depression Scale and a short version of the Cook-Medley Hostility Scale have previously been analyzed as predictors of morbidity and mortality [10, 11]. Both scales have been shown to predict cardiovascular disease in the 1914 cohort, and there is a large literature on associations between cardiovascular factors and cognitive decline [12]. Consequently, associations between the two scales and age-related cognitive decline may be hypothesized.

Several findings in nonclinical samples suggest that the Obvious Depression Scale primarily reflects stable aspects of neuroticism and to a smaller extent symptoms of depressive states. In the 1914 cohort 10- and 30-year retest correlations were 0.71 and 0.48 for the Obvious Depression Scale [13], and in another Danish sample of 584 healthy twins, the Obvious Depression Scale was demonstrated to correlate 0.69 with the Neuroticism Scale of the NEO-PI-R [14]. Trait anxiety and trait depression are core components of neuroticism as a broad dimension of personality, and consequently effects on cognitive decline of state anxiety and state depression must be separated from effects of personality. In a cross-sectional study the NEO personality factors explained up to 7% of the variance in cognition, while the state anxiety and state depression scales of the State-Trait Personality Inventory explained very little additional variance [15]. However, a study including a 3-year followup observed no associations between neuroticism and cognitive performance [16].

Hostility may be associated with a tendency to perceive the social environment as stressful and to elicit antagonistic reactions from other people [17]. However, few studies have investigated associations between hostility and age-related cognitive decline. A study using an abbreviated version of the Cook-Medley Hostility Scale found that hostility, in particular hostile attributions, predicted cognitive decline [18]. A more recent study of a community sample used 8 cynicism items from the Cook-Medley Hostility Scale and found that hostility was associated with baseline level of cognitive functioning, but did not influence decline over a 6-year period [19]. However, it is still possible that hostility would influence decline over a longer followup period, and the main aim of the present study was to investigate the obvious depression and Cook-Medley hostility scores at age 50 as predictors of cognitive decline over the following three decades of the lifespan.

Many previous studies have focused on tests of specific cognitive functions, such as reaction time [20], perceptual speed [21], and memory [22]. Studies of the Glostrup 1914 cohort incorporated the full Wechsler Adult Intelligence Scale (WAIS) and consequently, the data provide a unique opportunity to evaluate potential associations between personality and age-related decline in general intelligence. Previous analysis of the 1914 cohort has shown substantially more decline for the performance than for the Verbal IQ [23, 24], and consequently we expected the Performance IQ to be more sensitive to any effects that personality may have on age-related cognitive decline.

Measures of intelligence are usually strongly associated with demographic factors such as education and social status and to some extent this may also be the case for personality measures of depressive traits and hostility. Both intelligence and personality traits may also be associated with lifestyle factors [25], and consequently any observed association between personality and decline in intelligence may reflect confounding by demographic and lifestyle factors. Fortunately, the available data for the 1914 cohort made it possible to control for a range of these potentially confounding factors.

2. Materials and Methods

2.1. Participants. In 1964, the Copenhagen County Hospital and the County Mental Hospital initiated a population study of all people born in 1914 and living in a predefined administrative area close to the two hospitals in Glostrup. A total of 976 individuals were eligible for the study, and of these 802 50-year olds participated in the medical and 698 in the psychological part of the study. Follow-up studies were conducted during the next 45 years, the most recent being a 95-year followup.

In 1964 673 of the 698 participants (384 men and 289 women) completed both the WAIS and the Danish version of the MMPI. The present study sample comprises these 673 individuals and the subsamples participating in the 60-, 70- and 80-year followups conducted in 1974 ($n = 513:293$ men and 220 women), 1984 ($n = 136:71$ men and 65 women), and 1995 ($n = 184:91$ men and 93 women). Details about the medical [26] and psychological studies [9] of the cohort are provided elsewhere.

2.2. Measures

2.2.1. Cognitive Assessment. In the 50-, 60-, and 80-year studies the complete WAIS [27] was administered to all participants. When the 50-year-baseline study of the Glostrup

1914 cohort was initiated in 1964, the original version of the WAIS had just been translated into Danish. It consists of six verbal subtests (information, comprehension, similarities, arithmetic, digit span, vocabulary) and five performance subtests (digit-symbol, picture completion, block design, picture arrangement, and object assembly). Testing procedures and scoring criteria have previously been described in detail [28, 29]. To permit comparison between successive WAIS followups, all IQs are based on the Danish 50-year norms [30]. Only one tester was available for the 70-year followup, and consequently the complete WAIS was only administered to 141 participants, of whom 136 had completed the MMPI and were included in the present study sample. At the 80-year followup 329 of the 698 50-year participants were still alive, and of these 189 participated in the followup (184 had completed the MMPI and are included in the present study sample). As described previously, the 189 participants in the 80-year study obtained higher mean full-scale IQ at the 50-year baseline than the remaining participants in the 50-year study [23].

2.2.2. Obvious Depression Scale. The Danish version of the MMPI [31] consists of 408 true-false items, although "don't know" is a third answer category in the Danish version. The Obvious Depression Scale comprises 40 items: 8 items potentially reflecting physical health and 32 items reflecting mood, feelings of well-being, and self-esteem [11]. Coefficient alpha for the Danish 50-year sample was 0.78 for the Obvious Depression Scale.

2.2.3. Cook-Medley Hostility Scale. The Danish version of the MMPI did not include all the 566 items of the complete inventory. Consequently, the present study included only 27 of the 39-item abbreviated Cook-Medley Hostility Scale: 11 items on cynicism, 9 on hostile attributions, 4 on aggressive responding, and 3 items on hostile affect [32]. Coefficient alpha for the Danish 50-year sample was 0.82 for the 27 item Hostility Scale.

2.2.4. Demographic Covariates. These included sex, education, and social status assessed at the 50-year study. School education was coded on a 3-point scale (primary to upper secondary) and vocational training on a 5-point scale (no vocational training to academic). The two scores were combined into an overall ordinal index of educational level with a 2–8 point range [23]. Social status was ranked in 6 ordinal levels based on educational level, job position, and number of subordinates [33].

2.2.5. Lifestyle Factors. These included measurement of systolic blood pressure, smoking (as a binary variable), physical activity at work and at leisure (both four-level ordinal measures, recoded into three categories) [11], obesity (measured by body mass index (BMI)), and measures of total serum cholesterol, triglycerides, and insulin [26] analyzed in blood samples obtained in the morning after a 13-hour fast.

2.3. Data Analysis. Mixed-effects models were used to test associations between the two personality traits and level of WAIS performance and to test associations between personality traits and change in cognitive function. Data were analyzed using the xtmixed procedure of Stata version 12 (StataCorp LP, College Station, TX, USA). At the 50-year baseline, information on BMI, blood pressure, total serum cholesterol, triglycerides, and insulin was missing for 2, 13, 27, 29, and 27 individuals, respectively. To avoid diluting the sample in multivariate analyses including these variables, the relatively few missing values were imputed using the multivariate normal regression imputing facilities of Stata.

A basic growth curve model, including time since the 50-year baseline as both a fixed and random effect and assuming both random intercept and slope, was used in preliminary analyses of the WAIS full-scale IQ. Since decline in WAIS IQs was nonlinear, time squared was included to allow for non-linear change. Sex, education, and social status were considered core confounders explaining substantial variance in full-scale IQ, and these variables were included in a series of models, which for each continuous covariate tested linear and quadratic regression, and for all covariates tested the significance of the interaction with the time since baseline variable. None of the interactions with the time variable was significant, and significant quadratic effects were only observed for social status and insulin level. Consequently, mean-centered squared variables were included in models with these two variables.

For the obvious depression and hostility scales both main effects and interactions with the time variable were tested in the following models: Model 1 was the basic model including time since the baseline (and the squared time variable). Model 2 also included the sociodemographic variables of sex, education, and social status, including the centered squared status variable. Finally, model 3 further included the lifestyle variables of systolic blood pressure, serum cholesterol, triglycerides, insulin (including a quadratic term), BMI, work and leisure physical activity, and smoking. All three models were analyzed with the full-scale, verbal, and Performance IQs as outcome and with time since the 50-year baseline as both a fixed and random effect and assuming both random intercept and slope, corresponding to assuming random variation in level and form of the individual growth curves.

There was some evidence of selective attrition, and consequently the main analyses were repeated on a reduced longitudinal sample comprising the 184 individuals who participated in both the 50-year and 80-year studies.

The growth curve models provide random effect estimates of interindividual variance in level and slope of the decline curves. By comparing variance estimates for models with and without the obvious depression or the Cook-Medley Hostility Scale, it is possible to calculate the reduction in variance associated with including each of the MMPI scales in the models.

All statistical tests were two-sided and determined significant at the 5% level.

3. Results

The sample characteristics for the 50-year baseline and the three followups are shown in Table 1. The percentage of men and smokers decreased at the later followups, and the mean systolic blood pressure and triglycerides level fell. Notably, the mean educational level was higher at the 80-year followup, while the mean social status was lower. For all these variables, significant differences were observed when the 50-year baseline values of the 80-year sample was compared with the baseline values of the remaining 50-year sample. This difference was not significant for any of the remaining variables in Table 1.

Table 2 presents means and standard deviations for the two MMPI scales at the 50-year baseline. For both scales most of the possible score range was used. The distributions were reasonably symmetric with a positive skewness of 0.80 for the Obvious Depression Scale and 0.22 for the abbreviated Cook-Medley Hostility Scale. Women scored significantly higher than men on the Obvious Depression Scale and significantly lower than men on the Cook-Medley Hostility Scales.

Table 3 displays the observed mean IQs at baseline and the three full followup samples as well as means for the subsample comprising the 184 individuals who participated in both the 50- and 80-year studies. Table 3 also presents the mean difference between the results of the 50-year baseline and the 80-year followup. The relatively large standard deviations of this difference illustrate the substantial individual differences in decline which have previously been described [23], and which were further confirmed by the variance in slope (decline in intelligence) observed in all growth-curve models in the present study. Table 3 also shows the high retest correlations which should be compared with the 20-year retest correlations reported previously (for the full-scale IQ, the retest correlations were 0.94 from 50 to 60 years and 0.90 from 50 to 70 years) [9, 24].

For all three WAIS IQs, little decline was observed from age 50 to age 60, but decline was obviously increasing and was substantial from age 70 to age 80, particularly for the Performance IQ. Thus, the means in the table indicate that any model describing cognitive development during the 30-year followup period should include a quadratic trend.

Table 4 presents the analyses of the Obvious Depression Scale. The table shows coefficients for the scale in models only including a term for the main effect and in models adding a term for the interaction between the scale and the time since baseline variable. The table shows relatively large effects of obvious depression on all three IQs in the unadjusted models, corresponding to a 5-6 percent reduction in the estimated variance of the curve level. However, the effects became dramatically smaller (and nonsignificant for Verbal IQ) when adjusted for demographic background variables (1 percent or less reduction in curve level variance), while adjustment for the set of lifestyle factors hardly changed the estimates. None of the tests of interaction with the time since baseline variable was approaching significance, and these models accordingly showed negligible reduction in the estimates of slope variance. Thus, it must be concluded that obvious depression did not influence the form of the cognitive decline curve, while it was associated with the level of the curve (see Figure 1).

Table 5 presents the analyses of the Cook-Medley Hostility Scale. Compared with obvious depression smaller effects of Hostility on all three IQs were observed in the unadjusted models, corresponding to about 3 percent reduction in the estimated variance of the curve level. Although the coefficients became smaller when adjusted for demographic background variables, they remained significant for all three IQs both in models without and with adjustment for the lifestyle factors. For these models, the inclusion of the Cook-Medley Hostility Scale was associated with about 2 percent reduction in curve level variance. None of the tests of interaction with the time since baseline variable was approaching significance, and these models showed negligible reduction in the estimates of slope variance. Thus, scores on the Cook-Medley Hostility Scale were associated with the level of the cognitive performance, but did not influence the form of the decline curve (see Figure 2).

The models in Tables 4 and 5 only tested the linear effects of obvious depression and hostility. However, models including a quadratic term and testing both its main effect and interaction with time since baseline found no significant quadratic effects of either scale. Correlation coefficients can be used to express the size of the linear associations between the MMPI scales and intelligence. In the 50-year-baseline sample the bivariate correlations of the Obvious Depression Scale were −0.24, −0.22, and −0.24 with the full-scale, the verbal and the Performance IQs, but when adjusted for demographic variables, the corresponding partial correlations were only −0.09, −0.05 and −0.10. For the Cook-Medley Hostility Scale, the correlations were −0.19, −0.17, and −0.17, and the adjusted partial correlations were −0.15, −0.13, and −0.13, confirming a stronger adjusted association with WAIS performance for this scale compared with the Obvious Depression Scale.

The correlation between the Obvious Depression Scale and the Cook-Medley Hostility Scale was 0.30. When both MMPI scales were included in the same model, only the main effect of the Cook-Medley Hostility Scale remained significant in all models. Thus, the regression coefficients for the two scales were −0.10 ($P = 0.25$) and −0.27 ($P = 0.003$) in the fully adjusted model while the regression coefficients were −0.19 ($P = 0.023$) and −0.31 ($P < 0.001$) in the corresponding models including either the Obvious Depression Scale or the Cook-Medley Hostility Scale.

Since significant sex differences were observed on both scales, it is possible that the influence of obvious depression and hostility is different in men and women. If this were the case, the three-factor interaction between sex, time since baseline, and each of the two personality scales should be significant. However, this interaction was not found to be significant in supplementary analyses adjusting for demographic variables and also analyses adjusting for lifestyle factors.

The supplementary analyses based on the reduced longitudinal sample showed fewer significant associations

TABLE 1: Sample characteristics at 50-year baseline and the three followups[1].

Variable	50-year baseline	60-year followup	70-year followup	80-year followup
Number of participants	673	513	136	184
Demographic variables				
Men (%, n)	57 (384)	57 (293)	52 (71)	49 (91)*
Education (mean, SD)	3.6 (1.4)	3.6 (1.4)	3.6 (1.3)	3.8 (1.4)*
Social status (mean, SD)	4.5 (1.1)	4.5 (1.1)	4.5 (0.9)	4.3 (1.0)*
Lifestyle factors				
Smokers (%, n)	69 (461)	67 (339)*	66 (90)	55 (101)*
Sedentary work activity (%, n)[2]	27 (183)	27 (139)	24 (32)	32 (58)
Sedentary leisure activity (%, n)	18 (124)	17 (89)	15 (20)	17 (31)
BMI (mean, SD)	25.2 (4.0)	25.2 (3.8)	25.4 (4.1)	25.0 (3.3)
Systolic BP (mean mmHG, SD)	138.7 (20.4)	137.9 (19.4)	134.9 (18.2)*	135.2 (18.0)*
Total cholesterol (mean mg/dL, SD)	285.7 (49.5)	285.6 (49.9)	286.0 (47.9)	288.9 (47.7)
Fasting insulin (mean units/mL, SD)	22.6 (7.1)	22.5 (7.2)	23.4 (8.6)	22.7 (7.8)
Triglycerides (mean mM/liter, SD)	111.2 (68.4)	110.0 (70.5)	113.0 (76.1)	101.6 (50.9)*

[1]An* indicates that there was a significant difference on the variable between the followup subsample and the remaining part of the 50-year baseline sample.
[2]This percentage includes about 11% of the participants who reported no work.

TABLE 2: Score distributions on obvious depression and Cook-Medley Hostility Scales at age 50.

MMPI scale	N	Mean	SD	Range
Obvious depression scale[1]	673	11.48	5.38	1–34
Men	384	10.21	4.99	1–34
Women	289	13.18	5.42	4–30
Cook-Medley hostility scale[2]	673	10.43	4.92	0–25
Men	384	10.97	5.04	1–23
Women	289	9.72	4.67	0–25

[1]Women scored significantly higher than men ($P < 0.001$).
[2]Men scored significantly higher than women ($P = 0.001$).

between the MMPI scales and intelligence level, but otherwise showed essentially the same results as the analyses of the full sample.

4. Discussion

The present study based on multiple administrations of the full WAIS and a 30-year followup period showed that the personality traits obvious depression and hostility were associated with the level of WAIS performance, but did not influence the rate of decline in general intelligence during the 30-year followup period. The association with level of WAIS performance to some extent reflected confounding by demographic factors such as sex, education, and social status, but, except for Verbal IQ, the effects remained significant when these covariates were included in the statistical models. The effect estimates hardly changed when the models also included a wide range of lifestyle related variables.

While the low, but significant, negative correlation between obvious depression and intelligence is consistent with the relatively well-documented negative association between neuroticism and intelligence [8, 34], to our knowledge few—if any—studies exist on the relationship between personality and decline in general intelligence. Many studies have investigated depressive symptoms as a risk factor for dementia [7], while fewer studies have investigated associations between depressive symptoms and cognitive decline [35, 36]. A study based on a large sample and comprehensive assessment of cognitive functions observed no association [37], while another large-sample study observed an association between average depressive symptom score and cognitive decline over varying followup intervals with a mean length of 4.4 years [38]. Among the available studies, the present study is unique because of the young age of the participants at baseline, the long followup period, and the instruments used to assess depression and cognitive function: The participants were only 50 years old at baseline, the followup interval was exceptionally long, and our study used general intelligence as outcome. It is true that many studies have evaluated associations between depression and cognition, but these studies have typically assessed symptoms of depression within the last week in much older individuals, and they have typically focused on depression as a risk factor for dementia over much shorter followup intervals.

Personality traits reflect stable characteristics of an individual and the distinction between state and trait can

TABLE 3: Mean WAIS IQs during the lifespan from 50 to 80.

Followup	*N*	Full scale IQ		Verbal IQ		Performance IQ	
Full samples		Mean	SD	Mean	SD	Mean	SD
50-year baseline	673	98.96	14.40	98.19	14.21	99.12	14.22
60-year followup	513	98.84	14.33	99.21	14.59	97.65	13.80
70-year followup	136	94.90	14.12	96.22	13.71	93.40	14.37
80-year followup	184	87.66	15.49	92.27	15.64	83.46	14.78
80-year sample[1]	184						
50-year baseline		102.10	13.79	100.85	13.84	102.31	13.28
80-year followup		87.66	15.49	92.27	15.63	83.46	14.78
Difference		14.44	8.88	8.58	8.75	18.85	10.43
Retest correlation		0.82		0.83		0.73	

[1] Data are for the 184 participants who completed the WAIS at both the 50- and 80-year studies.

TABLE 4: Obvious depression scale: effects on WAIS IQs from 50 to 80.

Model	Coefficient[1]	95% CI	*P* for main effect	Interaction[2] coefficient	*P* for interaction
Full-scale IQ					
Model 1: unadjusted[3]	−0.639	(−0.83)–(−0.44)	<0.001	0.003	0.319
Model 2: demographics[4]	−0.184	(−0.35)–(−0.02)	0.029	0.003	0.291
Model 3: lifestyle factors[5]	−0.190	(−0.36)–(−0.03)	0.023	0.003	0.294
Verbal IQ					
Model 1: unadjusted[3]	−0.572	(−0.77)–(−0.38)	<0.001	0.002	0.638
Model 2: demographics[4]	−0.119	(−0.28)–(0.05)	0.156	0.002	0.613
Model 3: lifestyle factors[5]	−0.125	(−0.29)–(0.04)	0.131	0.002	0.616
Performance IQ					
Model 1: unadjusted[3]	−0.595	(−0.78)–(−0.41)	<0.001	0.005	0.227
Model 2: demographics[4]	−0.223	(−0.40)–(−0.05)	0.012	0.005	0.236
Model 3: lifestyle factors[5]	−0.228	(−0.40)–(−0.06)	0.009	0.005	0.236

[1] Fixed effect coefficient from a model only including the main effect of the depression scale. See Section 3 for description of the effects of obvious depression on the estimates of the random effects.
[2] Interaction coefficient from a model including a term for interaction between the obvious depression scale and time since baseline. Additionally all relevant main effects are included in the model.
[3] Model includes linear and quadratic time since baseline and the obvious depression scale.
[4] Model additionally includes sex, education, and social status.
[5] Model additionally includes sex, education, social status, systolic blood pressure, smoking, BMI, total cholesterol, triglycerides, insulin, and leisure and work physical activity.

only be made by empirical studies of stability over time. The high long-term stability of the obvious depression score described in the introduction suggests that this scale should primarily be considered a measure of depressive traits, but in addition there are important differences between the Obvious Depression Scale and scales assessing acute depressive states: typical measures of depressive symptomatology such as the SCL-90-R [39] and the CES-D [40] ask the respondent about symptoms within the last week, while the MMPI does not specify any time period, but asks the respondent to indicate whether the item is characteristic of the respondent which—in the context of items asking about self-confidence, being tense at work, liking parties, and about being happy most of time—is likely to be interpreted by the respondent as questions about his or her personality. Thus, the instruction to the respondent and the item content differentiate trait and state measures, and in the case of the Obvious Depression Scale make the high correlation with the Neuroticism Scale of the NEO-PI-R understandable [14].

For hostility, a recent study observed a measure of cynical hostility to be associated with lower cognitive function, but not with decline in cognition [19]. We observed essentially the same results with a longer followup period and with a measure of general intelligence as cognitive outcome.

Generally, few predictors of cognitive decline have been identified based on strong evidence [12] which may partly reflect complex methodological problems. In spite of the comprehensive assessment of intelligence, and in spite of the long followup period sample attrition is an obvious limitation of our study since, for each outcome, the study was based on 1506 observations, of which only 136 and 184 were from the 70- and 80-year followups. Thus, statistical power

Table 5: Abbreviated Cook-Medley hostility scale: effects on WAIS IQs from 50 to 80.

Model	Coefficient[1]	95% CI	P formain effect	Interaction[2] coefficient	P for interaction
Full Scale IQ					
Model 1: Unadjusted[3]	−0.524	(−0.74)–(−0.31)	<0.001	0.003	0.378
Model 2: Demographics[4]	−0.320	(−0.49)–(−0.15)	<0.001	0.003	0.386
Model 3: Lifestyle factors[5]	−0.311	(−0.48)–(−0.14)	<0.001	0.003	0.391
Verbal IQ					
Model 1: Unadjusted[3]	−0.496	(−0.71)–(−0.28)	<0.001	0.002	0.655
Model 2: Demographics[4]	−0.283	(−0.45)–(−0.11)	0.001	0.001	0.690
Model 3: Lifestyle factors[5]	−0.266	(−0.44)–(−0.10)	0.002	0.001	0.699
Performance IQ					
Model 1: Unadjusted[3]	−0.451	(−0.66)–(−0.24)	<0.001	0.005	0.269
Model 2: Demographics[4]	−0.295	(−0.48)–(−0.11)	0.002	0.005	0.272
Model 3: Lifestyle factors[5]	−0.297	(−0.48)–(−0.12)	0.001	0.005	0.280

[1]Fixed effect coefficient from a model only including the main effect of the hostility scale. See Section 3 for description of the effects of hostility on the estimates of the random-effects.
[2]Interaction coefficient from a model including a term for interaction between the abbreviated Cook-Medley Hostility Scale and time since baseline. Additionally all relevant main effects are included in the model.
[3]Model includes linear and quadratic time since baseline and the abbreviated Cook-Medley hostility scale.
[4]Model additionally includes sex, education and social status.
[5]Model additionally includes sex, education, social status, systolic blood pressure, smoking, BMI, total cholesterol, triglycerides, insulin and leisure and work physical activity.

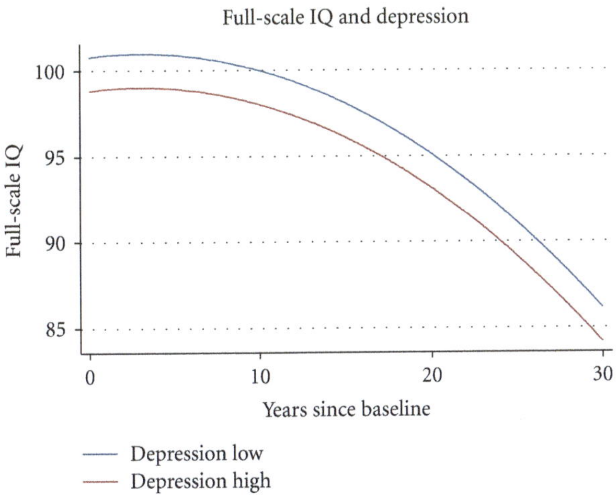

Figure 1: Obvious depression and decline in full-scale IQ from age 50 to age 80. The curves correspond to 1 SD below and above the mean on the Obvious Depression Scale. Adjusted for sex, education and social status.

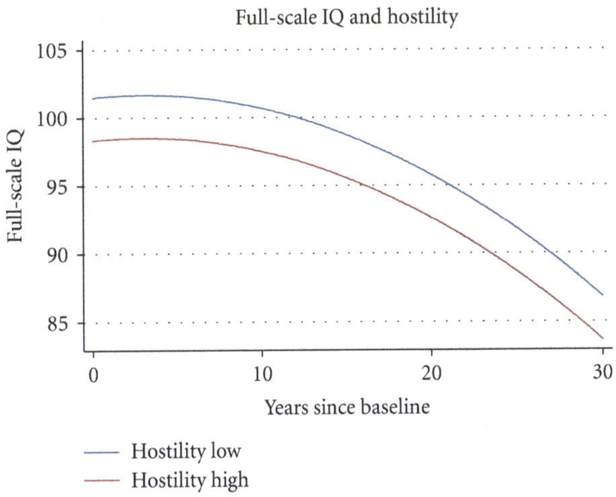

Figure 2: Hostility and decline in full-scale IQ age 50 to age 80. The curves correspond to 1 SD below and above the mean on the abbreviated Cook-Medley Hostility Scale. Adjusted for sex, education, and social status.

may not have been sufficient to detect weak associations between personality and decline in intelligence, particularly since cognitive change was only substantial at the last two followups.

If the negative findings with respect to influence of personality on the rate of cognitive decline reflect a statistical power problem, stronger effects may be expected on the outcome showing the most substantial decline. Over the 30-year followup period Table 3 shows about 1 standard deviation decline for Performance IQ, but only about half a standard deviation for Verbal IQ. Thus, clearer evidence of effects on decline was anticipated for the Performance IQ, but Tables 4 and 5 show no significant interactions for the Performance IQ. Furthermore, separate analyses of each of the WAIS subtests as outcome also showed no significant interactions between the MMPI scales and time since baseline (data not shown). However, potential effects of personality on age-related decline in specific cognitive functions should be further investigated.

The MMPI scales were not available for all followups, which is one of the reasons that we decided to conduct a prediction study based on the MMPI and covariate data from the 50-year baseline study. However, this may be considered a weakness of the study, to the extent that the traits assessed by the two MMPI scales may change during the long followup interval and to the extent that the 50-year scores were influenced by variance in the mental state of the participants. In particular, scores on the Obvious Depression Scale may reflect both trait and state components, although high retest correlations have previously been reported for this scale [13]. We observed substantial ten-year retest correlations from the 50-year baseline to the 60-year followup: 0.74 for the Cook-Medley Hostility Scale and 0.67 for the Obvious Depression Scale, and lack of stability is unlikely to be a major problem since the scales have previously been demonstrated to predict morbidity and mortality over long followup periods [10, 11].

Interpretations of the associations between low intelligence and traits such as obvious depression and hostility are ambiguous because they do not necessarily reflect effects of personality on intelligence or cognitive development since reverse causation—that is, effects of intelligence on personality or personality development—is also a possibility. Indeed, the associations need not reflect a causal relationship since both cognitive development and personality development may be related to factors such as adverse social conditions in childhood [41]. We were unable to control childhood history and social circumstances, but we did adjust for educational level and social status at the 50-year baseline. Tables 4 and 5 clearly show that a substantial part of the covariance between the MMPI scales and WAIS performance reflects association with education and social status. However, intelligence is likely to be one of the factors influencing achieved educational level, and therefore controlling for education may eliminate part of the variance in the association between personality and intelligence that is not due to confounding. In contrast, the tables show remarkably small effects of including a wide range of lifestyle-related factors in the statistical models. As discussed elsewhere, it has proven difficult to identify consistent effects of lifestyle factors on the rate of cognitive decline in the 1914 cohort [9], which is in line with the relatively small effects observed in major longitudinal cohort studies [42, 43].

To the extent that depression and hostility reflect stable personality characteristics, they are likely to be associated with stress and distress across the lifespan. This is the main rationale for the hypothesis that these personality traits influence cognitive decline since increased levels of stress may either influence brain functioning and cognition directly or indirectly through an association with cardiovascular dysfunction or disease [4, 19]. If effects of personality on decline in general intelligence cannot be demonstrated, this may be because the brain is less vulnerable to high levels of stress than expected, or because personality is only one out of a multitude of determinants of cognitive decline. Future studies should focus on the interaction between personality and other determinants of cognitive decline and track changes in personality and cognition across the lifespan to illuminate the direction of causality.

Acknowledgment

The authors thank the Glostrup 1914 Cohort participants, and staff at the Research Center for Prevention and Health, Glostrup University Hospital, for data collection.

References

[1] S. E. Hampson and H. S. Friedman, "Personality and health: a lifespan perspective," in *Handbook of Personality*, O. P. John, R. W. Robins, and L. A. Pervin, Eds., pp. 770–794, The Guilford Press, New York, NY, USA, 2008.

[2] C. D. Ryff, "Challenges and opportunities at the interface of aging, personality, and well-being," in *Handbook of Personality*, O. P. John, R. W. Robins, and L. A. Pervin, Eds., pp. 399–4184, The Guilford Press, New York, NY, USA, 2008.

[3] S. J. Lupien, B. S. McEwen, M. R. Gunnar, and C. Heim, "Effects of stress throughout the lifespan on the brain, behaviour and cognition," *Nature Reviews Neuroscience*, vol. 10, no. 6, pp. 434–445, 2009.

[4] M. Crowe, R. Andel, N. L. Pedersen, L. Fratiglioni, and M. Gatz, "Personality and risk of cognitive impairment 25 years later," *Psychology and Aging*, vol. 21, no. 3, pp. 573–580, 2006.

[5] N. Bolger and E. A. Schilling, "Personality and the problems of everyday life: the role of neuroticism in exposure and reactivity to daily stressors," *Journal of Personality*, vol. 59, no. 3, pp. 355–386, 1991.

[6] R. Kotov, W. Gamez, F. Schmidt, and D. Watson, "Linking "Big" personality traits to anxiety, depressive, and substance use disorders: A meta-analysis," *Psychological Bulletin*, vol. 136, no. 5, pp. 768–821, 2010.

[7] A. L. Byers and K. Yaffe, "Depression and risk of developing dementia," *Nature Reviews Neurology*, vol. 7, no. 6, pp. 323–331, 2011.

[8] P. L. Ackerman and E. D. Heggestad, "Intelligence, personality, and interests: evidence for overlapping traits," *Psychological Bulletin*, vol. 121, no. 2, pp. 219–245, 1997.

[9] E. L. Mortensen, "The aging intellect," in *Geropsychology—The Psychology of the Aging Person*, L. Larsen, Ed., pp. 65–95, Aarhus Universitetsforlag, Aarhus, Denmark, 2011.

[10] J. C. Barefoot, S. Larsen, L. von der Lieth, and M. Schroll, "Hostility, incidence of acute myocardial infarction, and mortality in a sample of older Danish men and women," *American Journal of Epidemiology*, vol. 142, no. 5, pp. 477–484, 1995.

[11] J. C. Barefoot and M. Schroll, "Symptoms of depression, acute myocardial infarction, and total mortality in a community sample," *Circulation*, vol. 93, no. 11, pp. 1976–1980, 1996.

[12] B. L. Plassman, J. W. Williams, J. R. Burke, T. Holsinger, and S. Benjamin, "Systematic review: factors associated with risk for and possible prevention of cognitive decline in later life," *Annals of Internal Medicine*, vol. 153, no. 3, pp. 182–193, 2010.

[13] J. C. Barefoot, E. L. Mortensen, M. J. Helms, K. Avlund, and M. Schroll, "A longitudinal study of gender differences in depressive symptoms from age 50 to 80," *Psychology and Aging*, vol. 16, no. 2, pp. 342–345, 2001.

[14] H. S. Hansen and E. L. Mortensen, "Dokumentation for den danske udgave af NEO PI-R og NEO PI-R kort version," in *NEO PI-R*, E. L. Mortensen and H. S. Hansen, Eds., pp. 53–85, Dansk Psykologisk Forlag, Copenhagen, Denmark, 2004.

[15] J. Booth, J. Schinka, L. Brown, J. Mortimer, and A. Borenstein, "Five-factor personality dimensions, mood states, and cognitive performance in older adults," *Journal of Clinical and*

Experimental Neuropsychology, vol. 28, no. 5, pp. 676–683, 2006.

[16] M. Jelicic, H. Bosma, R. W. H. M. Ponds, M. P. J. Van Boxtel, P. J. Houx, and J. Jolles, "Neuroticism does not affect cognitive functioning in later life," *Experimental Aging Research*, vol. 29, no. 1, pp. 73–78, 2003.

[17] J. C. Barefoot and S. H. Boyle, "Hostility and proness to anger," in *Handbook of Individual Differences in Social Behavior*, M. R. Leary and R. H. Hoyle, Eds., pp. 210–226, New York Guildford Press, New York, NY, USA, 2009.

[18] P. P. Vitaliano, D. Echeverria, J. Yi, P. E. M. Phillips, H. Young, and I. C. Siegler, "Psychophysiological mediators of caregiver stress and differential cognitive decline," *Psychology and Aging*, vol. 20, no. 3, pp. 402–411, 2005.

[19] L. L. Barnes, C. F. M. de Leon, J. L. Bienias, R. S. Wilson, S. A. Everson-Rose, and D. A. Evans, "Hostility and change in cognitive function over time in older blacks and whites," *Psychosomatic Medicine*, vol. 71, no. 6, pp. 652–658, 2009.

[20] R. H. Pietrzak, P. Maruff, M. Woodward et al., "Mild worry symptoms predict decline in learning and memory in healthy older adults: a 2-year prospective cohort study," *American Journal of Geriatric Psychiatry*, vol. 20, no. 3, pp. 266–275, 2012.

[21] A. A. M. Bielak, D. Gerstorf, K. M. Kiely, K. J. Anstey, and M. Luszcz, "Depressive symptoms predict decline in perceptual speed in older adulthood," *Psychology and Aging*, vol. 25, no. 3, pp. 576–583, 2011.

[22] R. S. Wilson, D. A. Fleischman, R. A. Myers et al., "Premorbid proneness to distress and episodic memory impairment in Alzheimer's disease," *Journal of Neurology, Neurosurgery and Psychiatry*, vol. 75, no. 2, pp. 191–195, 2004.

[23] E. L. Mortensen and P. Høgh, "A gender difference in the association between APOE genotype and age-related cognitive decline," *Neurology*, vol. 57, no. 1, pp. 89–95, 2001.

[24] E. L. Mortensen and M. Kleven, "A WAIS longitudinal study of cognitive development during the life span from ages 50 to 70," *Developmental Neuropsychology*, vol. 9, pp. 115–130, 1993.

[25] I. J. Deary, J. Corley, A. J. Gow et al., "Age-associated cognitive decline," *British Medical Bulletin*, vol. 92, no. 1, pp. 135–152, 2009.

[26] M. Schroll, "A ten-year prospective study, 1964–1974, of cardiovascular risk factors in men and women from the Glostrup population born in 1914," *Danish Medical Bulletin*, vol. 29, no. 5, pp. 213–252, 1982.

[27] D. Wechsler, *The Measurement and Appraisal of Adult Intelligence*, Williams & Wilkins, Baltimore, Md, USA, 1958.

[28] G. Hess, *WAIS anvendt på 698 50-årige*, Akademisk Forlag, Copenhagen, Denmark, 1974.

[29] G. Hess, *WAIS. Retesting af 528 60-årige*, Dansk Psykologisk Forlag, Copenhagen, Denmark, 1983.

[30] M. Kyng, *WAIS anvendt på 70-årige*, Dansk Psykologisk Forlag, Copenhagen, Denmark, 1978.

[31] S. R. Hathaway and J. C. McKinley, *Manual for the Minnesota Multiphasic Personality Inventory*, Psychological Corporation, New York, NY, USA, 1943.

[32] J. C. Barefoot, K. A. Dodge, B. L. Peterson, W. G. Dahlstrom, and R. B. Williams, "The Cook-Medley hostility scale: item content and ability to predict survival," *Psychosomatic Medicine*, vol. 51, no. 1, pp. 46–57, 1989.

[33] K. Svalastoga, *Prestige, Class and Mobility*, Gyldendal, Copenhagen, Denmark, 1959.

[34] J. Moutafi, A. Furnham, and I. Tsaousis, "Is the relationship between intelligence and trait neuroticism mediated by test anxiety?" *Personality and Individual Differences*, vol. 40, no. 3, pp. 587–597, 2006.

[35] R. S. Wilson, C. F. M. de Leon, D. A. Bennett, J. L. Bienias, and D. A. Evans, "Depressive symptoms and cognitive decline in a community population of older persons," *Journal of Neurology, Neurosurgery and Psychiatry*, vol. 75, no. 1, pp. 126–129, 2004.

[36] J. Chodosh, D. M. Kado, T. E. Seeman, and A. S. Karlamangla, "Depressive symptoms as a predictor of cognitive decline: MacArthur studies of successful aging," *American Journal of Geriatric Psychiatry*, vol. 15, no. 5, pp. 406–415, 2007.

[37] M. Ganguli, Y. Du, H. H. Dodge, G. G. Ratcliff, and C. C. Chang, "Depressive symptoms and cognitive decline in late life: a prospective epidemiological study," *Archives of General Psychiatry*, vol. 63, no. 2, pp. 153–160, 2006.

[38] V. M. Dotson, S. M. Resnick, and A. B. Zonderman, "Differential association of concurrent, baseline, and average depressive symptoms with cognitive decline in older adults," *American Journal of Geriatric Psychiatry*, vol. 16, no. 4, pp. 318–330, 2008.

[39] L. R. Derogatis, *SCL-90-R: Symptom Checklist-90-R. Administration, Scoring and Procedures Manual*, National Computer Systems, Minneapolis, Minn, USA, 3rd edition, 1994.

[40] L. Radloff, "The CES-D scale: a self report depression scale for research in the general population," *Applied Psychological Measurement*, vol. 1, pp. 385–401, 1977.

[41] G. E. Miller, E. Chen, and K. J. Parker, "Psychological stress in childhood and susceptibility to the chronic diseases of aging: moving toward a model of behavioral and biological mechanisms," *Psychological Bulletin*, vol. 137, pp. 959–997, 2011.

[42] I. J. Deary, L. J. Whalley, and J. M. Starr, *A Lifetime of Intelligence. Follow-Up Studies of the Scottish Mental Surveys of 1932 and 1947*, American Psychological Association, Washington, DC, USA, 2009.

[43] K. W. Schaie, *Developmental Influences on Adult Intelligence. The Seattle Longitudinal Study*, Oxford University Press, New York, NY, USA, 2005.

23

Measuring Fluid Intelligence in Healthy Older Adults

Mohammed K. Shakeel[1] and Vina M. Goghari[2]

[1]*Department of Psychology, University of Calgary, 2500 University Drive NW, Calgary, AB, Canada T2N 1N4*
[2]*Department of Psychology, University of Toronto, 1265 Military Trail, Toronto, ON, Canada M1C 1A4*

Correspondence should be addressed to Mohammed K. Shakeel; mohammed.kalathil@ucalgary.ca

Academic Editor: Elke Bromberg

The present study evaluated subjective and objective cognitive measures as predictors of fluid intelligence in healthy older adults. We hypothesized that objective cognitive measures would predict fluid intelligence to a greater degree than self-reported cognitive functioning. Ninety-three healthy older (>65 years old) community-dwelling adults participated. Raven's Advanced Progressive Matrices (RAPM) were used to measure fluid intelligence, Digit Span Sequencing (DSS) was used to measure working memory, Trail Making Test (TMT) was used to measure cognitive flexibility, Design Fluency Test (DFT) was used to measure creativity, and Tower Test (TT) was used to measure planning. The Cognitive Failures Questionnaire (CFQ) was used to measure subjective perceptions of cognitive functioning. RAPM was correlated with DSS, TT, and DFT. When CFQ was the only predictor, the regression model predicting fluid intelligence was not significant. When DSS, TMT, DFT, and TT were included in the model, there was a significant change in the model and the final model was also significant, with DFT as the only significant predictor. The model accounted for approximately 20% of the variability in fluid intelligence. Our findings suggest that the most reliable means of assessing fluid intelligence is to assess it directly.

1. Introduction

There has been a lot of interest in recent years in the use of subjective reports of cognitive functioning to predict the likelihood that a person will suffer from dementia [1]. However, the findings have been equivocal [2]. This may be in part because people are poor judges of their own mental functions [3], and this may be especially true of those who already have poor cognitive functioning [4]. This view has important implications for the use of subjective reports in dementias, which are characterized by cognitive, as well as metacognitive, deficits [5, 6]. There is a lack of empirical studies on the usefulness of making inferences about complex mental functions by assessing other, related mental functions (subjectively or objectively). This also has important implications for diagnosis, because it is often not feasible to administer time-consuming tests for complex functions (like intelligence) in a clinical setting, and may also require specific training in administration and interpretation. In contrast, though widely used, research has demonstrated that asking patients about their own mental functions may not be a fruitful approach [7, 8].

In the present study, we aimed to investigate, in healthy older adults, whether subjective and objective measures predicted complex cognitive functioning, namely, fluid intelligence. Fluid intelligence involves reasoning and problem solving for problems to which familiar solutions are not available. Fluid intelligence tends to decline with age [9] and is impaired in dementia [10]. Hence, fluid intelligence serves as an ideal candidate to investigate the usefulness of subjective and objective predictors for a complex cognitive function. However, as with many complex functions, it is not possible to reliably assess fluid intelligence using subjective reports. Therefore, we relied on using the Cognitive Failures Questionnaire, which requires the participant to answer questions that assess memory [11], attention [11], and executive functioning, which are related to fluid intelligence [12–14].

We also wanted to assess how well subjective reports of cognitive functioning perform compared to objective measures like working memory [15], cognitive flexibility [16],

Table 1: Sociodemographic information ($n = 93$).

	Mean (standard deviation) or percentage
Age	70.12 (4.61)
Handedness (% right)	84.9
Sex (% female)	65.6
Ethnicity	
Caucasian (%)	89.2
Asian (%)	8.6
Others (%)	2.2
Education (years)	15.79 (3.51)
Employment status	
Retired (%)	83.9
Full time employed (%)	3.3
Part time employed (%)	8.7
Others (%)	4.4

creativity [17], and planning [18], which are related to fluid intelligence [16, 19–22]. However, there is no consensus on the strength of the association between fluid intelligence and these variables (see, e.g., [19, 20, 23–25]), and it also remains to be determined whether the association holds for older adults as it does for other age groups.

Furthermore, for this study, we specifically chose objective measures that are neither time-consuming nor difficult to administer in a clinical setting. To avoid redundancy, we also ensured that the subjective and objective measures assessed nonoverlapping constructs related to fluid intelligence. We hypothesized that objective measures of related cognitive processes would predict fluid intelligence better than subjective report of cognition.

2. Materials and Methods

2.1. Participants. Sociodemographic information is presented in Table 1. The sample consisted of healthy older community-dwelling adults aged between 65 and 86 years, recruited from Calgary, Alberta. All participants were proficient in English. To reduce the effects of other factors that could affect cognitive functions or the ability to adequately perform the tasks, participants were excluded if they had a head trauma, brain fever, neurological illness, dementia or altered consciousness, history of recent (3 months) use of benzodiazepines or illicit drugs, current visual, auditory, or motor impairment, cardiovascular conditions, breathing problems or pathologies associated with cognitive impairment such as stroke, Parkinson's disease, intracranial hemorrhage, tumors, and normal pressure hydrocephalus, or a score of less than 27 on the Mini Mental State Examination [26]. Informed written consent was obtained from all participants. The study was approved by the University of Calgary Conjoint Faculties Research Ethics Board and is in accordance with the ethical standards of the Helsinki Declaration [27].

2.2. Measures. All data was collected in a single session held at the University of Calgary.

2.2.1. Raven's Advanced Progressive Matrices (RAPM) [28]. Raven's Advanced Progressive Matrices were used as a measure of fluid intelligence. The task requires participants to examine a series of images and select one out of 8 possible images to complete the pattern. The test has 36 items of progressively increasing difficulty. The total correct score obtained was used for the present analysis.

2.2.2. Digit Span Sequencing (DSS). Digit Span Sequencing was used to measure working memory [29]. The test is part of the Wechsler Adult Intelligence Scale-IV (WAIS-IV). In this task, the participant has to mentally rearrange a series of verbally presented digits and recall them in sequential order. The total raw score was used for the present analysis.

2.2.3. Trail Making Test (TMT). Trail Making Test Condition 4 was used as a measure of cognitive flexibility. Trail Making Test is part of the Delis-Kaplan Executive Function System (D-KEFS) [30]. For this task, the participant has to connect circles as quickly as possible while sequentially switching between circles which contain numbers and letters. The total raw score was used for the present analysis.

2.2.4. Design Fluency Test (DFT). Design Fluency Test Condition 3 was used as a measure of creativity. It also measures problem solving ability and inhibition. It is part of the D-KEFS [30]. In this task the participant is presented with squares containing 10 dots, 5 empty and 5 filled in. The participant has to draw designs by connecting dots in the square while constantly switching between empty and filled dots. The participant is also asked to generate unique designs for each square without repeating any of the designs. The total raw score was used for the present analysis.

2.2.5. Tower Test (TT). Tower Test was used as a measure of planning. Tower Test is part of the D-KEFS [30]. In this test, the participant has to move 5 colored disks of different sizes across 3 pegs to match a position shown by the investigator. The participant is asked to complete the task with as few moves as possible, moving only one disk at a time and without placing a larger disk over a smaller disk. The task gets progressively more difficult as the trials increase. Completing the trial in fewer moves results in higher achievement scores (as long as the task is completed within the time limit; for details, see [30]). The total achievement score was used for the present analysis.

2.2.6. Cognitive Failures Questionnaire (CFQ) [31]. Subjective evaluation of cognitive function in everyday life was assessed using the Cognitive Failures Questionnaire. Cognitive Failures Questionnaire is a 25-item self-report measure that evaluates difficulties in attention, memory, distractibility, and executive functions. The questionnaire has good validity and reliability [31]. An analysis of data from the Royal Navy showed that Cognitive Failures Questionnaire scores are also correlated with real world outcomes like accident proneness, human error, and psychological strain [32]. The participant has to read sentences and indicate how often in the past 6 months they have had any of the mentioned experiences. Examples of questions are "Do you leave important letters unanswered for days?"; "Do you fail to see what you want in a supermarket (although it is there)?"; "Do you start doing one thing at home and get distracted into doing something else (unintentionally)?"; "Do you say something and realize afterwards that it might be taken as insulting?"; "Do you find you cannot think of anything to say?"; and so forth. Higher scores on Cognitive Failures Questionnaire indicate more problems. The test showed good internal consistency in our sample (Spearman-Brown Coefficient for split-half reliability was .91). The total score was used for the present analysis.

2.3. Statistical Analysis. Complete data was available for 92 participants. The data was analyzed using correlational and hierarchical multiple regression analyses. Bayesian analysis was additionally used to evaluate the correlation between Cognitive Failures Questionnaire and Raven's Advanced Progressive Matrices. Five univariate outliers (with z-scores > 3.3) were excluded from the variables Cognitive Failures Questionnaire, Digit Span Sequencing, Design Fluency Test, and Trail Making Test. The final sample for analysis consisted of 93 participants. All assumptions for linear regression analysis were met.

3. Results

To observe the interrelationships between variables, Pearson's bivariate correlation analysis was conducted. Raven's Advanced Progressive Matrices were significantly correlated with Digit Span Sequencing ($r(91) = .22$, $p = .03$; $t(91) = 2.15$, $p = .03$), Trail Making Test ($r(91) = -.30$, $p < .003$; $t(91) = -3.0$, $p = .003$), and Design Fluency Test ($r(91) = .39$, $p < .01$; $t(91) = 4.04$, $p < .001$), but not with Cognitive Failures Questionnaire or Tower Test. Digit Span Sequencing was significantly correlated with Trail Making Test ($r(91) = -.24$, $p = .02$; $t(91) = -2.36$, $p = .02$) and Tower Test ($r(90) = .27$, $p = .01$; $t(91) = 2.66$, $p = .009$). Trail Making Test was significantly correlated with Design Fluency Test ($r(91) = -.41$, $p < .001$; $t(91) = -4.29$, $p < .001$) and Tower Test ($r(90) = -.21$, $p = .04$; $t(90) = -2.04$, $p = .04$). Design Fluency Test was significantly correlated with Tower Test ($r(90) = .31$, $p = .003$; $t(90) = 3.10$, $p = .002$) (Tables 2 and 3).

Cognitive Failures Questionnaire was not correlated with fluid intelligence ($r(91) = -.08$, $p = .45$; $t(91) = -0.76$, $p = .45$) or any other measure. The correlation between Cognitive Failures Questionnaire and fluid intelligence was also examined by estimating a Bayes factor. The results showed that the correlation had a JZS BF_{10} of 0.19. This demonstrates that the data was over 5 times more likely to occur under a model where Cognitive Failures Questionnaire was not related to Raven's Advanced Progressive Matrices, rather than a model in which they were related. No other significant correlations were present.

3.1. Regressions. Means and standard deviations for all variables are presented in Table 4. Hierarchical linear regression with Raven's Advanced Progressive Matrices as the dependent variable and Cognitive Failures Questionnaire as the independent variable in block 1 showed that the Cognitive Failures Questionnaire did not significantly predict the score on Raven's Advanced Progressive Matrices ($F(1, 90) = 0.49$, $p = .49$). When Digit Span Sequencing, Trail Making Test, Design Fluency Test, and Tower Test were included in block 2, it resulted in a significant final model ($F(5, 86) = 4.48$, $p = .001$) which accounted for over 20% of the variability in Raven's Advanced Progressive Matrices ($R^2 = .21$; adjusted $R^2 = .16$). However, the only significant predictor in the final model was the Design Fluency Test ($B = 0.33$, $\beta = .29$, $t(86) = 2.68$, $p = .009$, and $pr^2 = .28$) (Table 5).

A follow-up exploratory regression analysis was conducted to determine whether age was a potential contributing factor. Hierarchical regression analysis with Raven's Advanced Progressive Matrices as the dependent variable

TABLE 2: Correlations among variables ($n = 93$).

	RAPM	CFQ	DSS	TMT	DFT
RAPM					
CFQ	−.08				
DSS	.22*	.06			
TMT	−.30**	−.08	−.24*		
DFT	.39**	−.01	.20	−.41**	
TT	.18	.01	.27**	−.21*	.31**

RAPM = Raven's Advanced Progressive Matrices; CFQ = Cognitive Failures Questionnaire; DSS = Digit Span Sequencing; TMT = Trail Making test; DFT = Design Fluency Test; TT = Tower Test.
*$p < .05$.
**$p < .01$.

TABLE 3: Covariance among variables ($n = 92$).

	RAPM	CFQ	DSS	TMT	DFT	TT
RAPM	7.29					
CFQ	−2.84	205.38				
DSS	1.24	1.50	3.81			
TMT	−22.91	−30.70	−12.70	746.49		
DFT	2.53	−0.41	0.95	−26.69	5.72	
TT	1.94	0.86	2.13	−23.29	3.00	16.40

RAPM = Raven's Advanced Progressive Matrices; CFQ = Cognitive Failures Questionnaire; DSS = Digit Span Sequencing; TMT = Trail Making test; DFT = Design Fluency Test; TT = Tower Test.

TABLE 4: Mean (standard deviation) of measures ($n = 93$).

	Mean (standard deviation)
RAPM	8.02 (2.69)
CFQ	35.37 (14.29)
DSS	9.16 (1.95)
TMT	86.90 (27.22)
DFT	7.59 (2.38)
TT	16.65 (4.05)

RAPM = Raven's Advanced Progressive Matrices; CFQ = Cognitive Failures Questionnaire; DSS = Digit Span Sequencing; TMT = Trail Making test; DFT = Design Fluency Test; TT = Tower Test.

Table 5: Hierarchical regression analysis of Digit Span Sequencing, Trail Making Test, Design Fluency Test, and Tower Test on Raven's Advanced Progressive Matrices after controlling for Cognitive Failures Questionnaire ($n = 92$).

	B	SE	β	pr^2
Block 1				
Intercept	8.53	0.75		
CFQ	−0.01	0.02	−.07	−.07
R	.07			
Block 2				
Intercept	5.62	2.26		
CFQ	−0.02	0.02	−.09	−.10
DSS	0.19	0.14	.14	.14
TMT	−0.02	0.01	−.16	−.16
DFT	0.33	0.12	.29**	.28
TT	0.01	0.07	.02	.02
R	.45			
R^2	.21			

RAPM = Raven's Advanced Progressive Matrices; CFQ = Cognitive Failures Questionnaire; DSS = Digit Span Sequencing; TMT = Trail Making test; DFT = Design Fluency Test; TT = Tower Test; B = B-value; SE = Standard Error; β = Beta; pr^2 = partial r^2.
$^{**}p < .01$.

and participant's age as the independent variable in block 1 showed that age did not significantly predict the score on Raven's Advanced Progressive Matrices ($F(1, 90) = 3.18$, $p = .78$). When the cognitive variables (Cognitive Failures Questionnaire, Digit Span Sequencing, Trail Making Test, Design Fluency Test, and Tower Test) were included in block 2, the results remained similar to the first regression analysis with the cognitive variables resulting in a significant final model ($F(6, 85) = 3.78$, $p = .002$) of Raven's Advanced Progressive Matrices.

4. Discussion

These results demonstrated that measures of working memory, cognitive flexibility, and creativity were significantly associated with fluid intelligence, but planning and subjective report of cognitive functioning were not. We also found that creativity was the only significant predictor of fluid intelligence in the regression model, which included subjective report of cognitive functioning, as well as working memory, cognitive flexibility, and planning as predictors.

Our finding that subjective reports are poor predictors of objective cognitive functioning is in agreement with previous studies. For instance, one meta-analysis [2] reported that, in cross-sectional community settings, people who report subjective memory impairments only have a 20% chance of actually suffering from dementia, while 60% of people with dementia do not report any memory problems. This discrepancy between subjective judgements and the actual status of cognitive functions has also been demonstrated in basic cognition literature [3, 4]. Our findings extend this view to inferring the level of fluid intelligence based on subjective report of cognitive functions like attention, memory, distractibility, and executive functions. Subjective report of cognitive functioning was not associated with any of the objective measures either. This may be because the Cognitive Failures Questionnaire primarily assesses memory, attention, and executive functions, while the objective measures assess working memory (DSS), cognitive flexibility (TMT), creativity (DFT), and planning (TT), and there may be little overlap in the cognitive functions that the subjective and objective measures assess.

Our results showed that objective measures of cognitive functioning (working memory, cognitive flexibility, and creativity) are significantly associated with fluid intelligence. However, the final regression model only accounted for around 20% of the variability in fluid intelligence, and the test of creativity was the only significant predictor in the final model. By most standards, a linear regression model accounting for 20% variability is acceptable; however, the purpose of the present analysis was to determine whether the predictors could be used as substitutes for assessing fluid intelligence directly, hence saving time and effort in clinical settings. With that goal in mind, five tasks accounting for 20% of the variability are unfortunately not practically useful. Moreover, the test of creativity was the only significant predictor.

There is no consensus in the literature on the nature of the relationship between creativity and fluid intelligence; while some studies have found them to be strongly related [19, 20], others have only reported a weak association [23] or no relation [24]. Our findings provide partial support to the view that creativity and fluid intelligence are positively related. However, it must be noted that creativity only made a modest contribution to predicting fluid intelligence in our analysis and hence further studies are required to fully understand the strength and nature of the relation between these constructs.

There have been studies that have shown fluid intelligence to be associated with working memory [21], cognitive flexibility [16], and planning [22], although the strength of the association between fluid intelligence and other cognitive functions has been disputed (see, e.g., [25]). Unlike studies with mostly younger participants, we did not find working memory, cognitive flexibility, or planning to be significant individual predictors of fluid intelligence in our sample of healthy older adults. However, we did find an overall combined association of these variables with fluid intelligence.

One limitation of our study was including only a single self-report measure while multiple objective measures were used. Self-report measures of cognitive functioning in everyday life tend to assess several cognitive domains simultaneously and there is considerable overlap of constructs assessed by the Cognitive Failures Questionnaire with constructs assessed by other measures like Perceived Deficits Questionnaire [33], Patient-Reported Outcomes in Cognitive Impairment [34], and so forth. Hence, the use of multiple self-report measures of cognition in everyday life would be redundant. To control for multiple comparisons, individual predictors were analyzed only in the presence of a significant final model. However, we acknowledge that the use of a single self-report measure is a limitation of this study.

5. Conclusion

The aim of the present study was to investigate whether subjective or objective measures that are associated with fluid intelligence can be used as substitutes to measuring fluid intelligence directly. Given that subjective reports were not able to predict fluid intelligence and objective measures did not substantially account for fluid intelligence, we conclude that neither subjective nor objective measures used in this study can be used as substitutes to measuring fluid intelligence directly, at least in older adults. This does not rule out the possibility that future studies may identify other subjective/objective measures that can be reliably used as proxy measures, but our findings suggest that the only reliable way to assess complex cognitive functions is to assess them directly. We further recommend the use of the shorter version of Raven's Advanced Progressive Matrices, which takes around half the time as the full version yet adequately predicts scores on the full version [35].

Competing Interests

The authors declare no conflict of interests.

Acknowledgments

This work was supported by the Natural Sciences and Engineering Research Council of Canada Discovery Grant. Dr. Goghari was supported by a Canadian Institutes of Health Research New Investigator Award.

References

[1] B. Schmand, C. Jonker, C. Hooijer, and J. Lindeboom, "Subjective memory complaints may announce dementia," *Neurology*, vol. 46, no. 1, pp. 121–125, 1996.

[2] A. J. Mitchell, "The clinical significance of subjective memory complaints in the diagnosis of mild cognitive impairment and dementia: a meta-analysis," *International Journal of Geriatric Psychiatry*, vol. 23, no. 11, pp. 1191–1202, 2008.

[3] R. E. Nisbett and T. D. Wilson, "Telling more than we can know: verbal reports on mental processes," *Psychological Review*, vol. 84, no. 3, pp. 231–259, 1977.

[4] J. Kruger and D. Dunning, "Unskilled and unaware of it: how difficulties in recognizing one's own incompetence lead to inflated self-assessments," *Journal of Personality and Social Psychology*, vol. 77, no. 6, pp. 1121–1134, 1999.

[5] R. J. Perry and J. R. Hodges, "Attention and executive deficits in Alzheimer's disease. A critical review," *Brain*, vol. 122, no. 3, pp. 383–404, 1999.

[6] C. Derouesne, S. Thibault, S. Lagha-Pierucci, V. Baudouin-Madec, D. Ancri, and L. Lacomblez, "Decreased awareness of cognitive deficits in patients with mild dementia of the Alzheimer type," *International Journal of Geriatric Psychiatry*, vol. 14, no. 12, pp. 1019–1030, 1999.

[7] E. P. Feher, G. J. Larrabee, A. Sudilovsky, and T. H. Crook, "Memory self-report in Alzheimer's disease and in age-associated memory impairment," *Journal of Geriatric Psychiatry and Neurology*, vol. 7, no. 1, pp. 58–65, 1994.

[8] D. B. Carr, S. Gray, J. Baty, and J. C. Morris, "The value of informant versus individual's complaints of memory impairment in early dementia," *Neurology*, vol. 55, no. 11, pp. 1724–1726, 2000.

[9] A. S. Kaufman and J. L. Horn, "Age changes on tests of fluid and crystallized ability for women and men on the Kaufman Adolescent and Adult Intelligence Test (KAIT) at ages 17–94 years," *Archives of Clinical Neuropsychology*, vol. 11, no. 2, pp. 97–121, 1996.

[10] C. L. Grady, J. V. Haxby, B. Horwitz, G. Berg, and S. I. Rapoport, "Neuropsychological and cerebral metabolic function in early vs late onset dementia of the Alzheimer type," *Neuropsychologia*, vol. 25, no. 5, pp. 807–816, 1987.

[11] J. C. Wallace, S. J. Kass, and C. J. Stanny, "The cognitive failures questionnaire revisited: dimensions and correlates," *Journal of General Psychology*, vol. 129, no. 3, pp. 238–256, 2002.

[12] J. A. Mogle, B. J. Lovett, R. S. Stawski, and M. J. Sliwinski, "What's so special about working memory? An examination of the relationships among working memory, secondary memory, and fluid intelligence: research report," *Psychological Science*, vol. 19, no. 11, pp. 1071–1077, 2008.

[13] E. Hunt, J. W. Pellegrino, and P. L. Yee, "Individual differences in attention," *Psychology of Learning and Motivation*, vol. 24, pp. 285–310, 1989.

[14] N. P. Friedman, A. Miyake, R. P. Corley, S. E. Young, J. C. DeFries, and J. K. Hewitt, "Not all executive functions are related to intelligence," *Psychological Science*, vol. 17, no. 2, pp. 172–179, 2006.

[15] M. J. Kane, D. Z. Hambrick, and A. R. A. Conway, "Working memory capacity and fluid intelligence are strongly related constructs: comment on Ackerman, Beier, and Boyle (2005)," *Psychological Bulletin*, vol. 131, no. 1, pp. 66–71, 2005.

[16] L. S. Colzato, N. C. Van Wouwe, T. J. Lavender, and B. Hommel, "Intelligence and cognitive flexibility: fluid intelligence correlates with feature 'unbinding' across perception and action," *Psychonomic Bulletin & Review*, vol. 13, no. 6, pp. 1043–1048, 2006.

[17] M. Batey, A. Furnham, and X. Safiullina, "Intelligence, general knowledge and personality as predictors of creativity," *Learning and Individual Differences*, vol. 20, no. 5, pp. 532–535, 2010.

[18] N. A. Zook, D. B. Davalos, E. L. DeLosh, and H. P. Davis, "Working memory, inhibition, and fluid intelligence as predictors of performance on Tower of Hanoi and London tasks," *Brain and Cognition*, vol. 56, no. 3, pp. 286–292, 2004.

[19] E. C. Nusbaum and P. J. Silvia, "Are intelligence and creativity really so different? Fluid intelligence, executive processes, and strategy use in divergent thinking," *Intelligence*, vol. 39, no. 1, pp. 36–45, 2011.

[20] P. J. Silvia, "Another look at creativity and intelligence: exploring higher-order models and probable confounds," *Personality and Individual Differences*, vol. 44, no. 4, pp. 1012–1021, 2008.

[21] A. R. A. Conway, N. Cowan, M. F. Bunting, D. J. Therriault, and S. R. B. Minkoff, "A latent variable analysis of working memory capacity, short-term memory capacity, processing speed, and general fluid intelligence," *Intelligence*, vol. 30, no. 2, pp. 163–183, 2002.

[22] J. M. Unterrainer, B. Rahm, C. P. Kaller et al., "Planning abilities and the Tower of London: is this task measuring a discrete cognitive function?" *Journal of Clinical and Experimental Neuropsychology*, vol. 26, no. 6, pp. 846–856, 2004.

[23] K. H. Kim, "Can only intelligent people be creative? A meta-analysis," *Prufrock Journal*, vol. 16, no. 2-3, pp. 57–66, 2005.

[24] A. Furnham and V. Bachtiar, "Personality and intelligence as predictors of creativity," *Personality and Individual Differences*, vol. 45, no. 7, pp. 613–617, 2008.

[25] P. L. Ackerman, M. E. Beier, and M. O. Boyle, "Working memory and intelligence: the same or different constructs?" *Psychological Bulletin*, vol. 131, no. 1, pp. 30–60, 2005.

[26] M. F. Folstein, S. E. Folstein, and P. R. McHugh, "'Mini-mental state': a practical method for grading the cognitive state of patients for the clinician," *Journal of Psychiatric Research*, vol. 12, no. 3, pp. 189–198, 1975.

[27] World Medical Association, "Declaration of Helsinki: recommendations guiding medical doctors in biomedical research involving human subjects," in *Proceedings of the 18th World Medical Assembly*, Helsinki, Finland, 1964, revised in Tokyo, 1975. Venice, Italy in 1983.

[28] J. C. Raven, G. Foulds, and A. Forbes, *Advanced Progressive Matrices: Sets I and II: Plan and Use of the Scale with a Report of Experimental Work*, Lewis, London, UK, 1973.

[29] D. Wechsler, *Wechsler Adult Intelligence Scale*, Canadian Manual, Pearson, Toronto, Canada, 4th edition, 2008.

[30] D. C. Delis, E. Kaplan, and J. H. Kramer, *Delis-Kaplan Executive Function System (D-KEFS)*, Psychological Corporation, New York, NY, USA, 2001.

[31] D. E. Broadbent, P. F. Cooper, P. FitzGerald, and K. R. Parkes, "The cognitive failures questionnaire (CFQ) and its correlates," *British Journal of Clinical Psychology*, vol. 21, no. 1, pp. 1–16, 1982.

[32] A. J. Day, K. Brasher, and R. S. Bridger, "Accident proneness revisited: the role of psychological stress and cognitive failure," *Accident Analysis and Prevention*, vol. 49, pp. 532–535, 2012.

[33] M. J. Sullivan, K. Edgley, and E. Dehoux, "A survey of multiple sclerosis: I. Perceived cognitive problems and compensatory strategy use," *Canadian Journal of Rehabilitation*, 1990.

[34] L. Frank, J. A. Flynn, L. Kleinman et al., "Validation of a new symptom impact questionnaire for mild to moderate cognitive impairment," *International Psychogeriatrics*, vol. 18, no. 1, pp. 135–149, 2006.

[35] R. Hamel and V. D. Schmittmann, "The 20-minute version as a predictor of the Raven Advanced Progressive Matrices Test," *Educational and Psychological Measurement*, vol. 66, no. 6, pp. 1039–1046, 2006.

24

Effect of a Lifestyle-Based Intervention on Health-Related Quality of Life in Older Adults with Hypertension

Mei-Lan Chen,[1,2] **Jie Hu**,[3] **Thomas P. McCoy**,[4] **Susan Letvak**,[4] **and Luba Ivanov**[5]

[1]*Byrdine F. Lewis College of Nursing and Health Professions, Georgia State University, Atlanta, GA 30303, USA*
[2]*Gerontology Institute, Georgia State University, Atlanta, GA 30303, USA*
[3]*College of Nursing, The Ohio State University, Columbus, OH 43210, USA*
[4]*School of Nursing, University of North Carolina at Greensboro, Greensboro, NC 27402, USA*
[5]*College of Nursing, Chamberlain University, Downers Grove, IL 60515, USA*

Correspondence should be addressed to Mei-Lan Chen; mchen13@gsu.edu

Academic Editor: Carmela R. Balistreri

The purpose of this study was to examine the effect of a six-month lifestyle-based intervention on health-related quality of life (HRQOL) in older adults with hypertension. A secondary analysis of a randomized controlled trial was conducted to test the differences between the intervention and control groups on HRQOL ($N = 196$). The results indicated that there were no statistically significant differences between the intervention and control groups on change in HRQOL, but the final regression models were statistically significant. SF-36 mental component summary (MCS) score at baseline, stress at baseline, and change in stress were significant predictors for predicting change in the SF-36 MCS. SF-36 physical component summary (PCS) at baseline and change in stress were significant predictors for predicting change in the SF-36 PCS. The findings suggest that the development of an effective intervention in improving HRQOL should be considered within individual, interpersonal, societal, and cultural factors for future research and clinical practice.

1. Introduction

The older population is growing significantly in the United States and global society. In 2014, the number of Americans aged 65 and above was 46 million, representing 15% of the total U.S. population; by 2030, the older population is estimated to be about 21% of the total population and one in 13 will be older than 85 [1–3]. Older adults frequently experience aging-related functional declines and chronic diseases such as hypertension. Overall, one in three adults, an estimated 75 million adults, has hypertension in the United States and only about half have high blood pressure under control [4]. Hypertension is more prevalent among older adults than young adults. Among those 45 to 54 years of age, the prevalence of hypertension was 34.7%; the prevalence of hypertension was 64.7% among those 65 to 74 years of age; and the prevalence was 77.3% in older adults ≥75 years of age [5]. 82.9% of adults ≥60 years of age self-reported that they were taking antihypertensive medication [5]. However, the percentage of adults ≥60 years of age who had controlled hypertension was only 49.4% during 2015-2016 [6]. Hence, high prevalence and poor control of high blood pressure remain critical issues for older Americans.

The World Health Organization (WHO) has emphasized the importance of assessing and promoting people's quality of life [7]. One of the goals of Healthy People 2020 is promoting health-related quality of life (HRQOL) and well-being across all life stages [8]. It is referred to as HRQOL when quality of life is considered in the health-related context. HRQOL is a subjective and multidimensional concept which is related to physical, mental, emotional, and social functioning [8]. The term HRQOL is frequently used to measure the effects of interventions and treatments on health benefits in older adults. Trevisol et al. pointed out that patients with hypertension are likely to have lower quality of life than normotensive adults [9]. Studies also indicated that low HRQOL was associated with lower levels of treatment adherence in older adults with hypertension [10–12]. Hence, developing effective interventions to promote better HRQOL in older adults with hypertension is essential.

Studies suggested that stress and social support may impact HRQOL in older adults [13–16]. Frias and Whyne's study indicated that stress was negatively associated with HRQOL [13]. In addition, Gerber (2012) found that social support was not significantly associated with physical HRQOL, but lower levels of social support were significantly associated with lower levels of mental HRQOL [14]. Older adults can be more vulnerable to stressful life events. It is critically important to examine the influence of stress and its relation to HRQOL in older adults with hypertension. However, there is little research in this area. Studies also have shown that social support can impact older adults' HRQOL [17–20]. Based on existing literature, few studies have included a measure of both stress and social support in this population [21–25]. Healthy aging is largely determined by individual lifestyle choices [1, 26]. Lifestyle interventions have been found to promote physical functioning and mental health in older adults [27, 28]. However, few research studies tested the effects of lifestyle interventions in older adults with hypertension. The current study performed secondary data analysis to investigate the effect of a lifestyle-based intervention on HRQOL in this population.

2. Conceptual Framework and Hypotheses

The conceptual framework guiding the current study was derived from the Social Cognitive Theory [29] and literature review. This study assumes that there is a relationship between person (e.g., stress), environment (e.g., social support), and the outcome (e.g., HRQOL). Demographic factors (age, race, gender, education, and income) may determine stress (person) and social support (environment) and can influence HRQOL (outcome). Lifestyle-based interventions would significantly improve changes in stress (person), social support (environment), and HRQOL (outcome).

The purpose of this study was to test the effects of a 6-month lifestyle-based intervention on HRQOL in older American adults with hypertension, accounting for stress and social support as mediating variables. After receiving a 6-month lifestyle-based intervention, the intervention group was hypothesized to significantly improve in person (stress) and environment (social support) (H1) and outcome (HRQOL) (H2) in older adults with hypertension from pretest (baseline) to posttest (6 months) compared to the control group.

3. Materials and Methods

3.1. Data Source and Sample. This study was approved by the Institutional Review Board (IRB) of the University of North Carolina at Greensboro (study#: 14-0428). The sample in the current study was drawn from the Well Elderly 2 Study. The data from the Well Elderly 2 Study were provided by the Inter-university Consortium for Political and Social Research [28]. The research design, methods, and the intervention of the Well Elderly 2 Study have been previously described in detail by Clark, Carlson, Jackson, and their colleagues [27, 28, 30, 31]. Briefly, in the original study, a convenience sample was recruited from the urban Los Angeles area in California [28, 30, 31]. Independent-living older Americans who spoke either English or Spanish were included in the study. Participants were excluded from the study if they had signs of psychosis or were not able to complete the assessment battery. There were 460 older adults aged 60–95 enrolled in the study. Participants were randomly assigned into the 6-month lifestyle intervention group or the no-treatment control group. After 6 months, the control group received a delayed intervention (the same 6-month lifestyle intervention as the intervention group). The 6-month lifestyle-based intervention included weekly 2-hour group meetings, 10 individual 1-hour sessions in homes or community settings, and monthly community outings [27, 30]. The modular content of the intervention comprised "impact of everyday activity on health, time spending and energy conservation, transportation utilization, home and community safety, social relationship, cultural awareness, goal setting, and changing routines and habits" (30, p. 783; 31).

In the present secondary analysis, we used only data collected during the first 6 months of the study (baseline and the first 6-month time point). Participants who self-reported taking blood pressure medication at baseline in the Well Elderly 2 Study were selected as subjects.

3.2. Measures

3.2.1. Demographic Data and Medical History. Demographic characteristics and medical history obtained by participants' self-report included gender, age, race, educational level, prescription medications, over-the-counter medicine, and diagnosis.

3.2.2. Stress. Stress was measured using the adapted Perceived Stress Scale [32]. The Perceived Stress Scale (PSS) is one of the most widely used scales to examine levels of perceived stress in older adults [22, 33]. This instrument examines to what extent participants perceive the degree of their lives to be uncontrollable, unpredictable, and overloaded during the past month. The adapted PSS is an 18-item scale, and all items are rated on a 5-point Likert scale ranging from 1 (never) to 5 (very often). Scores theoretically range from 18 to 90; higher scores indicate higher levels of perceived stress. In this study, Cronbach's alpha coefficient of the adapted PSS was 0.85.

3.2.3. Social Support. Social support was assessed using the Lubben Social Network Scale (LSNS) [34]. The LSNS is one of most commonly used instruments to measure perceived social support in older adults [35–37]. It is a 10-item scale that assesses the level of perceived support received from family, friends, and neighbors. Scores of the LSNS range from 0 to 50; higher scores indicate higher levels of social support. In this study, Cronbach's alpha coefficient of the LSNS was 0.75.

Table 1: Characteristics of the sample at baseline ($N = 196$).

Characteristic/variables	Total ($N = 196$)	Intervention group ($n = 103$)	Control group ($n = 93$)	p
Education, n (%)				0.284
Less than high school graduate	57 (29)	36 (35)	21 (23)	
High school graduate	48 (25)	24 (23)	24 (26)	
Some college or technical school	71 (36)	33 (32)	38 (41)	
Four years of college or more	20 (10)	10 (10)	10 (11)	
Gender, n (%)				0.083
Male	72 (37)	32 (31)	40 (43)	
Female	124 (63)	71 (69)	53 (57)	
Race, n (%)				0.275
White	64 (33)	31 (30)	33 (36)	
African American	79 (40)	46 (45)	33 (36)	
Hispanic/Latino	33 (17)	19 (18)	14 (15)	
Asian	5 (3)	3 (3)	2 (2)	
Others	14 (7)	4 (4)	10 (11)	
Age (years), mean ± SD	74.8 ± 7.7	74.2 ± 7.7	75.3 ± 7.7	0.304
Monthly income, n (%)				0.564
\$0–\$999	104 (54)	56 (54)	48 (53)	
\$1,000–\$1,999	44 (23)	20 (19)	24 (27)	
\$2,000–\$2,999	24 (12)	15 (15)	9 (10)	
\$3,000 or more	21 (11)	12 (12)	9 (10)	
Other medications used, n (%)				
Diabetes medication	62 (32)	33 (32)	29 (31)	0.898
Antidepressant medication	21 (11)	14 (14)	7 (8)	0.170
Antipsychotic medication	39 (20)	22 (21)	17 (18)	0.590
Cholesterol reducer medication	95 (49)	49 (48)	46 (50)	0.792
Stress (PSS)	43.7 ± 10.7	43.8 ± 11.0	43.6 ± 10.5	0.885
Social support (LSNS)	27.2 ± 9.1	27.1 ± 8.5	27.3 ± 9.7	0.907
HRQOL : MCS	46.7 ± 11.4	46.1 ± 12.3	47.5 ± 10.4	0.405
HRQOL : PCS	39.6 ± 10.1	39.1 ± 10.1	40.2 ± 10.0	0.459

Note. SD: standard deviation; PSS: perceived stress scale; LSNS: Lubben Social Network Scale; HRQOL: health-related quality of life; MCS: mental component summary; PCS: physical component summary.

3.2.4. Health-Related Quality of Life (HRQOL). HRQOL was measured using the 36-Item Short-Form Health Survey (SF-36, version 2.0) [38, 39]. The SF-36 is frequently used to measure HRQOL in older adults [10, 40, 41]. It is a multi-domain that measures physical and mental components of HRQOL with eight subscales. The 8 subscales contribute to two resulting component summaries: a mental component summary (MCS) and a physical component summary (PCS). Both PCS and MCS scores range from 0 to 100, representing worst to best health. Higher scores indicate better HRQOL [42]. In this study, reliability coefficients of the SF-36 PCS and MCS were 0.83 and 0.85, respectively.

3.3. Data Analysis. Descriptive statistics were initially calculated using means and standard deviations or frequencies and percentages. Continuous variables were checked for outliers and normality in univariate analysis. To test hypotheses *H*1 and *H*2, multiple linear regression using a hierarchical regression model building approach was performed to test the effect of the intervention and make predictions on criterion variables [43, 44]. Demographic variables (age, race, gender, education, and income), stress at baseline, and the intervention group (intervention versus control) as independent variables were entered for modeling the change in stress. Similarly, demographic variables, social support at baseline, and the intervention group as independent variables were entered for separately modeling the change in social support. Finally, the change in HRQOL was modeled using independent variables including demographic variables, HRQOL at baseline, stress at baseline, change in stress, social support at baseline, change in social support, and the intervention group through hierarchical multiple regression analysis. A two-sided p value < 0.05 was considered statistically significant. All analyses were performed using SPSS version 23 (IBM corp., Armonk, IL).

4. Results

4.1. Sample Characteristics. There were a total of 196 participants in this study. Of the 196 participants, 103 were randomly assigned to the intervention group and 93 to the control group. Table 1 presents baseline characteristics of the participants and descriptive statistics. At baseline, the mean age of participants was 74.8 ± 7.7 years; 63% were women. Most participants were White (33%) and African American (40%); the majority reported having a high school education or more (71%). Also, more than half (54%) reported a monthly income less than \$1,000. In addition to taking hypertension medication, 32% of the participants reported that they also took diabetes medication and 49% used

Table 2: Hierarchical multiple regression analyses predicting change in stress (post – baseline) after lifestyle-based intervention (N = 169).

Independent variable	ΔR^2	β^a
Step 1: demographic variables	0.05	
Education		
Less than high school graduate[b]		
High school graduate		0.07
Some college or technical school		0.11
Four years of college or more		0.22*
Gender		
Male[b]		
Female		0.08
Race		
White[b]		
African American		0.11
Hispanic/Latino		0.20*
Asian		−0.03
Others		0.10
Age (years)		−0.04
Monthly income		
\$0–\$999[b]		
\$1,000–\$1,999		−0.08
\$2,000–\$2,999		−0.04
\$3,000 or more		0.09
Step 2	0.20***	
Stress at baseline (points)		−0.49***
Step 3	<0.01	
Control group[b]		
Intervention group		0.03
Total R^2	0.25***	

Note. [a]β shown is for the last step. [b]Reference category. $^{*}p < 0.05$; $^{**}p < 0.01$; $^{***}p < 0.001$.

Table 3: Hierarchical multiple regression analyses predicting change in social support (post – baseline) after lifestyle-based intervention (N = 168).

Independent variable	ΔR^2	β^a
Step 1: demographic variables	0.07	
Education		
Less than high school graduate[b]		
High school graduate		0.07
Some college or technical school		0.05
Four years of college or more		−0.05
Gender		
Male[b]		
Female		−0.07
Race		
White[b]		
African American		0.15
Hispanic/Latino		0.07
Asian		−0.02
Others		0.13
Age (years)		−0.03
Monthly income		
\$0–\$999[b]		
\$1,000–\$1,999		0.13
\$2,000–\$2,999		0.06
\$3,000 or more		0.01
Step 2	0.11***	
Social support at baseline (points)		−0.37***
Step 3	<0.01	
Control group[b]		
Intervention group		−0.06
Total R^2	0.18**	

Note. [a]β shown is for the last step. [b]Reference category. $^{*}p < 0.05$; $^{**}p < 0.01$; $^{***}p < 0.001$.

antihyperlipidemic agents. The intervention and control groups did not statistically significantly differ on any sample characteristics (all $p \geq 0.05$).

At baseline, the average stress score was 43.7 ± 10.7, and the average of social support score was 27.2 ± 9.1. The mean scores of the SF-36 mental component summary (MCS) and physical component summary (PCS) were 46.7 ± 11.4 and 39.6 ± 10.1, respectively. As shown in Table 1, there were no significant differences between the intervention and control groups on these measures at baseline ($p \geq 0.05$).

4.2. Effects of a Lifestyle-Based Intervention in Changes in Stress and Social Support. Table 2 indicates the results of the predictor variables at each step and in the final model for predicting change in stress (post – baseline) after lifestyle-based intervention. There was not a statistically significant difference between the intervention and control groups on change in stress, but the final regression model was statistically significant ($p < 0.001$). In the final hierarchical regression model, demographic variables (education, gender, race, age, and monthly income), stress at baseline, and intervention versus control significantly accounted for 25% of the variance in change in stress (R^2 = 0.25). In addition, stress at baseline accounted for a significant amount of variance in change in stress after controlling for the effect of demographic variables based on the second step of the hierarchical model building (ΔR^2 = 0.20, $p < 0.001$). Four years of college or more, Hispanic/Latino versus White Americans, and stress at baseline were significant predictors. Adjusting for all other factors, participants who received four years of college or more education were associated with a 0.22 increase in standard deviation (*SD*) units of predicted change in stress compared to participants who received less than high school; Hispanic/Latino participants were associated with a 0.20 increase in *SD* units of predicted change in stress compared to White participants. For every 1 *SD* increase in stress at baseline, the predicted mean decrease in change in stress was 0.49 *SD* units, adjusting for all other factors.

Table 3 presents the results for the predictor variables at each step and in the final model for predicting change in social support (post – baseline) after lifestyle-based intervention. As shown in Table 3, there was no statistically significant difference between the intervention and control groups on change in social support, but the final regression model was statistically significant ($p < 0.01$). In the final hierarchical regression model, demographic variables, social support at baseline, and intervention versus control significantly accounted for 18% of the variance in change in social support (R^2 = 0.18). Additionally, social support at baseline accounted for a significant amount of variance in

TABLE 4: Hierarchical multiple regression analyses predicting change in health-related quality of life (MCS; post − baseline) according to lifestyle-based intervention, stress, and social support ($N = 167$).

Independent variable	ΔR^2	β[a]
Step 1: demographic variables	0.05	
Education		
Less than high school graduate[b]		
High school graduate		0.03
Some college or technical school		0.13
Four years of college or more		0.10
Gender		
Male[b]		
Female		−0.13
Race		
White[b]		
African American		0.02
Hispanic/Latino		−0.01
Asian		0.01
Others		0.01
Age (years)		0.06
Monthly income		
\$0–\$999[b]		
\$1,000–\$1,999		0.03
\$2,000–\$2,999		0.00
\$3,000 or more		−0.01
Step 2	0.26***	
MCS at baseline (points)		−0.66***
Step 3	<0.01	
Control group[b]		
Intervention group		0.07
Step 4	0.08**	
Stress at baseline (points)		−0.27**
Change in stress		−0.28**
Social support at baseline (points)		0.07
Change in social support		0.05
Total R^2	0.39***	

Note. MCS: mental component summary. [a]β shown is for the last step. [b]Reference category. *$p < 0.05$; **$p < 0.01$; ***$p < 0.001$.

TABLE 5: Hierarchical multiple regression analyses predicting change in health-related quality of life (PCS; post − baseline) according to lifestyle-based intervention, stress, and social support ($N = 167$).

Independent variable	ΔR^2	β[a]
Step 1: demographic variables	0.03	
Education		
Less than high school graduate[b]		
High school graduate		−0.04
Some college or technical school		−0.04
Four years of college or more		−0.07
Gender		
Male[b]		
Female		−0.03
Race		
White[b]		
African American		−0.01
Hispanic/Latino		−0.01
Asian		−0.03
Others		0.03
Age (years)		0.06
Monthly income		
\$0 - \$999[b]		
\$1,000 - \$1,999		−0.01
\$2,000 - \$2,999		0.12
\$3,000 or more		0.04
Step 2	0.10***	
PCS at baseline (points)		−0.38***
Step 3	<0.01	
Control group[b]		
Intervention group		0.04
Step 4	0.05	
Stress at baseline (points)		−0.13
Change in stress		−0.18*
Social support at baseline (points)		0.12
Change in social support		0.07
Total R^2	0.18*	

Note. PCS: physical component summary. [a]β shown is for the last step. [b]Reference category. *$p < 0.05$; **$p < 0.01$; ***$p < 0.001$.

change in social support, after controlling for the effect of demographic variables ($\Delta R^2 = 0.11$, $p < 0.001$). The only significant predictor was social support at baseline, where for every 1 *SD* increase in social support at baseline, the predicted mean decrease in change in social support was 0.37 *SD* units, adjusting for all other factors.

4.3. Effects of a Lifestyle-Based Intervention in Changes in HRQOL. Table 4 indicates the results of the associations with the predictor variables at each step in predicting change in the SF-36 mental component summary (MCS; post − baseline) according to lifestyle-based intervention, stress, and social support. There was no statistically significant difference between the intervention and control groups on change in the SF-36 MCS, but the final regression model was statistically significant ($p < 0.001$). In the final hierarchical regression model, demographic variables, SF-36 MCS score at baseline, intervention versus control, stress at baseline, change in stress, social support at baseline, and change in social support significantly accounted for 39% of variance in change in the SF-36 MCS ($R^2 = 0.39$). The SF-36 MCS at baseline accounted for a significant amount of variance in change in the SF-36 MCS, after controlling for the effect of demographic variables in the second step of modeling ($\Delta R^2 = 0.26$, $p < 0.001$). In the last step, stress at baseline, change in stress, social support at baseline, and change in social support accounted for a significant amount of variance in change in the SF-36 MCS after controlling for the effect of demographic variables, SF-36 MCS score at baseline, and the effect of intervention ($\Delta R^2 = 0.08$, $p < 0.01$). The SF-36 MCS score at baseline, stress at baseline, and change in stress were significant predictors in the final model. For every 1 *SD* increase in the SF-36 MCS at baseline, the predicted mean decrease in the change in the SF-36 MCS was 0.66 *SD* units; for every 1 *SD* increase in stress at baseline, the predicted mean decrease in change in the SF-36 MCS was 0.27 *SD* units; for every 1 *SD* increase in change in stress, the predicted mean decrease in change in the SF-36 MCS was 0.28 *SD* units, adjusting for all other factors.

Table 5 shows the results for the associations with the predictor variables at each step for predicting change in the

SF-36 physical component summary (PCS; post – baseline) according to lifestyle-based intervention, stress, and social support. As shown in Table 5, there was no statistically significant difference between the intervention and control groups on change in the SF-36 PCS, but the final regression model was statistically significant ($p < 0.05$). In the final hierarchical regression model, demographic variables, SF-36 PCS score at baseline, intervention versus control, stress at baseline, change in stress, social support at baseline, and change in social support significantly accounted for 18% of the variance in change in the SF-36 PCS ($R^2 = 0.18$). The SF-36 PCS score at baseline accounted for a significant amount of variance in the change in the SF-36 PCS after controlling for the effect of demographic variables ($\Delta R^2 = 0.10$, $p < 0.001$). The SF-36 PCS at baseline and change in stress were significant predictors of change in PCS scores in the final model. For every 1 *SD* increase in the SF-36 PCS at baseline, the predicted mean decrease in the change in the SF-36 PCS was 0.38 *SD* units; for every 1 *SD* increase in change in stress, the predicted mean decrease in change in the SF-36 PCS was 0.18 *SD* units, adjusting for all other factors.

5. Discussion

This secondary analysis examined the effectiveness of a lifestyle-based intervention on HRQOL in older adults with hypertension and investigated stress and social support as mediating variables. As many older adults suffer from hypertension, developing effective interventions to enhance older adults' HRQOL is necessary for healthy aging. The results of this analysis provide empirical evidence, advance the scientific knowledge, and propose intervention recommendations for future research and clinical practice in older adults with hypertension.

The findings of the study indicated that there were no statistically significant intervention effects on stress, social support, and HRQOL, but the final regression models were statistically significant in the last step of the hierarchical multiple regression analysis. According to Baron and Kenny (1986) criteria for a mediation analysis, social support and stress failed to function as mediators in the current study [45]. This result is inconsistent with previous research. Previous studies revealed that social support and stress can mediate lifestyle practices and health-related quality of life in older adults [17–20]. Additionally, in the original study, the 6-month intervention was an activity-based lifestyle intervention which emphasized the importance of activity participation and developing new health-related habits (28; 31, p. 92). However, for older adults, stress and lack of social support can come from chronic illness, financial difficulties, retirement, change in living situation, family problems, or aging-related physical impairments [20, 24, 46]. Therefore, this lifestyle intervention may not have significant effects on changes in stress, social support, and HRQOL. Also, many stressors are chronic and long term in older adults [24, 46]. The 6-month duration of the intervention may not be sufficient for changing stress and HRQOL. Hence, this study suggests that further interventions should consider how to reduce stress and increase social support for older adults with hypertension.

In this study, stress at baseline and change in stress were significant predictors in predicting the mental component of HRQOL; change in stress was a significant predictor in predicting the physical component of HRQOL. Gerber also found that higher perceived stress was significantly associated with poorer mental HRQOL in older adults [14]. In addition, Frias and Whyne revealed that stress was negatively associated with HRQOL in community-dwelling older adults [13]. Gerber indicated that there were significant interactions between perceived stress and social support on mental HRQOL [14]. However, synergistic effects of stress and social support on HRQOL remain unclear. These findings suggest that stress should be considered as a significant predictor for changes on HRQOL in older adults with hypertension.

Aging is a multifaceted process and is related to reduced functional capacity and chronic diseases [47–49]. Many older adults have at least one chronic disease such as hypertension, diabetes, or cardiovascular diseases. However, there has been little research to investigate the effects of lifestyle-based interventions in older adults with chronic diseases. The result of this study showed the presence of comorbidities in participants with hypertension. The effects of comorbidities on HRQOL remain unclear. Thus, comorbidities should be considered as a factor for future studies, and the conceptual framework should be expanded to include comorbidities. Finally, there is no common language on what is the dose-response effect of lifestyle-based programs in older adults with hypertension. How much is enough for older adults with hypertension? Further research should focus on older adults with hypertension in exposure to lifestyle interventions and racial differences in response to lifestyle interventions.

The current study has several limitations. First, the effect of the lifestyle-based intervention was tested from pretest (baseline) to posttest (the 6-month time point). Hence, the lifestyle intervention may not have significant short-term effects on change in social support, stress, and HRQOL [28, 31, 50, 51]. Second, some confounding factors were not available in the dataset that may impact the intervention effect on HRQOL, such as frailty, chronic pain, and sleep quality. Also, details on the hypertensive status of patients were not available in the dataset. Additionally, most participants were women and reported low income. Lastly, the sample was urban, community-dwelling older adults and cannot be generalized to older adults who live in rural areas and nursing homes.

6. Conclusions

There is limited research to test the effects of lifestyle interventions on HRQOL in older adults with hypertension. In this study, the results revealed that the regression model is statistically significant in predicting changes in HRQOL according to lifestyle-based intervention, stress, and social support. Educational levels, race, stress at baseline are significant predictors for predicting change in stress; social support at baseline is the significant predictor for predicting change in social support. In addition, SF-36 MCS score at baseline, stress at baseline, and change in stress are significant predictors of change in MCS scores in the final model. SF-36 PCS score at baseline and change in stress are significant predictors for predicting change in the SF-36 PCS. As many older adults have high blood pressure and reduced HRQOL, developing effective interventions in promoting hypertension self-management and improving HRQOL for older adults with hypertension is essential. This secondary analysis suggests that stress management and social support resources should be included in the lifestyle intervention for future research and clinical practice. The results indicate that the development of an effective intervention in improving HRQOL should be considered within individual, interpersonal, societal, and cultural factors when implementing the lifestyle-based interventions.

Conflicts of Interest

The authors declare that there are no conflicts of interest regarding the publication of this paper.

References

[1] Centers for Disease Control and Prevention, *FastStats: Older Persons' Health*, Centers for Disease Control and Prevention, Atlanta, GA, USA, 2015, http://www.cdc.gov/nchs/fastats/older-american-health.htm.

[2] National Center for Health Statistics, *Older Americans 2016: Key Indicators of Well-Being. Federal Interagency Forum on Aging-Related Statistics*, U.S. Government Printing Office, Washington, DC, USA, 2016.

[3] U.S. Census Bureau, *An Aging Nation: The Older Population in the United States*, U.S. Census Bureau, Suitland, MD, USA, 2014, http://www.census.gov/prod/2014pubs/p25-1140.pdf.

[4] Centers for Disease Control and Prevention, *High Blood Pressure Facts*, Centers for Disease Control and Prevention, Atlanta, GA, USA, 2016, https://www.cdc.gov/bloodpressure/facts.htm.

[5] E. J. Benjamin, M. J. Blaha, S. E. Chiuve et al., "Heart disease and stroke statistics—2017 update: a report from the American Heart Association," *Circulation*, vol. 135, no. 10, pp. e146–e603, 2017.

[6] National Center for Health Statistics, *Hypertension Prevalence and Control Among Adults: United States, 2015–2016, NCHS Data Brief, 289*, National Center for Health Statistics, Hyattsville, MD, USA, 2017.

[7] World Health Organization, "The World Health Organization Quality of Life Assessment (WHOQOL): position paper from the World Health Organization," *Social Science and Medicine*, vol. 41, no. 10, pp. 1403–1409, 2005.

[8] Office of Disease Prevention and Health Promotion, *Healthy People 2020: Health-Related Quality of Life and Well-Being*, Office of Disease Prevention and Health Promotion, Washington, DC, USA, 2015, https://www.healthypeople.gov/2020/about/foundation-health-measures/Health-Related-Quality-of-Life-and-Well-Being.

[9] D. J. Trevisol, L. B. Moreira, A. Kerkhoff, S. C. Fuchs, and F. Fuchs, "Health- related quality of life and hypertension: a systematic review and meta-analysis of observational studies," *Journal of Hypertension*, vol. 29, no. 2, pp. 179–188, 2011.

[10] E. W. Holt, P. Muntner, C. J. Joyce, L. Webber, and M. A. Krousel-Wood, "Health-related quality of life and antihypertensive medication adherence among older adults," *Age and Ageing*, vol. 39, no. 4, pp. 481–487, 2010.

[11] D. J. Trevisol, L. B. Moreira, S. C. Fuchs, and F. Fuchs, "Health-related quality of life is worse in individuals with hypertension under drug treatment: results of population-based study," *Journal of Human Hypertension*, vol. 26, no. 6, pp. 374–380, 2012.

[12] R. B. Trivedi, B. Ayotte, D. Edelman, and H. B. Bosworth, "The association of emotional well-being and marital status with treatment adherence among patients with hypertension," *Journal of Behavioral Medicine*, vol. 31, no. 6, pp. 489–497, 2008.

[13] C. M. de Frias and E. Whyne, "Stress on health-related quality of life in older adults: the protective nature of mindfulness," *Aging and Mental Health*, vol. 19, no. 3, pp. 201–206, 2015.

[14] E. J. Gerber, *The Relations of Social Support and Perceived Stress to Health-Related Quality of Life in Older Adults*, University of Maryland, Baltimore, MD, USA, 2012.

[15] C. L. Keyes, B. Michalec, R. Kobau, H. Zahran, M. M. Zack, and E. J. Simoes, "Social support and health-related quality of life among older adults: Missouri, 2000," *Morbidity and Mortality Weekly Report*, vol. 54, no. 17, pp. 433–437, 2005, http://www.cdc.gov/mmwr/preview/mmwrhtml/mm5417a4.htm.

[16] A. M. Sherman, S. A. Shumaker, W. J. Rejeski, T. Morgan, W. B. Applegate, and W. Ettinger, "Social support, social integration, and health-related quality of life over time: results from the Fitness and Arthritis in Seniors Trial (FAST)," *Psychology and Health*, vol. 21, no. 4, pp. 463–480, 2006.

[17] J. A. Carlson, J. F. Sallis, T. L. Conway et al., "Interactions between psychosocial and built environment factors in explaining older adults' physical activity," *Preventive Medicine*, vol. 54, no. 1, pp. 68–73, 2012.

[18] B. Fernandez, E. Montenegro, N. Knoll, and R. Schwarzer, "Self-efficacy, action control, and social support explain physical activity changes among Costa Rican older adults," *Journal of Physical Activity and Health*, vol. 11, no. 8, pp. 1573–1578, 2014.

[19] R. E. Taylor-Piliae, J. M. Fair, W. L. Haskell et al., "Validation of the Stanford Brief Activity Survey: examining psychological factors and physical activity levels in older adults," *Journal of Physical Activity and Health*, vol. 7, pp. 87–94, 2010.

[20] K. Yoshiuchi, S. Inada, R. Nakahara et al., "Stressful life events and habitual physical activity in older adults: 1-year accelerometer data from the Nakanojo Study," *Mental Health and Physical Activity*, vol. 3, no. 1, pp. 23–25, 2010.

[21] M. Hamer, "Psychosocial stress and cardiovascular disease risk: the role of physical activity," *Psychosomatic Medicine*, vol. 74, no. 9, pp. 896–903, 2012.

[22] K. H. Kwag, P. Martin, D. Russell, W. Franke, and M. Kohut, "The impact of perceived stress, social support, and home-based physical activity on mental health among older adults," *International Journal of Aging and Human Development*, vol. 72, no. 2, pp. 137–154, 2011.

[23] A. L. Paukert, J. W. Pettit, M. E. Kunik et al., "The roles of social support and self-efficacy in physical health's impact on depressive and anxiety symptoms in older adults," *Journal of Clinical Psychology in Medical Settings*, vol. 17, no. 4, pp. 387–400, 2010.

[24] U. Rimmele, R. Seiler, B. Marti, P. H. Wirtz, U. Ehlert, and M. Heinrichs, "The level of physical activity affects adrenal and cardiovascular reactivity to psychosocial stress," *Psychoneuroendocrinology*, vol. 34, no. 2, pp. 190–198, 2009.

[25] L. M. Warner, J. P. Ziegelmann, B. Schüz, S. Wurm, and R. Schwarzer, "Synergistic effect of social support and self-efficacy on physical exercise in older adults," *Journal of Aging and Physical Activity*, vol. 19, no. 3, pp. 249–261, 2011.

[26] W. J. Chodzko-Zajko, *ACSM's Exercise for Older Adults*, Wolters Kluwer/Lippincott Williams & Wilkins, Philadelphia, PA, USA, 2014.

[27] M. Carlson, J. Jackson, D. Mandel et al., "Predictors of retention among African American and Hispanic older adult research participants in the Well Elderly 2 randomized controlled trial," *Journal of Applied Gerontology*, vol. 33, no. 3, pp. 357–382, 2014.

[28] F. Clark, *Well Elderly 2, Los Angeles, California, 2004-2008: ICPSR33641-v1*, Inter-University Consortium for Political and Social Research, Ann Arbor, MI, USA, 2012.

[29] A. Bandura, *Social Foundations of Thought and Action: A Social Cognitive Theory*, Prentice Hall, Englewood Cliffs, NJ, USA, 1985.

[30] F. Clark, J. Jackson, M. Carlson et al., "Effectiveness of a lifestyle intervention in promoting the well-being of independently living older people: results of the Well Elderly 2 randomised controlled trial," *Journal of Epidemiology of Community Health*, vol. 66, no. 9, pp. 782–790, 2012.

[31] J. Jackson, D. Mandel, J. Blanchard et al., "Confronting challenges in intervention research with ethnically diverse older adults: the USC Well Elderly II trial," *Clinical Trials*, vol. 6, no. 1, pp. 90–101, 2009.

[32] S. Cohen, T. Kamarck, and R. Mermelstein, "A global measure of perceived stress," *Journal of Health and Social Behavior*, vol. 24, no. 4, pp. 385–396, 1983.

[33] R. S. White, J. Jiang, C. B. Hall et al., "Higher perceived stress scale scores are associated with higher pain intensity and pain interference levels in older adults," *Journal of the American Geriatrics Society*, vol. 62, no. 12, pp. 2350–2356, 2014.

[34] J. E. Lubben, "Assessing social networks among elderly population," *Family and Community Health: The Journal of Health Promotion and Maintenance*, vol. 11, no. 3, pp. 42–52, 1988.

[35] D. Burnette and S. Myagmarjav, "Translation and validation of the 18-item Lubben Social Network Scale with older adults in Mongolia," *International Psychogeriatrics*, vol. 25, no. 9, pp. 1493–1502, 2013.

[36] J. Gray, J. Kim, J. R. Ciesla, and P. Yao, "Rasch analysis of the Lubben Social Network Scale–6 (LSNS-6)," *Journal of Applied Gerontology*, vol. 35, no. 5, pp. 508–528, 2014.

[37] J. Lubben, E. Blozik, G. Gillmann et al., "Performance of an abbreviated version of the Lubben Social Network Scale among three European community-dwelling older adult populations," *Gerontologist*, vol. 46, no. 4, pp. 503–513, 2006.

[38] J. E. Ware, *Construction of the SF-36. SF-36 Health Survey Update*, 2013, http://www.sf-36.org/tools/SF36.shtml.

[39] J. E. Ware and C. D. Sherbourne, "The MOS 36-item short form health survey (SF-36): conceptual framework and item selection," *Medical Care*, vol. 30, no. 6, pp. 473–483, 1992.

[40] J. Hu, K. J. Gruber, and K. H. Hsueh, "Psychometric properties of the Chinese version of the SF-36 in older adults with diabetes in Beijing, China," *Diabetes Research and Clinical Practice*, vol. 88, no. 3, pp. 273–281, 2010.

[41] Z. Yang, W. Li, X. Tu et al., "Validation and psychometric properties of the Chinese version of SF-36 in patients with hypertension, coronary heart diseases, chronic gastritis and peptic ulcer," *International Journal of Clinical Practice*, vol. 66, no. 10, pp. 991–998, 2012.

[42] J. E. Ware, M. Kosinski, and S. D. Keler, *SF-36 Physical and Mental Health Summary Scales: A User's Manual*, The Health Institute, Boston, MA, USA, 1994.

[43] G. M. Fitzmaurice, N. M. Laird, and J. H. Ware, *Applied Longitudinal Analysis*, Wiley-Interscience, Hoboken, NJ, 2011.

[44] D. F. Polit, *Statistics and Data Analysis for Nursing Research*, Pearson Education Inc., Upper Saddle River, NJ, USA, 2nd edition, 2010.

[45] R. M. Baron and D. A. Kenny, "The moderator–mediator variable distinction in social psychological research: conceptual, strategic, and statistical considerations," *Journal of Personality and Social Psychology*, vol. 51, no. 6, pp. 1173–1182, 1986.

[46] R. Rueggeberg, C. Wrosch, and G. E. Miller, "The different roles of perceived stress in the association between older adults' physical activity and physical health," *Health Psychology*, vol. 31, no. 2, pp. 164–171, 2012.

[47] M. L. Chen, "The growing costs and burden of family caregiving of older adults: a review of paid sick leave and family leave policies," *Gerontologist*, vol. 56, no. 3, pp. 391–396, 2016.

[48] M. L. Chen and J. Hu, "Health disparities in Chinese Americans with hypertension: a review," *International Journal of Nursing Sciences*, vol. 1, no. 3, pp. 318–322, 2014.

[49] J. Sheffler and N. Sachs-Ericsson, "Racial differences in the effect of stress on health and the moderating role of perceived social support," *Journal of Aging and Health*, vol. 28, no. 8, pp. 1362–1381, 2016.

[50] R. A. Fielding, W. J. Rejeski, S. Blair et al., "The lifestyle interventions and independence for elders study: design and methods," *Journals of Gerontology Series A: Biological Sciences and Medical Sciences*, vol. 66, no. 11, pp. 1226–1237, 2011.

[51] W. J. Rejeski, S. L. Mihalko, W. T. Ambrosius, L. B. Bearon, and J. W. McClelland, "Weight loss and self-regulatory eating efficacy in older adults: the cooperative lifestyle intervention program," *Journals of Gerontology Series B: Psychological Sciences and Social Sciences*, vol. 66, no. 3, pp. 279–286, 2011.

25

Perspectives of Older Adults on Aging Well: A Focus Group Study

Hadeel Halaweh,[1,2] **Synneve Dahlin-Ivanoff**,[1,3] **Ulla Svantesson**,[1] **and Carin Willén**[1]

[1]*Department of Health and Rehabilitation, Institute of Neuroscience and Physiology, University of Gothenburg, Gothenburg, Sweden*
[2]*Department of Physiotherapy & Rehabilitation, Faculty of Health Professions, Al-Quds University, Jerusalem, State of Palestine*
[3]*Centre for Ageing and Health, AGECAP, University of Gothenburg, Gothenburg, Sweden*

Correspondence should be addressed to Hadeel Halaweh; hadeel.halaweh@neuro.gu.se

Academic Editor: Carmela R. Balistreri

Background. With increasing number of older adults worldwide, promoting health and well-being becomes a priority for aging well. Well-being and physical and mental health are closely related, and this relation may become more vital at older ages as it may contribute to aging well. The state of well-being is a multifaceted phenomenon that refers to an individual's subjective feelings, and exploring perspectives of older adults on aging well is developing to be an important area of research. Therefore, the aim of this study was to explore perceptions on aging well among older adult Palestinians ≥60 years. *Methods.* A qualitative research design in the context of focus group discussions was used; seven focus groups were conducted including fifty-six participants (aged 63–81 years). Data were analyzed using a qualitative interpretative thematic approach described by Braun and Clarke. *Results.* Three major themes were identified, *"sense of well-being," "having good physical health,"* and *"preserving good mental health."* The participants perceived that aging well is influenced by positive feelings such as being joyous, staying independent, having a life purpose, self-possessed contentment, and financially secured, in addition to be socially engaged and enjoying good physical and mental health. *Conclusion.* This study contributes to get a better insight concerning older adults' perspectives on aging well. Enhancing physically active lifestyle, participation in social and leisure activities, healthy eating habits, having a purpose in life, and being intellectually engaged are all contributing factors to aging well. Vital factors are to be considered in developing strategic health and rehabilitative plans for promoting aging well among older adults.

1. Introduction

Worldwide, the age group of sixty years old and older is growing faster than any other age group [1]. With this remarkable increase of older adults; promoting health and well-being becomes a priority for aging well [2]. Aging well is conceptualized using different contemporary theoretical frameworks in the last decades, including healthy aging, positive aging, productive aging, active aging, and successful aging [3, 4]. These theoretical frameworks integrate both biological and social sciences, considering social participation, psychology, lifestyles, activities, finances, and other domestic and environmental factors as well [4]. The WHO defines *active aging* [1] *as* "the process of optimizing opportunities for health, participation, and security in order to enhance quality of life as people age including those who are frail, disabled, and in need of care." As a policy framework [1, 5], active aging allows people to realize their potential for physical, social, and mental well-being throughout the life course and to participate in society. The concept of active aging can be applied for promoting aging well in both developed and developing countries and this is consistent with our study setting in the West Bank/Palestine.

The state of well-being is a multifaceted phenomenon in the older population which generally involves happiness, self-contentment, satisfying social relationships, and autonomy [6]. The sense of well-being refers to an individual's feelings, in this case, based on how older persons perceive the concept of well-being. Thus, the term "subjective well-being" is frequently used [7]. Well-being is also subject to other persons' feelings about oneself whether that is positive or negative. According to McNulty et al. [8], well-being is determined jointly by the interplay between individual characteristics and qualities of people's social environments.

With advanced age, well-being might be adversely influenced by declining physical health and functioning due to age-related changes [9, 10]; older adults may consequently encounter more challenges in pursuing aging well [7, 11, 12]. Maintaining good physical health and functioning plays an important role in facilitating mobility and enables older adults to perform more integrated functional tasks which include activities of daily living, fulfillment of social roles, and recreational activities [7, 13]. Evidence suggests that better physical functioning is associated with physical activity, an interaction that is positively reflected on physical and functional well-being [14–16]. In addition, good physical functioning contributes to decrease falls' incidence [17–19] and prevent the negative impact of falling consequences including social isolation and activity restriction in older adults [20, 21].

Older adults are strongly concerned about cognitive health in terms of keeping a good memory and prevent cognitive decline. Therefore, cognitive functioning was addressed as a primary contributor to aging well [22, 23]. Good cognitive health is linked to social connectedness, independence, and life activities, and it might be preserved and enhanced by maintaining an intellectually engaged and physically active lifestyle [24, 25]. Furthermore, having positive mental attitudes towards aging and one's capabilities may contribute to healthier mental health, higher level of satisfaction, and lower levels of anxiety and depression among older adults [26].

Well-being and physical and mental health are closely linked and the link may become more important at older ages, a connection that contributes to aging well in terms of life satisfaction, feelings of happiness, having sense of purpose, and meaning in life [27–30]. In the West Bank/Palestine, about one-third of adult Palestinians ≥18 years reported low levels of well-being; this was influenced by different socioeconomic factors including marital status, living standard, and community participation [31]. These contributing factors to well-being can be more prominent among older adult Palestinians, a marginalized growing population age group with a high rate of poverty, unemployment, and chronic diseases that requires further studies and research [32, 33]. To our knowledge, this is the first qualitative study exploring perceptions of older adult Palestinians on aging well. Thus, the aim of this study was to explore perceptions about aging well among older adult Palestinians who were 60 years old and older at the time of the data collection.

2. Methods

2.1. Study Design. Focus group method was used to acquire data about perceptions of older adults towards aging well. Focus groups are defined as "carefully planned series of discussions designed to obtain perceptions on a defined area of interest in a permissive, nonthreatening environment" [34]. Group interaction is a fundamental part of this method, in which the vital group discussions among the participants produce the data of the studied topic [35, 36].

2.2. Participants. A convenient sample was selected from previous related cross sectional studies [16, 19], addressing physical activity and physical functioning among older adults (n = 176). The inclusion criteria were being community dwelling older adults (aged ≥60 years), living in the West Bank (Palestine), being able to walk with or without walking aids, and having no communication deficits that would make interviewing and discussions impossible.

In order to obtain a broader view of the participants' perceptions about aging well; heterogeneity was taken into consideration [34, 35] through inviting older adults with different age and levels of education. Issues related to heterogeneity and homogeneity within the groups were considered during groups' formation in order to enhance an interactive discussion and to get a broad range of experience that covering a wide scope of the studied topic [34, 35].

All participants were given verbal and written information about the aim of the study and they signed an informed consent form. The participants were ensured confidentiality and informed that participation was voluntary and that they could drop out of the study at any time. The study received ethical approval from the research Ethics Committee of Al-Quds University, Palestine (Ref No: 1/REC/13), which complies with the Declaration of Helsinki.

2.3. Procedure. All focus groups were arranged by the first author as a moderator. Focus group sessions were conducted in familiar, comfortable, and accessible settings for the participants and took place in community and physiotherapy centers in the West Bank (Palestine).

The moderator started the group sessions by welcoming the participants and clarifying the purpose of the study. Subsequently, the participants were invited to introduce themselves and were given a chance to ask if they had any inquiry regarding the study.

The moderator clarified that the discussion would be carried out involving the participants themselves as knowledgeable and expert persons of the studied topic and that the moderator would not contribute to answer the questions. The moderator guided the discussion and encouraged all participants to share and ensured giving sufficient time for each participant to express his or her own view; in addition, comprehension probes were used if needed to clarify responses.

The sessions were initiated with a starting question "*How do you describe aging well*," followed by these questions:

> *What do you think about older adults' lifestyles in our community?*
>
> *How do you think aging well can be achieved? Meaning how aging well can be facilitated?*
>
> *What obstacles stand in the way of aging well?*

The focus groups lasted from 90 to 120 minutes; the interviews were digitally audio-recorded. All interviews were transcribed verbatim by the first author and translated from Arabic to English by the first author in collaboration with a bilingual translator.

2.4. Data Analysis. The analyzing process was conducted using the interpretative thematic analysis described by Braun and Clarke [37]. The initial phase of the analysis "becoming familiar with the data" was initiated with reading and rereading the transcripts for several times. Repeated reading contributed to get a better understanding and enhanced researchers' familiarity with the data. Following the initial stage, "generating initial codes (coding)" from the data set that had a reoccurring pattern was performed in the second phase. Coding was carried out through systematic way of organizing and gaining meaningful characteristics of data related to the research question. The first author began the process of initial coding; all transcriptions were coded one by one. Research team meetings were held to discuss the generating initial codes; exchanges that helped create an interpretative space for testing the findings and confirming coding analyses. This process was repeated until coding consensus was reached. The software NVivo 10 [38] was used as a helpful tool for analysis. The third phase *"searching for themes"* focused on a broader level of analysis and involved the researchers identifying suitable themes to which codes could be attributed, initial codes pertinent to research question were integrated into themes considering how relationships were formed between codes and potential themes. To visualize and explore trends and relationships in the source data, codes, and themes, a tree mapping was formulated using NVivo wizards. Derived themes were reviewed in phase four of the analysis, through cyclical process that involves back and forth movements between phases of data analysis until consensus was reached on the final themes. Consequently, in phase five, "Defining and naming themes" was completed, through refining existing themes and subthemes that will be presented in the final analysis.

3. Results

3.1. Descriptive Information. A total of 56 participants were recruited in this study, the mean age was 68.3 ± 4.72, ranged between 63 and 81 years old. The participants were assigned into different groups according to their place of residency and their preferences to participate in groups that consisted of only women, only men, or women and men together in one group. Accordingly, seven focus groups were formulated: four women groups, two men groups, and one group of women and men together. Participants in all seven groups ranged from 5 to 10 participants. The developed groups were homogenous in terms of independence level and place of residency. The majority of the participants (78%) had one or more chronic diseases, and all participants who lived alone (16%) were women. Participants' demographic and clinical characteristics are illustrated in Table 1. The participants' names were changed to preserve the anonymity of the participants.

3.2. Perceptions on Aging Well. Three major themes were identified, and twelve interrelated subthemes were derived. These themes and subthemes were elicited from the discussions for all focus groups combined within the scope to which they were supported by the qualitative data. Themes and subthemes are presented in the following sections.

3.2.1. Sense of Well-Being. Sense of well-being was highlighted through discussions in different focus groups as an important attribute to aging well. This theme was categorized into four related subthemes; feeling joyous, self-possessed contentment, satisfying social relationships, and staying independent.

(1) Feeling joyous was viewed as a catalyst to go on in life "joy extends life span," "joy makes you energetic"; in these words, the participants expressed on the importance of being happy. They have connected happiness with living to advanced age, it was important for them to keep sweet flavor to their lives, no matter how difficult their circumstances were.

> *Nelly (F, 65y): Despite life is full with troubles and blues, I continue.*
>
> *Nadia (F, 73y): I try to be happy, means one accepts everything, no matter bad or good.*
>
> *Nelly: Yes, we need something taking us out of our concerns and make us happy.*
>
> *Shafiq (M, 68y): Absolutely right, being happy is very important for us in this age.*

The participants found ways to add joys to their lives through different strategies such as gatherings, spending time with grandchildren, and sharing activities with others. For them, having leisure activities was of great importance in the context of aging well for older adults.

> *Fatima (F, 70y): We get together from time to time, where we joke and laugh, listening traditional songs or singing together, this encourages us and makes us happy.*
>
> *Sara (F, 64y): For me, the sweetest thing I do is playing with grandson.*
>
> *Ibrahim (M, 67y): Yes, grandsons are dearest of sons, they refresh my heart.*
>
> *Sara: I feel energized; I play with them as a young girl.*

(2) Self-possessed contentment was apparently viewed as an important concern for older adults. Throughout the participants' discussions, feeling secured and being satisfied were frequently mentioned, self-contentment was manifested in the necessity of having access to needed resources in terms of health services and daily-life requirements. In this context, feeling financially secured contributed to the state of self-contentment and was described as a facilitating mean to manage life pressures for being able to age well:

> *Zeinab (F, 65y): When you get old and there is no income, you may be in destitution.*
>
> *Ribhieh (F, 67y): Financial status plays a big role in our life.*
>
> *Zeinab: This brings you many worries and occupies your mind.*
>
> *Ibrahim (M, 67y): Yes, the fact if one at ease can eat better can dress better, can live better, this reflects on the state of well-being for us as old people.*

TABLE 1: Demographic and clinical characteristics of the participants (n = 56).

Variables	All groups n = 56	Group 1 n = 10	Group 2 n = 8	Group 3 n = 7	Group 4 n = 9	Group 5 n = 5	Group 6 n = 10	Group 7 n = 7
Gender								
Women, n (%)	40 (71)	10		7	9		7	7
Men, n (%)	16 (29)		8			5	3	
Marital status								
Married, n (%)	41(73)	7	8	6	4	5	7	4
Single, n (%)	3 (5)				2		1	
Widowed, n (%)	12 (22)	3		1	3		2	3
Living status								
With family, n (%)	47 (84)	7	8	6	8	5	7	6
Alone, n (%)	9 (16)	3		1	1		3	1
Diagnosed disease, n (%)								
Yes	44 (78)	8	6	6	7	4	9	4
No	12 (22)	2	2	1	2	1	1	3
Hypertension	30 (54)	6	6	3	4	2	7	2
Diabetes	14 (25)	4	1	2	3		3	1
Musculoskeletal	24 (43)	6		4	5	2	4	3
Use assistive aid, n (%)								
Glasses	33 (59)	5	4	4	6	4	5	5
Walking aid (cane)	5 (9)	1		2		1	1	
Self-rated fitness, n (%)								
Poor	5 (9)	1		2	1			1
Quite good	22 (39)	4	1	3	3	2	7	2
Good	22 (39)	5	4	1	4	2	3	3
Very good	7 (13)		3	1	1	1		1

(3) Satisfying social relationships were viewed as an attribute to aging well at both familial and community levels. Among different groups' discussions, the participants talked about how important it was for them to be accepted and involved in an area of life. They reflected on how being isolated and lonely might be a serious obstacle to aging well. This subtheme was mostly prominent among women:

> *Nayfeh (F, 66y): I live alone, nobody knocks my door, that's hard.*
>
> *Mariam (F, 70y): I live alone too, but my son lives in the first floor (same building). My daughter lives in town, and they are always around, that helps a lot, they don't let me alone at all.*
>
> *Huda (F, 65y): Yes, It's hard to live alone, but I go out, I share in different occasions, social participation is a good motivator for us as we growing old.*

Staying socially active was described in different phrases and was manifested about "having good neighbors and visiting friends," "highly motivated person towards life," and "not being dismal." Participation in community events was described by some participants as a helpful tool for older adults to stay socially active. Additionally, being socially active was connected with community voluntary work. The participants, both men and women commented on how vital for them it was to do voluntary activities, which helped them as older adults to efficiently spend their free time by doing something sensible to serve their own community. The participants reflected on how voluntary work or being involved in charitable work may enhance their state of well-being.

(4) Staying independent was viewed as a major characteristic of aging well. Apart from the participants' living status (alone or with family), the importance of being independent was connected with the autonomous status of the older adults. A major concern that was frequently mentioned was not being or becoming a burden to others. Along the interactive discussions in all groups, the participants reflected on the necessity of staying independent in performing their daily life activities including both personal and instrumental activities.

> *Seham (F. 65y): I am taking care of myself, my health is good, I need to stay healthy and mentally oriented, so I won't seek anybody help.*
>
> *Hannah (F, 81y): I live alone, I have a big house. I do everything by myself; nobody brings me even a glass of water.*

3.2.2. Throughout the Second Theme "Having Good Physical Health". Throughout the second theme "having good physical health," the participants have considered maintaining physical health as an important component of aging well, through our analysis, having good physical health was categorized into five related subthemes; staying active, free from debilitated illness, healthy eating habits, fall prevention, and having a good physical appearance.

(1) Staying active was connected to aging well, the participants prominently commented on the importance of staying active by keep on moving. The participants viewed staying active as a key factor for good health. Frequently, the

participants talked about staying active in terms of walking which was viewed as a useful tool for aging well; walking was the most prevalent mode of physical activity and has been mentioned repeatedly as a routine activity. Staying active was also connected to good physical functioning, helping older adults to maintain good physical functioning, and keeping good health.

> *Hannah (F, 81y): I like going out even I have pain in my legs, if I stay home, I will be destructed.*
>
> *Salwa (F, 66y): Me too, I' am taking care of my health, I walk a lot.*
>
> *Zarifeh (F, 67y): You know, I have a brother in law, he is 81 years old, he is still working and going out everywhere by feet.*

Staying active was also revolved around continuing to work, which was described differently by the participants; men talked more about income generating and community work, while women talked about household and charitable work. Despite there were different perspectives on the concept of "continuing to work," still it was considered as an important attribute for good physical health and for aging well throughout women and men expressions.

In other circumstances, staying active has been linked to gardening. The participants expressed on the importance of doing some gardening in order to stay active and energetic.

> *Salem (M, 72y): I work in my garden, and I see myself more active than my sons.*
>
> *Nelly (F, 65y): Ohh, I love gardening a lot, I spend like two hours caring of my plants, digging around them. Always my plants look good, my whole garden is tidy, and that keeps me active and energetic.*

(2) Free from debilitated illness, staying healthy in terms of absence of debilitated diseases was highlighted during group discussions as an important attribute to good physical health and consequently to aging well. The participants described how occurrences of illness may influence their physical health and their daily-life activities.

> *Ribhieh (F,67y): Illness sometimes over shadow, I try to forget it, but it is dominated.*
>
> *Fatima (F, 70y): After rheumatism, I am not able to walk like before, that affected me a lot.*
>
> *Ribhieh: Yes, it caused me gloominess sometimes.*
>
> *Nelly (F, 65y): Ahh, you know, I underwent two surgeries, and I've suffered a lot, but I've challenged every pain and every disease, I try to live my life.*

(3) Healthy eating habits were evoked and being discussed in all groups, the participants reflected on this by focusing on the importance of taking healthy foods. Culturally, ideas regarding the Palestinian diet, which consists mainly of olives oil and lots of vegetables, were mentioned frequently. The participants related healthy diet with good physical health and longevity.

Within this subtheme, promoting healthy eating habits related to aging well were addressed. The participants talked about healthy habits to be taken as well as unhealthy eating style to be skipped. In this context, overeating or getting a full stomach was described as a source of disease, a behavior that has to be prevented in order to maintain good health. Unhealthy eating habits like skipping breakfast and excessive use of salt and sugar were viewed as aggravating factors for some disease symptoms.

(4) Falls prevention was a persistent topic that has been discussed among the participants as an important contributor to good physical health. For them, it was vital to stay active but constantly they were concerned about falling. They have viewed falling at this age as a devastating problem, thinking about fall consequences both physically and socially. The participants connected their concern of falling with the associated physical decline.

> *Majida (F, 70y): I prefer using a cane rather than falling down.*
>
> *Wardeh (F,77y): Yah, me too, I pay attention to prevent slipping or falling.*
>
> *Majida: Before I got sick, there was no problem, I didn't never ever catch any handrails.*
>
> *Mariam (F, 70y): Yes I see, it is hard to fall and get fracture at this age, healing is not granted.*

(5) Having a good physical appearance was viewed as an important trait to age well. The participants talked about how vital it was for them to keep in good physical appearance; this was connected with "keeping good shape," "having good stature," and "maintaining external appearance." Others pointed out that older persons who are aging well "maintaining good external appearance and dressed well."

3.2.3. Preserving Good Mental Health. The vitality of maintaining good mental health was viewed as an important attribute to aging well. This theme was categorized into three related subthemes: staying alert, having a positive attitude, and modes to keep good mental health.

(1) Staying alert: participants valued their state of mental alertness related to being independent, having control over their own affairs, and being self-governing. Being mentally alert and having a good memory was mentioned frequently as an imperative dimension of aging well.

> *Salma (F, 68y): I was living with my mother in law, she reached her nineties, and she had a clear mind, everyone respected her, and I've learned a lot from her.*
>
> *Ribhieh (F, 66y): Yes I agree, If the brain is still good, you will be fine.*

(2) Having a positive attitude emerged as an important attribute to aging well, and it was diversely characterized as follows: "my spirit is strong, I just follow my mind," "I don't

let anybody put me down," and "I'm in any way, I want to live." The participants commented on the importance of getting this impulse of life by staying positive. In this context, having positive attitudes towards own capabilities as older adults was reflected by fulfilling own ambitions and having a life purpose in pursuit of one's aspiration.

Being positive was also connected with spiritual merits, having faith, praying, and trust in God; these traits have been mentioned frequently through discussions in different groups. The participants commented on the importance of reaching a state of serenity and tranquility as an important attribute to aging well.

(3) Modes to keep good mental health including actions such as reading newspapers and books, watching TV and listening to the radio, eating certain foods like nuts, staying active, and playing mental games. All these statements were mentioned to describe taken activities by the participants in order to keep good mental health and to age well:

> *Farida (F, 64y): I read newspaper every day, that keeps me oriented.*
>
> *Nayfeh (F, 66y): For me, I can't read well, watching TV and hearing radio amuses me and keeps me alert.*
>
> *Hannah (F, 81y): I work with letters and numbers, Sudoku is good if you manage to deal with it.*
>
> *Farida: Ohh, That's good too.*

Willingness to learn new skills was also considered by some participants as a way to keep a good mind; the new skills were mostly revolving around computer uses, handcrafts, and simple maintenance work.

4. Discussion

Happiness, self-contentment, satisfying social relationships, and independence are primary characteristics of the state of well-being that contribute to aging well in the older population [6]. A study by Tamir and Ford [39] indicated that people who generally wanted to feel more happiness and less anger experienced greater well-being. Corresponding with our results, as illustrated in the first theme, the participants have considered joy and happiness an important tool to age well. Feeling joyous was viewed as a catalyst to go on in life and was connected with living to advanced age. When older adults experience well-being, they are also experiencing the sense of self-contentment which is connected to the feeling of being happy and satisfied. Self-contentment in this study was manifested in feeling financially secured and in the necessity of having access to needed resources in terms of health services and daily-life requirements. The findings are consistent with a similar study [40], where financial security appeared to be an essential contributor to aging well.

Well-being is also subject to how a person feels that other people in their surroundings perceive them, whether this is positive or negative [8]. The findings are corresponding with our results in the subtheme "satisfying social relationships," and the participants commented on the importance of having social connections at both familial and community levels. These findings are in harmony with the concept of active aging [1], which enables older people to realize their diverse potentials for well-being. However, the well-being of a person does not only depend on the individual, rather well-being has a social component as well, and it is determined jointly by the interplay between individual characteristics and qualities of people's social environments [39].

The participants reflected on how sensible for them it was not to be ignored and isolated at this age, and they thought being isolated and lonely as a serious obstacle to aging well. This concern was mostly prominent among older women who are more likely to spend their later stage of their lives alone [32]. Related to literature, living alone and low social participation were found to be significant risk factors for later disability onset [41]. Older adults who live alone report more fatigue and more health difficulties than older adults who do not live lonely [42, 43], issues that are negatively contributing to aging well.

Our findings revealed that autonomy and independence were viewed as primary attributes to age well. Concern of being a burden to others was very prominent throughout participants' expression. Older adults in other cultural circumstances as well placed a high value on personal independence and self-reliance, where staying independent was viewed as a major trait for aging well [24, 44]. The participants related their level of independence to their physical and mental health; a sensible understandable relation as a higher level of physical functioning enables older adults to perform more integrated functional tasks which include activities of daily living and the fulfillment of social roles as well as recreational activities [7], issues that are essential to age well.

Throughout the second theme "having a good physical health," the participants connected their good physical health with staying active. Often, they have talked about staying active in terms of walking. This can be explained as walking was viewed as one of the most popular forms of physical activity among older adults and can easily be adapted into daily lifestyle [45].

In this study, walking was connected to good physical functioning and has been mentioned repeatedly as a routine activity, helping older adults to maintain good physical functioning and keeping good health. Findings are consistent with similar studies indicating that walking is positively associated with physical and functional well-being in older adults [14, 15].

Physical health was addressed according to Phelan et al. as being in good health and absence of chronic diseases [46]. In Rowe and Kahn's model, it was addressed as avoiding disease and maintaining high cognitive and physical function [47]. In this study, the majority of the participants, about 78% had one or more chronic diseases. For them, the concern about physical health in term of diseases was more prominently about being free from debilitated illness that may incapacitate their abilities and limit their daily-life activities. Results that are consistent with a related study showed that participants with higher prevalence of chronic diseases recorded lower level of physical activity [15].

Promoting healthy eating habits related to aging well was also addressed in this study. The participants related healthy diet with good physical health and consequently to aging well, a subtheme that was also found among perceptions of older Japanese adults in a study towards aging well [40].

Additionally, falls prevention was a persistent topic that has been discussed among the participants as an important contributor to good physical health. For them, especially women, it was imperative to stay active but constantly they were concerned about falling. This can be attributed to the fact that higher incidence of falls is associated with higher age, and women tend to fall more frequently than men [48, 49]. Participants have viewed falling at this age as a big problem, thinking about fall consequences both physically and socially. A subtheme is consistent with other studies [17–19], which have shown that good physical health and physical functioning play an important role in decreasing falls' incidence and fear of falling and, in turn, prevent the negative impact of falling consequences including social isolation, activity restriction, and enhance state of well-being in older adults [20, 21].

In this study, preserving good mental health and staying alert were viewed as important attributes to aging well, and good mental health was connected to staying independent and being self-governing. In a study by Laditka et al. [24], maintaining good cognitive health was linked to social connectedness, independence, and life activities that are difficult to maintain with poor cognitive health. Within the second theme, "having a positive attitude" was described as an attribute to good mental health and to age well. This can be understandable as having positive attitudes towards aging and owns capabilities may contribute to healthier mental health. More positive attitudes were associated with higher level of satisfaction and lower levels of anxiety and depression in older adults [26].

Within this theme, participants related having a positive attitude to spiritual merits, having faith, praying, and trust in God. These traits have been mentioned frequently in different groups where the participants commented on the importance of reaching a state of serenity and tranquility that can be achieved through spiritual dimension as an important attribute to aging well. A spirituality dimension of aging well was found in similar studies [24, 40] as well under categories such as faith, religion, blessings, and internal peace.

The state of well-being is positively influenced by having a life purpose that can motivate older adults to sustain independence, social life, and make life meaningful for older adults [29]. The feeling of having a purpose in life was also contributing to aging well in our study that was manifested by fulfilling ambitious and having a life goal in pursuit of one's aspiration.

Evidence suggests that cognitive functioning may be preserved and enhanced by maintaining an intellectually engaged and physically active lifestyle. Meaningful social engagement is also an important factor of better maintenance of cognitive functioning in old age [25]. Keeping good mental health was an important concern for older adults in this study; different modes were described to maintain good mental health including being mentally engaged (reading, playing mental games), taking good foods for the brain like nuts and staying physically active.

4.1. Strengths and Limitations. The aim of this study was to explore perceptions about aging well among older adults, as the state of aging well refers to an individual's subjective feelings and is basically dependent on the older adults' views [7, 50]. Therefore, a qualitative research design in the context of focus group discussions was used; this qualitative thematic analysis approach contributed to get better insight into older adults' perceptions and experiences that cannot be elicited through quantitative studies.

Using focus group discussion as a method of data collection has enabled the researchers to get both individual and interactive opinions by the participants. This method is effectively used in research on aging [51, 52], and it is considered appropriate for collecting the views and experiences of a selected group through dynamic interaction and vital group discussion of a studied topic [35, 36]. In addition, focus group method was used, because it is a friendly respectful research method and not a condescending method [53] to be used with older adult participants. To assure permissive and nonthreatening environment for conducting this study [34], participants were assigned into different groups according to their place of residency and their preferences to participate in groups that consist of only women, only men, or women and men together. This procedure contributed to a relaxed discussion atmosphere through having familiar, comfortable, and accessible settings for the participants.

The groups' size in this study was determined based on the research question, taking into consideration that small groups with less than five participants may limit the range of interactive discussions, while large groups meaning more than ten participants can be hard to be managed by the moderator and may bound the participants' opportunities to share their thoughts and experiences [34, 54].

The relationship between the researcher (first author) and the participants has been developed progressively through several interviews. Our sample was selected conveniently from previous related cross-sectional studies [16, 19], addressing physical activity, physical functioning, and fall-related efficacy among older adults. Familiarity of researcher with the participants gave a chance to create a comfortable interviewing atmosphere, which helped the researcher build a trusting connection with the participants and encouraged the participants to talk more freely.

This study addresses aging well in a holistic manner that includes state of well-being, physical and mental health, independence, and social participation [3, 55]. This helped us in giving a better understanding about the interaction between different physical, social, and mental functioning dimensions regarding the state of well-being among older adults. However, further studies addressing each dimension in more depth may add additional evidence towards a better understanding of the concept of aging well.

A possible limitation of this study could be that we recruited older adults who are relatively independent and functioning and living in the community at own homes within a family or alone, and most of them rated their self-fitness between good and very good. Further studies are needed to explore perspectives on aging well among older adults living in institutions with lower level of functioning and independence.

5. Conclusion

This study gives in-depth understanding of the dynamic multidimensional physical, social, and mental functioning on the state of well-being among older adults. Findings contribute to get better insight about older adults' perspectives on aging well. Aging well is positively influenced by feeling joyous, staying independent, self-possessed contentment, and being financially secured, in addition to being socially engaged and enjoying good physical and mental health. Enhancing a physically active lifestyle, social participation, and leisure activities as well as healthy eating habits and having a purpose in life and intellectually engagement are all important factors to promote aging well. Vital factors are to be considered in developing strategic health and rehabilitative plans for promoting aging well among older adults.

Conflicts of Interest

The authors declare that they have no conflicts of interest.

Acknowledgments

This study is based on a doctoral thesis [56], which was supported by Gothenburg University and Al-Quds University. The authors would like to thank all the participants for their valuable contributions to this study.

References

[1] World Health Organization, *Active Ageing, A Policy Framework*, World Health Organization, Geneva, Switzerland, 2002.

[2] World Health Organization, "Facts about ageing," September 2014, http://www.who.int/ageing/about/facts/en/.

[3] L. Foster and A. Walker, "Active and successful aging: a European policy perspective," *Gerontologist*, vol. 55, no. 1, pp. 83–90, 2015.

[4] L. Buys and E. Miller, *Active Ageing: Developing a Quantitative Multidimensional Measure, Active Ageing, Active Learning*, Springer, Berlin, Germany, 2012.

[5] A. Kalache and A. Gatti, "Active ageing: a policy framework," *Advances in Gerontology*, vol. 11, pp. 7–18, 2003.

[6] U. Kunzmann, T. D. Little, and J. Smith, "Is age-related stability of subjective well-being a paradox? Cross-sectional and longitudinal evidence from the Berlin aging study," *Psychology and Aging*, vol. 15, no. 3, pp. 511–526, 2000.

[7] W. W. Spirduso, K. L. Francis, and P. G. Macrae, *Physical Dimensions of Aging*, Human Kinetics, Champaign, IL, USA, 2005.

[8] J. K. Mcnulty and F. D. Fincham, "Beyond positive psychology? Toward a contextual view of psychological processes and well-being," *American Psychologist*, vol. 67, no. 2, pp. 101–110, 2012.

[9] O. Fusco, A. Ferrini, M. Santoro, M. R. Lo Monaco, G. Gambassi, and M. Cesari, "Physical function and perceived quality of life in older persons," *Aging Clinical and Experimental Research*, vol. 24, no. 1, pp. 68–73, 2012.

[10] N. Garatachea, O. Molinero, R. Martinez-Garcia, R. Jimenez-Jimenez, J. Gonzalez-Gallego, and S. Marquez, "Feelings of well being in elderly people: relationship to physical activity and physical function," *Archives of Gerontology and Geriatrics*, vol. 48, no. 3, pp. 306–312, 2009.

[11] N. Steverink and S. Lindenberg, "Which social needs are important for subjective well-being? What happens to them with aging?," *Psychology and Aging*, vol. 21, no. 2, pp. 281–290, 2006.

[12] Y. Liu, M. Dijst, and S. Geertman, "The subjective well-being of older adults in Shanghai: the role of residential environment and individual resources," *Urban Studies*, vol. 54, no. 7, pp. 1692–1714, 2017.

[13] H. Halaweh, U. Svantesson, and C. Willen, "Experiences of habitual physical activity in maintaining roles and functioning among older adults: a qualitative study," *Rehabilitation Research and Practice*, vol. 2016, Article ID 1459597, 8 pages, 2016.

[14] H. Hörder, I. Skoog, and K. Frändin, "Health-related quality of life in relation to walking habits and fitness: a population-based study of 75-year-olds," *Quality of Life Research*, vol. 22, no. 6, pp. 1213–1223, 2013.

[15] H. Halaweh, C. Willen, A. Grimby-Ekman, and U. Svantesson, "Physical activity and health-related quality of life among community dwelling elderly," *Journal of Clinical Medicine Research*, vol. 7, no. 11, pp. 845–852, 2015.

[16] H. Halaweh, C. Willén, and U. Svantesson, "Association between physical activity and physical functioning in community-dwelling older adults," *European Journal of Physiotherapy*, vol. 19, no. 1, pp. 40–47, 2017.

[17] T. Yamashita, H. Jeon, A. J. Bailer, I. M. Nelson, and S. Mehdizadeh, "Fall risk factors in community-dwelling elderly who receive Medicaid-supported home- and community-based care services," *Journal of Aging and Health*, vol. 23, no. 4, pp. 682–703, 2011.

[18] K. Delbaere, N. Van Den Noortgate, J. Bourgois, G. Vanderstraeten, W. Tine, and D. Cambier, "The physical performance test as a predictor of frequent fallers: a prospective community-based cohort study," *Clinical Rehabilitation*, vol. 20, no. 1, pp. 83–90, 2006.

[19] H. Halaweh, C. Willen, A. Grimby-Ekman, and U. Svantesson, "Physical functioning and fall-related efficacy among community-dwelling elderly people," *European Journal of Physiotherapy*, vol. 18, no. 1, pp. 11–17, 2015.

[20] K. Legters, "Fear of falling," *Physical Therapy*, vol. 82, no. 3, pp. 264–272, 2002.

[21] M. E. Tinetti, C. F. Mendes De Leon, J. T. Doucette, and D. I. Baker, "Fear of falling and fall-related efficacy in relationship to functioning among community-living elders," *Journals of Gerontology*, vol. 49, no. 3, pp. M140–M147, 1994.

[22] H. M. Fillit, R. N. Butler, A. W. O'connell et al., "Achieving and maintaining cognitive vitality with aging," *Mayo Clinic Proceedings*, vol. 77, no. 7, pp. 681–696, 2002.

[23] K. J. Bourassa, M. Memel, C. Woolverton, and D. A. Sbarra, "Social participation predicts cognitive functioning in aging adults over time: comparisons with physical health, depression, and physical activity," *Aging and Mental Health*, vol. 21, no. 2, pp. 133–146, 2017.

[24] S. B. Laditka, S. J. Corwin, J. N. Laditka et al., "Attitudes about aging well among a diverse group of older americans: implications for promoting cognitive health," *Gerontologist*, vol. 49, no. 1, pp. S30–S39, 2009.

[25] C. Hertzog, A. F. Kramer, R. S. Wilson, and U. Lindenberger, "Enrichment effects on adult cognitive development: can the functional capacity of older adults be preserved and enhanced?," *Psychological Science in the Public Interest*, vol. 9, no. 1, pp. 1–65, 2008.

[26] C. Bryant, B. Bei, K. Gilson, A. Komiti, H. Jackson, and F. Judd, "The relationship between attitudes to aging and physical and mental health in older adults," *International Psychogeriatrics*, vol. 24, no. 10, pp. 1674–1683, 2012.

[27] C. D. Ryff, "Psychological well-being in adult life," *Current Directions in Psychological Science*, vol. 4, no. 4, pp. 99–104, 1995.

[28] V. Mitchell and R. M. Helson, "The place of purpose in life in women's positive aging," *Women & Therapy*, vol. 39, no. 1-2, pp. 213–234, 2016.

[29] J. Irving, S. Davis, and A. Collier, "Aging with purpose: systematic search and review of literature pertaining to older adults and purpose," *International Journal of Aging and Human Development*, vol. 85, no. 4, pp. 403–437, 2017.

[30] A. Steptoe, A. Deaton, and A. A. Stone, "Subjective wellbeing, health and ageing," *The Lancet*, vol. 385, no. 9968, pp. 640–648, 2015.

[31] N. Harsha, L. Ziq, R. Ghandour, and R. Giacaman, "Well-being and associated factors among adults in the occupied Palestinian territory (oPt)," *Health and Quality of Life Outcomes*, vol. 14, no. 1, p. 122, 2016.

[32] Palestinian Central Bureau of Statistics, "Dissemination and analysis of census findings: the conditions and requirements of elderly care in the Palestinian territory 1997-2007," December 2017, http://www.pcbs.gov.ps/Portals/_PCBS/Downloads/book1647.pdf.

[33] Palestinian Central Bureau of Statistics, "On the eve of world elderly day," December 2017, http://www.pcbs.gov.ps/post.aspx?lang=en&ItemID=1755.

[34] R. A. Krueger and M. A. Casey, *Focus groups: A practical Guide for Applied Research*, Sage Publications, Thousand Oaks, CA, USA, 4th edition, 2009.

[35] J. Kitzinger, "The methodology of focus groups: the importance of interaction between research participants," *Sociology of Health & Illness*, vol. 16, no. 1, pp. 103–121, 1994.

[36] S. D. Ivanoff and J. Hultberg, "Understanding the multiple realities of everyday life: basic assumptions in focus-group methodology," *Scandinavian Journal of Occupational Therapy*, vol. 13, no. 2, pp. 125–132, 2006.

[37] V. Braun and V. Clarke, "Using thematic analysis in psychology," *Qualitative Research in Psychology*, vol. 3, no. 2, pp. 77–101, 2006.

[38] B. Edhlund, *NVivo 10 Essentials*, Form & Kunskap AB, Sweden, Stallarholmen, 2012.

[39] M. Tamir and B. Q. Ford, "Should people pursue feelings that feel good or feelings that do good? Emotional preferences and well-being," *Emotion*, vol. 12, no. 5, pp. 1061–1070, 2012.

[40] G. Y. Iwamasa and M. Iwasaki, "A new multidimensional model of successful aging: perceptions of Japanese American older adults," *Journal of Cross-Cultural Gerontology*, vol. 26, no. 3, pp. 261–278, 2011.

[41] R. Lund, C. J. Nilsson, and K. Avlund, "Can the higher risk of disability onset among older people who live alone be alleviated by strong social relations? A longitudinal study of non-disabled men and women," *Age Ageing*, vol. 39, no. 3, pp. 319–326, 2010.

[42] J. L. Deng, J. M. Hu, W. L. Wu, B. R. Dong, and H. M. Wu, "Subjective well-being, social support, and age-related functioning among the very old in China," *International Journal of Geriatric Psychiatry*, vol. 25, no. 7, pp. 697–703, 2010.

[43] H. Gilmour, "Social participation and the health and well-being of Canadian seniors," *Health Reports*, vol. 23, no. 4, pp. 23–32, 2012.

[44] R. Shaw and M. Langman, "Perceptions of being old and the ageing process," *Ageing International*, vol. 42, no. 1, pp. 115–135, 2017.

[45] O. T. Atalay and U. Cavlak, "The impact of unsupervised regular walking on health: a sample of Turkish middle-aged and older adults," *European Review of Aging and Physical Activity*, vol. 9, no. 1, pp. 71–79, 2012.

[46] E. A. Phelan, L. A. Anderson, A. Z. Lacroix, and E. B. Larson, "Older adults' views of "successful aging"–how do they compare with researcher's definitions?," *Journal of the American Geriatrics Society*, vol. 52, no. 2, pp. 211–216, 2004.

[47] J. W. Rowe and R. L. Kahn, "Successful aging," *Gerontologist*, vol. 37, no. 4, pp. 433–440, 1997.

[48] J. Luk, T. Y. Chan, and D. K. Chan, "Falls prevention in the elderly: translating evidence into practice," *Hong Kong Medical Journal*, vol. 21, no. 2, pp. 165–171, 2015.

[49] A. Bergland, "Fall risk factors in community-dwelling elderly people," *Norsk Epidemiologi*, vol. 22, no. 2, pp. 151–164, 2012.

[50] A. L. Stewart and A. C. King, "Evaluating the efficacy of physical activity for influencing quality-of-life outcomes in older adults," *Annals of Behavioral Medicine*, vol. 13, no. 3, pp. 108–116, 1991.

[51] V. Finn and R. Ellis, "Media Review: Curry, L., Shield, R., & Wetle, T. (2006). Improving aging and public health research: qualitative and mixed methods. Washington, DC: American Public Health Association and the Gerontological Society of America," *Journal of Mixed Methods Research*, vol. 3, no. 4, pp. 414-415, 2006.

[52] E. Costello, M. Kafchinski, J. Vrazel, and P. Sullivan, "Motivators, barriers, and beliefs regarding physical activity in an older adult population," *Journal of Geriatric Physical Therapy*, vol. 34, no. 3, pp. 138–147, 2011.

[53] D. L. Morgan and R. A. Krueger, *Successful Focus Groups: Advancing the State of the Art*, SAGE Publications, Inc., Thousand Oaks, CA, USA, 1993.

[54] P. Gill, K. Stewart, E. Treasure, and B. Chadwick, "Methods of data collection in qualitative research: interviews and focus groups," *British Dental Journal*, vol. 204, no. 6, pp. 291–295, 2008.

[55] L. Foster and A. Walker, "Gender and active ageing in Europe," *European Journal of Ageing*, vol. 10, no. 1, pp. 3–10, 2013.

[56] H. Halaweh, "Active ageing a path towards ageing well. physical functioning, physical activity, falls self-efficacy and social participation in community-dwelling elderly," Doctoral Dissertation, University of Gothenburg, Gothenburg, Sweden, 2016.

26

Conceptions of Healthy Aging Held by Relatives of Older Persons in Isan-Thai Culture: A Phenomenographic Study

Pornpun Manasatchakun,[1] **Åsa Roxberg**,[2,3] **and Margareta Asp**[4]

[1]*Boromarajonani College of Nursing, Udon Thani, Thailand*
[2]*School of Health and Welfare, Halmstad University, Halmstad, Sweden*
[3]*VID Specialized University, Bergen, Norway*
[4]*School of Health, Care and Social Welfare, Mälardalen University, Eskilstuna, Västerås, Sweden*

Correspondence should be addressed to Pornpun Manasatchakun; pornpun.manasatchakun@gmail.com

Academic Editor: Arshad Jahangir

In Thailand, family nurses are expected to provide support for older persons and their family members to promote healthy aging. Family bonds are strong, and relatives are expected to take care of their older family members. However, there is limited research on how older persons' family members perceive healthy aging. This study aimed to describe the conceptions of healthy aging held by the children and grandchildren of older persons in northeast Thailand. In a phenomenographic study, 14 interviews were performed to qualitatively analyze different conceptions of healthy aging. Four descriptive categories emerged: being independent, not being afflicted by diseases or illnesses, being a giver and a receiver, and being wise. The conceptions of healthy aging entail both autonomy and interdependence. The relative's perspective needs to be considered when policies relating to healthy aging are implemented in the community and when family nurses provide support to families to promote healthy aging.

1. Introduction

Thailand's healthcare system emphasizes the importance of family participation in care for older persons [1]. A family nurse is the key person who works with older clients and their family members to provide care and support those people's health. In Thailand, a family nurse is defined as a person who takes responsibility for public health, holistic healthcare, and enhancing the quality of life among the population [2]. The roles of a family nurse include not only identifying health problems and managing chronic and acute medical conditions but also collaborating with families and providing health services [2]. These tasks encompass preventing diseases and promoting health for families [2]. Family nurses have traditionally been expected to provide support for older persons and their family members. Family members play a key role as the primary caregivers of older persons in Thai society, especially in the northeastern region of Thailand, also known as Isan. Thus, family nurses should value the role of family when engaging older persons in their care. With a growing aging population, the Thai government has developed health policies to maintain the older population's health and improve their quality of life [3]. The promotion of healthy aging is one of the key strategies adopted in the national agenda for meeting the challenges of caring for the older population [4].

The concept of healthy aging is adopted and studied throughout the world [5, 6]. In Thailand, studies of healthy aging have focused on older persons' perspectives [7–9]. The literature indicates that healthy aging is facilitated not only by older persons themselves but also by their families and culture [6, 10]. To promote healthy aging and encourage family members to work together with healthcare providers, family nurses must consider the relatives' perspective, as relatives contribute to the improvement of health among older persons. Understanding what healthy aging means to family members of older persons may be helpful when collaborating with them and their families in the promotion of health among people in the northeast of Thailand.

1.1. Healthy Aging: Positive Outcomes of Old Age and Policies for Responding to the Aging Situation in Thailand. There are many terms that can be used to explain the maintenance of well-being in older persons [6], such as successful aging [11], active aging [12], and healthy aging [6]. Healthy aging is a concept that covers the multidimensional aspects of older persons' lives and may help incorporate the overlapping concepts of active aging and successful aging [6]. Moreover, healthy aging is viewed as a complex concept that involves multiple dimensions and relates to physical, mental, and social well-being [8]. Previous studies have shown that healthy aging entails achieving positive health outcomes, maintaining well-being throughout one's life, and preventing long-term health conditions [6, 10].

Healthy aging has become a major consideration for global policy-makers aiming to preserve the health and improve the quality of life of the older population [13]. As in many countries worldwide, Thailand is currently facing the problem of an aging population [14]. Older persons, their families, and the government need to be aware of the increased risks of chronic diseases and disabilities associated with old age [15]. The Thai government is concerned about the aging of the Thai population. Therefore, healthy aging is one of the goals of the national plan for older persons, which aims to provide support for older individuals to enable them to maintain a healthy lifestyle and to reduce long-term care costs [3]. Implementation of this plan challenges family nurses to achieve the goal of promoting healthy aging.

1.2. Family: The Unit Responsible for the Informal Care of Older Persons in Northeast Thailand. Family is viewed as a unit of care [16] and represents the context for individual development, according to one dimension of family nurses [17]. The family has the primary responsibility for advocating the development of family members. The family serves as the context for a client's health, which means that the focus is on the client, and the family is viewed in the background of the client [17]. The individual's health influences the family, and the capability of the family has an impact on the health of individual members [17]. When caring for older persons and promoting their health, the family nurse should be concerned with both the older person and the family members.

In Thai society, family is highly valued [2]. The northeast of Thailand, also referred to as Isan, has a large population of older persons [18] and is afflicted by poverty, especially among the older population [19]. The children of the current generation of older persons remain an important support group in the northeast of Thailand [20, 21]. This importance may stem from the Isan culture's long tradition of paying respect to older persons and the cultural belief in the concept of repaying one's parents [20]. According to Isan cultural values, children are obliged to care for their parents based on Buddhist customs [20–23]. Children and other family members serve as informal caregivers who play an important role in supporting their parents both socially and financially [21]. Older persons still receive support from their family members (e.g., daughters, sons, and grandchildren) to fulfill their needs [21]. However, societal changes in Isan are affecting families and older persons' lives. In Isan, similar to other regions in Thailand, the family structure has shifted from the extended family to the nuclear family. Older persons and young persons have become separated. Young adults tend to move to larger cities featuring centers of commerce to seek economic opportunities [24, 25]. Some adults in Isan leave their own children with their parents and emigrate to the capital city or to other countries to work [21]. A previous study [26] showed that, compared with earlier generations, the current younger generation in the Isan region has fewer opportunities to stay with their older relatives. Sudnongbua et al. [26] reported that older persons in the Isan region felt abandoned because their children had migrated to other areas to work. The consequence of social change is a challenge for family nurses and provides an opportunity for family nurses to improve health among older persons and support their families who live in the northeast of Thailand.

1.3. Family Members of Older Persons and Healthy Aging in Northeast Thailand. A previous study of healthy aging in the Isan region showed that older persons' perspectives on healthy aging are related to the support that they receive from family members [7]. However, no studies focusing on the conceptions of healthy aging held by the relatives of older persons in the Isan region have been conducted. The understanding of healthy aging that is held by the relatives of older persons in Isan-Thai culture needs to be expanded. Such studies may enable family nurses to broaden their views regarding the meaning of healthy aging and provide a foundation for developing care practices consistent with healthcare policies. Therefore, the aim of this study was to describe the conceptions of healthy aging held by children and grandchildren caring for older persons in northeast Thailand.

2. Methodology

2.1. Study Design. This study has a descriptive and phenomenographic design with an epistemological basis in lifeworld theory, as suggested by Ashworth and Lucas [27, 28]. This methodology was used because phenomenography and lifeworld theory aim to explain how human beings derive meaning from their connections with the world around them [29, 30]. One's lifeworld is the everyday life that he or she experiences [29, 31], and each individual experiences things in his or her lifeworld as different phenomena [29]. Phenomenography uncovers different qualitative conceptions of specific phenomena [30, 32]. The phenomenon of interest in this study was the notion of healthy aging.

2.2. Study Setting and Participants. This study was set in Udon Thani Province, which is located in northeast Thailand and features a growing population of people aged 60 years or older. We selected this province as the setting because it exhibits both rural and urban characteristics and is an example of an area undergoing modernization and growth [33]. A purposive sampling technique was used to select the participants from a list of family members caring for 17 older persons from 17 families who participated in a previous study on healthy aging in the northeast region of Thailand [7].

Table 1: Participants' characteristics ($n = 14$).

Number	Sex	Age	Relation with older person	Education	Marital status	Occupation	Religion
1	F	16	Granddaughter	High school	Single	Student	Buddhism
2	F	42	Daughter	Elementary	Married	Housewife	Buddhism
3	F	45	Daughter	Elementary	Married	Farmer	Buddhism
4	F	34	Daughter	High school	Married	Housewife	Buddhism
5	M	41	Son	High school	Married	Employee	Buddhism
6	M	24	Grandson	High school	Single	Self-employed	Buddhism
7	M	46	Son	High school	Single	Self-employed	Buddhism
8	F	41	Daughter	Master degree	Single	Teacher	Buddhism
9	F	56	Daughter	Bachelor degree	Married	Teacher	Buddhism
10	F	40	Daughter	Master degree	Single	Teacher	Buddhism
11	F	54	Daughter	High school	Single	Employee	Buddhism
12	F	48	Daughter	Elementary	Married	Self-employed	Buddhism
13	F	40	Daughter	Elementary	Married	Farmer	Buddhism
14	F	42	Daughter	Elementary	Married	Employee	Buddhism

Various background characteristics, such as age, sex, marital status, and educational level, were used as inclusion criteria. To ensure that the conceptions of healthy aging were not drawn from older persons, this study included older persons' children and grandchildren aged < 60 years. Three family members were excluded because they were the spouses of the participants in a previous study on healthy aging who were aged > 60 years.

Twelve children and two grandchildren of older persons (11 women and three men) participated in this study, and the age range varied from 16 to 56 years. Five participants had an elementary school education, six had a high school education, one had a bachelor's degree, and two had a master's degree. Eight participants were married, and six participants were single. All participants were Buddhists. The participants' characteristics are described in Table 1.

2.3. Data Collection. The first author collected all data from September to October 2013 using semistructured, in-depth interviews and recorded the interviews to produce verbatim transcripts of each conversation. All the participants agreed to have their conversations recorded. The interviews were initiated using open-ended questions, such as "What is meant by healthy aging, in your opinion?," "Could you tell me about healthy aging?," and "What makes older persons healthy?" Then, the first author asked specific follow-up questions to prompt the participants to reflect on the meaning of the phrase "healthy aging" and on their own thoughts, such as "What do you mean when you say ...?" or "Please give me an example of ...." The lengths of the interviews varied, depending on the participants' responses, between 45 and 90 minutes. Each interview was transcribed verbatim, and each transcript was then translated from Thai to English by a professional Thai-English translator to ensure that the translations were accurate [34].

2.4. Data Analysis. The authors analyzed the transcribed interviews according to the steps suggested by Dahlgren and Fallsberg [35]. First, in the familiarization step, the first author read the transcriptions several times in both Thai and English to gain an overview of the relatives' conceptions of healthy aging. This step was necessary to verify the accuracy of the transcriptions in Thai and English. The first author confirmed that the transcriptions completely retained the meaning of the responses. The English transcripts were then used throughout the analysis process. The other authors read the English transcripts several times to familiarize themselves with the content. In the second step, the meaning units associated with healthy aging were condensed into short statements. In the third step, called the comparison step, similarities and differences in the dialogue excerpts were identified. Then, similar statements were grouped into descriptive categories in the fourth step. In the fifth step, or the articulating step, embedded conceptions in each group of meaning units were identified. The sixth step was the labeling step, in which the authors named the various categories. The final step was the contrasting step, in which the differences and similarities between categories were considered.

2.5. Ethical Approval. We followed the guidelines of the principles outlined in the Declaration of Helsinki [36], which emphasize showing respect for all participants and protecting their rights. The first author orally informed the participants about the study and then provided them with written information detailing the purpose of the study and its possible benefits. The participants could choose the time and place of the interview and were allowed to withdraw from the study at any time. The participants were also ensured that their information would remain confidential. Permission to conduct this study was granted by the Udon Thani Provincial Public Health Office Committee Board in Thailand and the Ethical Review Board of Research Involving Humans. This study was registered with the Research Ethical Review Board of Uppsala, Sweden (Dnr 2013/019).

3. Results

The participants' conceptions of healthy aging consisted of four qualitatively different descriptive categories: being independent, not being afflicted by diseases or illnesses, being a giver and a receiver, and being wise. Each descriptive category is presented and described in detail below.

3.1. Being Independent. Healthy aging means having a desire to do everything by oneself and to avoid relinquishing control or seeking assistance from family members. This category comprised the following two subcategories: "performing activities without the assistance of others" and "not being a burden to others."

3.1.1. Performing Activities without the Assistance of Others. Healthy aging means being able to care for oneself, to be free, and to participate in activities considered appropriate for one's age without needing assistance from relatives. Healthy aging also means having the ability to work after retirement to earn an adequate income as a means of supporting oneself financially. One participant described healthy aging as follows:

> *My mother is expected to do things by herself. Older persons should work and earn their own income. They can choose what they want to do. Some choose to eat vegetables or fish. Some like chili paste. You just live on your own.* (6)

Healthy aging means having the ability to adjust to different circumstances and having autonomy, which fosters a sense of freedom that prevents individuals from being forced to perform unwanted activities.

3.1.2. Not Being a Burden to Others. According to the participants, healthy aging means not being dependent on family members. Specifically, healthy aging means that one's needs are sufficiently met such that he or she demands nothing. Thus, one who ages healthily lives a sufficient life and does not strive for unnecessary things, offend anyone, or interfere in others' business. One participant described this idea as follows:

> *She does what she can and doesn't impose a burden on her children and grandchildren. Someone always expresses concern that our family spoils her. But my mother isn't like that. We don't have to worry about her.* (2)

This statement indicates that healthy aging means not being a burden to others and that one should not impose oneself on one's children or grandchildren.

3.2. Not Being Afflicted by Diseases or Illnesses. Healthy aging was described as a lack of degeneration of the body and mind. This concept means that one does not suffer or worry about living with chronic diseases or illnesses. In this state, one has the ability to maintain the functions of his or her body and mind. Healthy aging means having a considerably strong, age-appropriate body and mind, the strength of which is visually apparent to oneself and to others. This category encompassed the subcategories "living with diseases or illnesses" and "exhibiting physical and mental strength."

3.2.1. Living with Diseases or Illnesses. Healthy aging means having the ability to live with serious diseases or illnesses and to continue performing daily life activities. One relative noted the following:

> *My mother is free from illness. Older persons can have some diseases, but not many. Although they have diseases, they effectively live with them. As long as they can simply live according to their routine, they are fine.* (12)

The participants stated that even individuals who have some chronic diseases can exhibit healthy aging, although these individuals must find a way to live with their health conditions and thus live an ordinary life.

3.2.2. Exhibiting Physical and Mental Strength. Healthy aging means being in good physical and mental conditions and free of diseases or illnesses that can limit one's ability to perform daily life activities. Healthy aging also means having a good memory, which is particularly desirable among older persons. Such individuals are able to manage their emotions and are as strong as others of the same age.

> *They must be healthy, both physically and mentally, and free of diseases or illnesses. If you have a strong body, you also have a good mind. If you are well on the inside, your physical body is also well. If you are healthy physically, everything is healthy. When you have a positive state of psychological health, everything is fine. If you are calm people around you feel cool.* (9)

Healthy aging means being strong and being a psychologically healthy person. Healthy individuals' bodily functions are clearly connected to their mental functions, linking their inner and outer states.

3.3. Being a Giver and a Receiver. The participants conceived of healthy aging as giving and receiving help from others and stated that happiness and satisfaction derive from these exchanges. Furthermore, healthy aging means being generous and performing good deeds in accordance with Buddhist beliefs, resulting in satisfaction, and delight from Buddhist practices. This category comprised the following two subcategories: "giving assistance and receiving support" and "devoting oneself to and being delighted by Buddhist practices."

3.3.1. Giving Assistance and Receiving Support. Healthy aging means having family members available to provide help, as well as helping children and others by acting as a giver. In this context, healthy individuals are good parents who have raised and provided for their family members but who also receive help from their children and grandchildren.

> *She makes bamboo sticks for grilled sticky rice for her son. He sells grilled sticky rice in town, and she helps him. She is happy to do it. I help take care of her bed and her mosquito net. My aunt sells grilled eggs in town. She always buys delicious food for my grandmother when she visits.* (4)

In this context, healthy aging means providing cooking materials for family members and receiving support from family members. It means asking for help, for example, to meet one's daily needs. Healthy aging also means helping family members in their work to support them.

3.3.2. Devoting Oneself to and Being Delighted by Buddhist Practices. Healthy aging means devoting oneself to the beliefs of Buddhism and attaining peace as a result of Buddhist practices. Healthy individuals live virtuous and positive lives, and perform noble deeds. In return, these individuals experience happy lives and good health. Dedicating oneself to Buddhism involves making merit and practicing the Buddhist doctrine.

> *She likes to go to temple. The temple is her society. Sometimes, she cuts the grass for the abbot and the monks. The monks support her, and my mother supports them. She offers to make merit in religious ceremonies. My mother lives in the community and adheres to Dharmic principles. Making merit is a sign that one's mind is peaceful and that one's health is also good.* (9)

Healthy aging means that one is dedicated to the act of making merit in accordance with Buddhist teachings. Making merit entails not only doing something good for others but also receiving merit in return, such as happiness, positive energy, peace, and enjoyment.

3.4. Being Wise. Healthy aging means being wise, which entails understanding one's own life and life situations that occur. In particular, being wise means having the inner strength to address life's challenges and the knowledge to prevent diseases and take care of oneself. This category consisted of the following two subcategories: "experiencing life as a journey" and "preparing for old age."

3.4.1. Experiencing Life as a Journey. Healthy aging means having sufficient knowledge—although not necessarily educational knowledge or an educational degree—to address problems in life. In the context of healthy aging, this subcategory refers to life experiences, which are derived from one's lifestyle. Healthy individuals regularly engage in positive practices in their everyday life to gain experiences that can help them make necessary decisions.

> *She understands what she needs to do because her life experience helps her. She learns from what she does. If it is good for her, she will continue to do it. She learns from her behavior. My mother has lived long enough to have experienced good and bad events in her life.* (12)

The participants stated that healthy aging means having the ability to learn through life experiences and to experience life as a journey.

3.4.2. Preparing for Aging. Healthy aging means preparing oneself for growing old, which includes being satisfied with one's present life and focusing on the moment. Preparing for aging involves practicing what is beneficial for one's health to continue feeling young.

> *People should prepare for what they have to confront when they get old. They have prepared themselves since they were young, that is, our age. My mother has been doing this. She does aerobic dance and jumps rope, for example.* (10)

Healthy aging is conceived of as preparing oneself to face the process of growing old. Preparing for aging includes preventing a decline in functions, for instance, by exercising and maintaining proper nutrition and hygiene.

4. Discussion

This study is the first to examine how the children and grandchildren of older persons in northeast Thailand conceive of healthy aging. The participants determined the meaning of healthy aging based on their lived experience of connecting to older persons they lived with and took care of in everyday life. The meaning of healthy aging consists of four descriptive categories: "being independent," "not being afflicted by diseases or illnesses," "being a giver and a receiver," and "being wise." The findings of this study reveal existential aspects of healthy aging. Additionally, the current study elucidates different conceptions of healthy aging that family nurses should consider when working together with the family members of older persons.

The family is viewed as the context, according to the focus of the family nursing perspective [17], which means that the older person is in the foreground and the family is in the background. Although the older person is the main focus of the promotion of healthy aging, family nurses should also consider the perspectives of older persons' family members. The family is an important unit since the family supports and provides for the older family member. Family nurses therefore need to integrate the conceptions of healthy aging held by the family members of older persons in their care. This does not mean changing their way of thinking but involves being aware that there is not only one conception of healthy aging when participating with the family members of older persons. To work with the family members of older persons, family nurses should respect and try to understand their conceptions of healthy aging. The challenge for family nurses and policy-makers is to find strategies to handle the different ways in which the relatives experience healthy aging. It is obvious that the family members of older persons conceive of healthy aging differently. As the results show, family nurses should equally emphasize the importance of being autonomous and depending on others. Moreover, healthy aging is related to disease and illness but is also focused on wisdom in old age. Therefore, family nurses should apply these perceptions when promoting healthy aging. Another challenge is to integrate the differences between the perspectives of older persons and family members when working with these groups of people. This practice may be useful for supporting good relationships among older persons, family members, and healthcare providers when implementing a plan to promote healthy aging.

A comparison of healthy aging from the perspectives of the children and grandchildren of older persons reveals similarities between healthy aging, successful aging, and active aging. These similarities demonstrate that the meaning of healthy aging relates to the ability to remain active and to maintain the overall functioning. This is in line with the definition of successful aging, which emphasizes healthy cognitive function and focuses on the state of functioning that makes an active life possible [11, 37]. When comparing the findings of this study with the concept of active aging, we found that both healthy aging and active aging refer to the ability to maintain autonomy as well as the importance of independence for the older person [12]. There is little difference between the concepts of healthy aging found in this study and a previous study [38]. That previous study on healthy aging also showed that healthy aging was defined as freedom from chronic illness and impairment [38]. However, in the present study, healthy aging is defined not only as the absence of disease or illness but also the importance of the ability to live with disease or illness.

Our results indicate the diversity of meanings of healthy aging, which is consistent with the characteristics of the ontological health concept [39], which is perceived as a movement toward wholeness and holiness [40]. The four descriptive categories are consistent with the three health levels in the ontological health concept: health as behavior, health as being, and health as becoming [39]. Herberts and Eriksson [39] described the first dimension of health as having health, which is a way of achieving health through certain behaviors that are considered healthy by the individual or society. The conceptions of healthy aging as being independent and not being afflicted by diseases or illnesses are related to the first dimension of health, that is, having health. Healthy aging also entails being independent, having the ability to care for oneself, being free from diseases or illnesses, and maintaining strong bodily and cognitive functions. Healthy aging is consistent with the idea of evaluating health using external objective criteria and focusing on illness-related problems [39].

A comparison of the meaning of healthy aging found in this study and that reported in other studies reveals explicit differences and similarities. Regarding the description of the nature of each category, the conceptions of healthy aging as being independent and not afflicted by diseases or illnesses are consistent with the ideas expressed by healthcare professionals in earlier studies of healthy aging in Western countries [5, 6]. We observed that being independent was a criterion for healthy aging, which may indicate that Thai cultural values have been influenced by Western traditions, in which individualism plays a prominent role [24, 41]. Thus, modern society may have an impact on people's beliefs and normative contexts. A previous study showed that, according to the perspective of older persons in the Isan region, healthy aging still depends on one's relatives [7]. Furthermore, older persons are dependent on caregivers [21, 42], whereas their younger relatives may value independence. While older persons still need assistance [21] because of changes in their bodily functions [43], the children and grandchildren of older persons conceptualize healthy aging with respect to the functional capacity of older persons and not being a burden on relatives. These conceptions may be partly related to ageism, the belief that older persons are inferior to younger people because of their age [44]. Children and grandchildren view older persons as being different from themselves, which may result in negative attitudes toward older persons. This study indicates that family nurses should be aware of these conceptions when collaborating with the children and grandchildren of older persons to promote healthy aging. Considering these aspects, policies should be developed according to the conception of healthy aging with respect to the burden of older persons on family members and the roles of older persons in society. Another suggestion is to support older persons when they lack the capacity to increase the value of their lives. Policy-makers and family nurses should emphasize the value of older persons to younger people.

Healthy aging is also defined as "being a giver and a receiver." This category is related to the second dimension of the ontological health concept, in which health is viewed as "being health" [39]. Health is characterized as the achievement of balance and harmony, whether between the body and soul; between physiological, psychological, and social factors; or between internal and external elements [39, 45]. When comparing that conception of healthy aging to the meaning found in this study, there are differences between the categories "being independent" and "being a giver and a receiver." Surprisingly, "being independent" and "being a giver and a receiver" seem to be contradictory. The meaning of healthy aging that focuses on healthy aging as a state characterized by independence may reflect the influence of the Western perspective [5]. In contrast, "being a giver and a receiver" stresses the importance of the relationships between older persons and their family members as an influential factor in healthy aging, which may be due to the values of Isan culture. Being a giver and a receiver is related to the dynamics of the relationships between children and grandchildren and older persons in Isan culture. This relationship reflects the idea that children are indebted to their parents because their parents raised them from birth [22, 42]. Thus, these relationships may be related to the concept of intersubjectivity, which is defined in phenomenological theory [29, 46, 47] as the idea that everyone relies on and exists in relation to others [48]. The children and grandchildren of older persons interact with older persons throughout their lives and use their own bodies to understand how the concept of healthy aging relates to the older persons with whom they live. Parents provide for their children, love them, and take care of them from early childhood, and children are taught that they should live with and repay their parents until the parents die [22]. This connection may be described as an obligation and a social norm in Isan-Thai culture, which is based on Buddhism. Although the Isan lifestyle has been changed by modernization [24], people in this region continue to have a strong belief in Buddhism [49]. Isan customs and Buddhist beliefs are passed down from generation to generation [50], and the cultural values tied to these customs and beliefs determine the individual person's thoughts and ideas [51]. Isan people cling to their culture through local customs [49]. Buddhists believe in the concept of karma [22, 52], which means that one receives what he or she gives to others; this means that whatever one does to others may also be done to him/herself in the future. This belief is illustrated by the practice of making merit, which, according to Buddha's teachings, brings happiness and peace [9]. Isan values are rooted in the interactions between an individual and others. Thus, this category is related to the interdependence [8, 53] that characterizes Isan society. This finding indicates that family nurses should endeavor to enhance the relationships between older people and their children and grandchildren to promote healthy aging.

In the final category, healthy aging is conceived of as "being wise." Comparisons between our results and those of previous studies regarding healthy aging [5, 6] indicate that the domains of one's experience, adaptation, and preparation are related to wisdom. Being wise is related to the last dimension of health, in which health is perceived as "becoming" [39], meaning that human beings are becoming something greater than themselves and/or becoming whole at a deeper level [39]. In this context, wholeness refers to physical, mental, and spiritual wholeness [39]. Furthermore, Eriksson [54] noted that health as becoming means that "the person strives to reconcile himself with the circumstances of life and to become whole in a deeper dimension of integration" (p. 76). Our findings indicate that being wise is linked to self-adjustment and to one's ability to face his or her problems and the changes associated with the aging process. People in society believe that older persons have gained important life experiences that enable them to face life's problems and thus consider these life experiences as valuable sources of wisdom [55]. Wisdom is believed to benefit older persons in facing life situations and is correlated with older age [56, 57]. Wisdom also underlies the respect shown to older persons by children and other relatives who greatly admire them [58]. Another explanation for this behavior is consistent with the idea of ego integrity [59, 60]. This category may be associated with the ability to integrate one's life experiences. This finding suggests that the life experiences and wisdom of older persons should be revealed in order to promote positive attitudes toward older persons. We observed that participants also defined healthy aging as preparation for aging.

The findings of this study represent a starting point for family nurses and/or policy-makers when considering the perspectives of young adults regarding healthy aging. For the future challenges of supporting healthy aging, we suggest that family nurses plan for the promotion of healthy aging with adults in parallel with the current older population, according to the findings of this study. For example, family nurses should serve the workforce and programs for preparing healthy aging in middle adulthood. These programs should be related to the prevention of health problems. Moreover, the promotion of healthy aging should be relevant to the different conceptions of healthy aging. The family members of older persons should be encouraged to brainstorm a list of the key determinant factors in supporting their health and advance care planning to promote healthy aging.

4.1. Methodological Considerations. Rigor in phenomenographic research is based on the study's validity and reliability [61]. The participants of this study were carefully selected using a strategy intended to obtain a varied and broad picture regarding the focus of the study—the conceptions of healthy aging held by the relatives of older persons. The number of participants recruited for this study was considered reasonable, but the participants included more women than men. Thus, the conceptions of healthy aging held by the men who participated in this study may not be fully representative. In-depth interviews exploring the conceptions of healthy aging were conducted by one person (the first author), which allowed probing for deeper elaboration and ensuring that all information was considered. Specific quotations were used to clarify the meaning of healthy aging. The rigorous approach used in this study also yielded findings that are transferable [62]. This study focused on the conceptions of healthy aging held only by the children and grandchildren of older persons who live in the Isan region of Thailand. This restriction may have influenced our findings, as cultural backgrounds may impact people's beliefs. However, the findings of this study may be used to transfer to the relatives of older persons with similar backgrounds, such as the children and grandchildren of older persons who live in the northeast of Thailand. Although the results of the present study can be related to the Western perspective on the meaning of healthy aging, data were drawn from the relatives of older persons in only one region of Thailand. The information about the meaning of healthy aging gathered from this group of family members of older persons cannot be applied to the entire world. The purposive sampling method may also limit the generalizability of our results. Moreover, all the participants were Buddhists. Although Buddhism is a main religion in Thailand, the conceptions of healthy aging held by Buddhists may differ from those held by members of other religions.

5. Conclusions

The key findings of this study are the conceptions of healthy aging represented as a set of categories: "being independent," "not being afflicted by diseases or illnesses," "being a giver and a receiver," and "being wise." Furthermore, the meaning of healthy aging is linked to older persons, their relatives, and the Buddhist religion, which emphasizes the importance of a holistic view of healthy aging. Although some relatives' conceptions of healthy aging were consistent with Western perspectives, traditional Isan-Thai cultural values still influence the meaning of healthy aging. This study highlights the need to be aware of the unique conceptions held by the children and grandchildren of older persons in the Isan region when promoting healthy aging.

Conflicts of Interest

The authors declare that they have no conflicts of interest with respect to this study or the authorship and/or publication of this article.

Acknowledgments

The authors would like to thank all the participants who participated in this study.

References

[1] W. Suwanrada, W. Pothisiri, V. Prachuabmoh et al., "Community-based integrated approach for older person's long-term care in Thailand," College of Population Studies Visid Prachuabmoh Building Chulalongkorn University, Bangkok, 2014, https://www.toyotafound.or.jp/international/2014/publications/data/2015-0430-1012.pdf.

[2] C. Wacharasin and S. Theinpichet, "Family nursing practice, education, and research: what is happening in Thailand?," *Journal of Family Nursing*, vol. 14, no. 4, pp. 429–435, 2008.

[3] S. Jitapunkul and S. Wivatvanit, "National policies and programs for the aging population in Thailand," *Ageing International*, vol. 33, no. 1–4, pp. 62–74, 2008.

[4] C. Williamson, "Policy mapping on aging in Asia and the Pacific: analytical report," HelpAge International, East Asia/Pacific Regional Office, Chiang Mai, Thailand, 2015, http://www.refworld.org/pdfid/55c9e6664.pdf.

[5] L. Hansen-Kyle, "A concept analysis of healthy aging," *Nursing Forum*, vol. 40, no. 2, pp. 45–57, 2005.

[6] L. Hung, G. I. J. M. Kempen, and N. K. De Vries, "Cross-cultural comparison between academic and lay views of healthy ageing: a literature review," *Ageing and Society*, vol. 30, no. 8, pp. 1373–1391, 2010.

[7] P. Manasatchakun, P. Chotiga, Å. Roxberg, and M. Asp, "Healthy ageing in Isan-Thai culture-a phenomenographic study based on older persons' lived experiences," *International Journal of Qualitative Studies on Health and Well-being*, vol. 11, no. 1, pp. 1–9, 2016.

[8] K. Thanakwang, K. Soonthorndhada, and J. Mongkolprasoet, "Perspectives on healthy aging among Thai elderly: a qualitative study," *Nursing and Health Sciences*, vol. 14, no. 4, pp. 472–479, 2012.

[9] L. Thiamwong, M. S. McManus, and J. Suwanno, "Development of the Thai healthy aging model: a grounded theory study," *Nursing and Health Sciences*, vol. 15, no. 2, pp. 256–261, 2013.

[10] L. L. Bryant, K. K. Corbett, and J. S. Kutner, "In their own words: a model of healthy aging," *Social Science and Medicine*, vol. 53, no. 7, pp. 927–941, 2001.

[11] J. W. Rowe and R. L. Kahn, "Successful aging," *Gerontologist*, vol. 37, no. 4, pp. 433–440, 1997.

[12] A. Walker, "A strategy for active ageing," *International Social Security Review*, vol. 55, no. 1, pp. 121–139, 2002.

[13] World Health Organization, "Multisectoral action for a life course approach to healthy aging: draft global strategy and plan of action on aging and health," May 2016. http://apps.who.int/gb/ebwha/pdf_files/WHA69/A69_17-en.pdf?ua=1.

[14] J. Knodel, B. Teerawichitchainan, V. Prachuabmoh, and W. Pothisiri, "The situation of Thailand's older population: an update based on the 2014 survey of older persons in Thailand," Tech. Rep. 35353, HelpAge International, Chiang Mai, Thailand, 2015.

[15] S. Jitapunkul, C. Kunanusont, W. Phoolcharoen, P. Suriyawongpaisal, and S. Ebrahim, "Disability-free life expectancy of elderly people in a population undergoing demographic and epidemiologic transition," *Age and Ageing*, vol. 32, no. 4, pp. 401–405, 2003.

[16] P. Martin, T. Duffy, B. Johnston, P. Banks, E. Harkess-Murphy, and C. R. Martin, "Family health nursing: a response to the global health challenges," *Journal of Family Nursing*, vol. 19, no. 1, pp. 99–118, 2013.

[17] H. Hanson, "Family health care nursing: an introduction," in *Family Health Care Nursing: Theory, Practice & Research*, S. H. Hanson, V. Gedaly-Duff, and J. R. Kaakinen, Eds., pp. 3–37, F.A. DAVIS, Philadelphia, PA, USA, 2005.

[18] J. Knodel and N. Chayovan, "Population aging and the well-being of older persons in Thailand," Tech. Rep. 08659, Institute for Social Research, University of Michigan, Ann Arbor, MI, USA, 2008.

[19] World Bank, "Thailand-Northeast economic development report," Tech. Rep. 35353, World Bank, Washington, DC, USA, 2005.

[20] R. A. Caffrey, "Caregiving to the elderly in northeast Thailand," *Journal of Cross-Cultural Gerontology*, vol. 7, no. 2, pp. 117–134, 1992.

[21] J. Rittirong, P. Prasartkul, and R. R. Rindfuss, "From whom do older persons prefer support? The case of rural Thailand," *Journal of Aging Studies*, vol. 31, pp. 171–181, 2014.

[22] T. Choowattanapakorn, "The social situation in Thailand: the impact on elderly people," *International Journal of Nursing Practice*, vol. 5, no. 2, pp. 95–99, 1999.

[23] S. Sasat and B. J. Bowers, "Spotlight Thailand," *Gerontologist*, vol. 53, no. 5, pp. 711–717, 2013.

[24] R. A. Caffrey, "Family care of the elderly in northeast Thailand: changing patterns," *Journal of Cross-Cultural Gerontology*, vol. 7, no. 2, pp. 105–116, 1992.

[25] J. Knodel, J. Kespichayawattana, C. Saengtienchai, and S. Wiwatwanich, "How left behind are rural parents of migrant children? Evidence from Thailand," *Ageing and Society*, vol. 30, no. 5, pp. 811–841, 2010.

[26] S. Sudnongbua, S. LaGrow, and J. Boddy, "Feelings of abandonment and quality of life among older persons in rural northeast Thailand," *Journal of Cross-Cultural Gerontology*, vol. 25, no. 3, pp. 257–269, 2010.

[27] P. Ashworth and U. Lucas, "What is the 'World' of phenomenography?," *Scandinavian Journal of Educational Research*, vol. 42, no. 4, pp. 415–431, 1998.

[28] P. Ashworth and U. Lucas, "Achieving empathy and engagement: a practical approach to the design, conduct and reporting of phenomenographic research," *Studies in Higher Education*, vol. 25, no. 3, pp. 295–308, 2000.

[29] K. Dahlberg, H. Dahlberg, and M. Nyström, *Reflective Lifeworld Research*, Studentlitteratur, Lund, Sweden, 2008.

[30] F. Marton and S. A. Booth, *Learning and Awareness*, Lawrence Erlbaum and Associates, Mahway, NJ, USA, 1997.

[31] J. Bengtsson, "With the lifeworld as ground. A research approach for empirical research in education-the Gothenburg

tradition," *Indo-Pacific Journal of Phenomenology*, vol. 13, pp. 1–18, 2013.

[32] F. Marton, "Phenomenography? Describing conceptions of the world around us," *Instructional Science*, vol. 10, no. 2, pp. 177–200, 1981.

[33] T. Phuttharak and A. Dhiravisit, "Rapid urbanization-its impact on sustainable development: a case study of Udon Thani, Thailand," *Asian Social Science*, vol. 10, no. 22, 2014.

[34] K. Regmi, J. Naidoo, and P. Pilkington, "Understanding the processes of translation and transliteration in qualitative research," *International Journal of Qualitative Methods*, vol. 9, no. 1, pp. 16–26, 2010.

[35] L. O. Dahlgren and M. Fallsberg, "Phenomenography as a qualitative approach in social pharmacy research," *Journal of Social and Administrative Pharmacy*, vol. 8, pp. 150–156, 1991.

[36] WMA, "World Medical Association declaration of Helsinki: ethical principles for medical research involving human subjects," *JAMA*, vol. 310, no. 20, pp. 2191–2194, 2013.

[37] L. Foster and A. Walker, "Active and successful aging: a European policy perspective," *Gerontologist*, vol. 55, no. 1, pp. 83–90, 2015.

[38] G. L. Burke, A. M. Arnold, D. E. Bild et al., "Factors associated with healthy aging: the cardiovascular health study," *Journal of the American Geriatrics Society*, vol. 49, no. 3, pp. 254–262, 2001.

[39] S. Herberts and K. Eriksson, "Nursing leaders' and nurses' view of health," *Journal of Advanced Nursing*, vol. 22, no. 5, pp. 868–878, 1995.

[40] U. Å. Lindström, L. Lindholm Nyström, J. E. Zetterlund, and K. Eriksson, "Theory of caritative caring," in *Nursing Theorists and Their Work*, M. R. Alliegood, Ed., pp. 171–201, Mosby, Maryland Heights, MO, USA, 2014.

[41] J. Knodel, N. Chayovan, and S. Siriboon, "The impact of fertility decline on familial support for the elderly: an illustration from Thailand," *Population and Development Review*, vol. 18, no. 1, pp. 79–103, 1992.

[42] N. Wongsawang, S. Lagampan, P. Lapvongwattana, and B. J. Bowers, "Family caregiving for dependent older adults in Thai families," *Journal of Nursing Scholarship*, vol. 45, no. 4, pp. 336–343, 2013.

[43] L. Ghahremani, S. Niknami, and M. Nazari, "The prediction of physical activity intention and behavior in elderly male residents of a nursing home: a comparison of two behavioral theories," *Iranian Journal of Medical Sciences*, vol. 37, no. 1, pp. 23–31, 2012.

[44] J. Angus and P. Reeve, "Ageism: a threat to "aging well" in the 21st century," *Journal of Applied Gerontology*, vol. 25, no. 2, pp. 137–152, 2006.

[45] K. Eriksson, "Theories of caring as health," in *Caring as Healing: Renewal Through Hope*, D. Gaut and A. Boykin Eds., pp. 3–20, National League for Nursing, New York, NY, USA, 1994.

[46] U. M. Kellett, "Heideggerian phenomenology: an approach to understanding family caring for an older relative," *Nursing Inquiry*, vol. 4, no. 1, pp. 57–65, 1997.

[47] K. M. Stroh, "Intersubjectivity of Dasein in Heidegger's being and time: how authenticity is a return to community," *Human Studies*, vol. 38, no. 2, pp. 243–259, 2015.

[48] L. Todres, K. Galvin, and K. Dahlberg, "Lifeworld-led healthcare: revisiting a humanising philosophy that integrates emerging trends," *Medicine, Health Care, and Philosophy*, vol. 10, no. 1, pp. 53–63, 2007.

[49] S. Wanlu, S. Chantachon, and B. Rachote, "An application of Isan local indigenous knowledge in suppression of social disputes," *Social Sciences*, vol. 4, pp. 180–185, 2009.

[50] D. Rattanamongkolgul, W. Sritanyarat, and L. Manderson, "Preparing for aging among older villagers in northeastern Thailand," *Nursing and Health Sciences*, vol. 14, no. 4, pp. 446–451, 2012.

[51] M. Leininger, "Cultural diversities of health and nursing care," *Nursing Clinics of North America*, vol. 12, no. 1, pp. 5–18, 1977.

[52] L. Ghose, "Karma and the possibility of purification: an ethical and psychological analysis of the doctrine of karma in Buddhism," *Journal of Religious Ethics*, vol. 35, no. 2, pp. 259–290, 2007.

[53] B. Ingersoll-Dayton, C. Saengtienchai, J. Kespichayawattana, and Y. Aungsuroch, "Psychological well-being Asian style: the perspective of Thai elders," *Journal of Cross-Cultural Gerontology*, vol. 16, no. 3, pp. 283–302, 2001.

[54] K. Eriksson, "Caring, spirituality, and suffering," in *Caring from the Heart: The Convergence of Caring and Spirituality*, M. S. Roach, Ed., pp. 68–83, Paulist Press, New York, NY, USA, 1997.

[55] A. Montgomery, C. Barber, and P. McKee, "A phenomenological study of wisdom in later life," *International Journal of Aging and Human Development*, vol. 54, no. 2, pp. 139–157, 2002.

[56] M. Ardelt, "Wisdom and life satisfaction in old age," *Journals of Gerontology. Series B: Psychological Sciences and Social Sciences*, vol. 52B, no. 1, pp. P15–2P7, 1997.

[57] M. Ardelt, "Antecedents and effects of wisdom in old age," *Research on Aging*, vol. 22, no. 4, pp. 360–394, 2000.

[58] T. Choowattanapakorn, R. Nay, and D. Fetherstonhaugh, "Nursing older people in Thailand: embryonic holistic rhetoric and the biomedical reality of practice," *Geriatric Nursing*, vol. 25, no. 1, pp. 17–23, 2004.

[59] E. H. Erikson, *Childhood and Society*, Vintage Book Company, London, UK, 1995.

[60] J. B. James and N. Zarrett, "Ego integrity in the lives of older women: a follow-up of mothers from the Sears, Maccoby, and Levin (1951) patterns of child rearing study," *Journal of Adult Development*, vol. 12, no. 4, pp. 155–167, 2005.

[61] S. Sin, "Considerations of quality in phenomenographic research," *International Journal of Qualitative Methods*, vol. 9, no. 4, pp. 305–319, 2010.

[62] E. G. Guba, "Criteria for assessing the trustworthiness of naturalistic inquiries," *Educational Communication and Technology*, vol. 29, pp. 75–91, 1981.

Successful Aging: A Psychosocial Resources Model for Very Old Adults

G. Kevin Randall,[1] Peter Martin,[2] Mary Ann Johnson,[3] and Leonard W. Poon[4]

[1] *CC Wheeler Institute, Bradley University, 05 Bradley Hall, 1501 W. Bradley Avenue, Peoria, IL 61625, USA*
[2] *Gerontology Program, Iowa State University, 1096 LeBaron Hall, Ames, IA 50011-1120, USA*
[3] *Department of Foods & Nutrition, The University of Georgia, 143 Barrow Hall, 115 DW Brooks Dr, Athens, GA 30602, USA*
[4] *Institute of Gerontology, College of Public Health, The University of Georgia, 255 E. Hancock Avenue, Athens, GA 30602-5775, USA*

Correspondence should be addressed to G. Kevin Randall, krandall@bradley.edu

Academic Editor: Roger A. Fielding

Objectives. Using data from the first two phases of the Georgia Centenarian Study, we proposed a latent factor structure for the Duke OARS domains: Economic Resources, Mental Health, Activities of Daily Living, Physical Health, and Social Resources. *Methods.* Exploratory and confirmatory factor analyses were conducted on two waves of the Georgia Centenarian Study to test a latent variable measurement model of the five resources; nested model testing was employed to assess the final measurement model for equivalency of factor structure over time. *Results.* The specified measurement model fit the data well at Time 1. However, at Time 2, Social Resources only had one indicator load significantly and substantively. Supplemental analyses demonstrated that a model without Social Resources adequately fit the data. Factorial invariance over time was confirmed for the remaining four latent variables. *Discussion.* This study's findings allow researchers and clinicians to reduce the number of OARS questions asked of participants. This has practical implications because increased difficulties with hearing, vision, and fatigue in older adults may require extended time or multiple interviewer sessions to complete the battery of OARS questions.

1. Introduction

Aging is often conceptualized as a developmental challenge to maintain balance between the gains and losses of resources necessary for adaptation to age-related change, with losses increasing over the lifespan [1, 2]. Yet, Von Faber and colleagues [3] reminded us that, "Successful aging as an optimal state implicates more than physical well-being and fits the World Health Organization's definition of health as a state of complete physical, mental, and social well-being and not merely the absence of disease or infirmity." These resources-material, social, or personal characteristics essential for successful aging-hold a prominent position in studies of older adults [4–6]. Consequently, the need for a valid, reliable, and efficient resource measure, designed for use in clinical and community settings with older adults, arose. In response, Fillenbaum [7] and associates developed the *Multidimensional Functional Assessment of Older Adults: The Duke Older Americans Resources and Services Procedures* (OARS hereafter). Since development of the OARS, advances in statistical methodology, computer technology, and software programs have made factor analytic procedures commonplace, enabling researchers to suggest less complex and shorter versions of measurement scales and to model measurement error in empirical studies. To date, we know of no studies that investigated the underlying, latent factor structure of the five OARS resources with data from older adults—the purpose of the present study.

Studies on multiple resources and successful aging among older adults have grown tremendously [8–11], spawning psychometric concerns regarding how and what to assess [12]. Researchers have demonstrated the need to expand investigations of multidimensional resources in older populations [13, 14]. This body of work was motivated not only by the increased prevalence of older adults but also by a growing concern among those assessing and caring for frail older adults. The OARS was developed by a multidisciplinary team who recognized that older adults' personal well-being encompasses many aspects or multiple functions [7]. Because older adults often present with chronic disabilities or ailments [15, 16], the developers of the OARS designed an assessment tool that focused primarily on adaptation and the maintenance of personal well-being in five resources: Social Resources, Economic Resources, Mental Health, Physical Health, and self-care capacity or functional health (including both instrumental activities of daily living (IADL) and activities of daily living (ADLs)). This instrument has received widespread use by a diverse group of geriatric practitioners, researchers, and service group providers such as epidemiologists characterizing particular populations, clinicians assessing patient status, resource allocators providing services, and program evaluators investigating the impacts of interventions [12, 17–19].

In addition, because clinical work and empirical research may be tiring and confusing for older participants, a reduced version of the five OARS resources as modeled by five latent variables would prove helpful in reducing the time required to assess older adults' resources. However, few studies have specified the OARS resources as latent variables [20–22]. Further, to date, no study was found that developed a measurement model for all five OARS resources.

The purpose of this study was to specify and test the latent factor structure of the five OARS resources administered to participants in their 60s, 80s, and 100s. We hypothesized that (a) the resource model proposed by Fillenbaum [7] can be obtained using data from old and very old individuals and (b) a reduced short version of the OARS will yield a satisfactory latent variable solution.

2. Methods

2.1. Procedure and Participants. Participants were selected through the assistance of the University of Georgia Survey Research Center, the Office of the Governor of Georgia, the media, and local older adult service organizations [23–25]. Selection criteria for the final sample of community-dwelling individuals included a score of 23 or higher on the Mini-Mental Status Examination (MMSE; [26]) or a score of 2 or lower on the Global Deterioration Scale [27].

The data collection at phase one included 321 older adults (217 women, 104 men), classified as sexagenarians ($n = 91$), octogenarians ($n = 93$), and centenarians ($n = 137$). At time two, 201 participants provided data for this longitudinal study: 70 sexagenarians, 63 octogenarians, and 68 centenarians. Those in their 60s and 80s were followed up within 60 months; due to mortality attrition, centenarians were followed up within 20 months. Almost one-third of the sample was African American (27.7% and 30.8% at Time 1 and Time 2, resp.). The majority of the sample was female (67.6%), well-educated (at least graduated from high school), and rated their health as excellent or good (Table 1).

Table 1: Sample demographic characteristics.

Variables	Time 1		Time 2		χ^2
	n	%	n	%	
Sex					1.59
Male	104	32.4	60	29.9	
Female	217	67.6	141	70.1	
Race					2.61
Black	89	27.7	62	30.8	
White	232	72.3	139	69.2	
Age group					18.86***
60s	91	28.3	70	34.8	
80s	93	29.0	63	31.3	
100s	137	42.7	68	33.8	
Education					6.19
0-8 years	90	28.2	55	28.8	
High school	84	26.3	42	22.0	
Business/trade school	23	7.2	14	7.3	
College	75	23.6	44	23.0	
Graduate school	47	14.7	36	18.8	
Self-rated health					4.7
Excellent	67	21.1	39	20.2	
Good	159	50.2	93	48.2	
Fair	79	24.9	52	26.9	
Poor	12	3.8	9	4.7	

Because of rounding, percentages may not add to 100.
***$P < .001$.

As noted earlier, in this sample of old and very old adults, mortality attrition resulted in a reduction of participants, particularly among the centenarians, from 321 at time 1 to 201 at time 2. Table 2 examines the differences for the OARS manifest variables and two measures of cognitive status. Overall, the sample at time 2 showed significantly higher scores relative to time 1.

2.2. Measures. Because the purpose of this study was to develop a latent variable model for the five OARS resources, in this section we provide a brief overview of the measures based upon Fillenbaum's [7] work. Details of our final latent variables and corresponding indicators are presented in Section 3. In addition, the appendix lists each resource and its indicators and associated questions, based on our final results.

2.2.1. Economic Resources. Six questions were asked; examples included "How well does the amount of money you have take care of your needs—very well, fairly well, or poorly?" and "Please tell me how well you think you are now doing financially as compared to other people your age—better, about the same, or worse?" These items were scaled from 0: poorly or worse to 2: very well or better.

2.2.2. Mental Health. Satisfaction (six items), sleep disturbance (two items), lethargy (6 items), and paranoid (three

TABLE 2: Differences between participants at Time 1 and participants at Time 1 and Time 2.

Variables	Time 1 Only		Time 1 and Time 2		t
	M	SD	M	SD	
Mini-Mental (MMSE)	25.30	2.72	26.31	3.01	−3.03**
Short Portable (SPMSQ)	8.63	1.58	9.04	1.38	−2.41*
Economic Resources	4.73	1.48	4.82	1.47	.48
Mental Health	5.12	1.33	5.27	1.24	.97
IADLs	4.81	1.30	5.25	1.19	3.02**
Physical Health	3.73	1.70	4.24	1.58	2.73**
Social Resources	4.49	1.55	4.57	1.47	.42

*$P < .05$. **$P < .01$.

items) comprised the four dimensions of Mental Health [7]. Examples of questions included (a) satisfaction: "In general, do you find life exciting, pretty routine, or dull?" scaled so that 0: dull, 1: pretty routine, and 2: exciting; (b) sleep disturbance: "Do you wake up fresh and rested most mornings?" scaled so that 0: no, 1: yes; (c) lethargy: "Have you had periods of days, weeks, or months when you couldn't take care of things because you couldn't "get going?" scaled so that 0: no, 1: yes; (d) paranoid: "Does it seem that no one understands you?" scaled so that 0: no, 1: yes.

2.2.3. ADLs. Two commonly used dimensions, instrumental activities of daily living (IADL; seven items) and physical activities of daily living (PADLs; six items), comprised the self-care capacity assessment. An example of an IADL question included "Can you do your housework?" scaled so that 2: without help (can clean floors, etc.); 1: with some help (can prepare some things but unable to cook full meals yourself) or 0: are you completely unable to prepare any meals? A PADL question was "Can you dress and undress yourself" scaled so that 2: without help (able to pick out clothes, dress and undress yourself) 1: with some help, or 0: are you completely unable to dress and undress yourself?

2.2.4. Physical Health. Three questions assessing subjective self-rated health were included. For example, participants responded to "How would you rate your overall health at the present time—excellent, good, fair, or poor?" scaled so that 0: poor and 3: excellent.

2.2.5. Social Resources. Social Resources were measured using seven questions. An example of a question focusing on the interaction aspect of social support was "How many people do you know well enough to visit with in their homes?" Participants chose from a scale of 0: none to 3: five or more. An assessment of dependability of social support included two questions. These questions were answered 1: yes and 0: no. For example, one question was "Do you have someone you can trust and confide in?" A third assessment of the affective domain of social support also included two questions, scaled 1: yes and 0: no. For example, one question was "Do you see your relatives and friends as often as you want to or not?"

2.3. Data Analysis. The analyses conducted to confirm a measurement model included the following steps for each resource: (a) specifying and testing Fillenbaum's subscales; (b) adapting Fillenbaum's recommendations when modeling difficulties were encountered; (c) employing exploratory factor analyses (i.e., principal axis factoring retaining three factors with oblique rotation) to assess relationships within the data and to posit possible indicators for latent constructs; (d) testing the measurement model by confirmatory factor analyses. We developed at least three indicators for each resource and then tested the latent variable measurement model via confirmatory factor analysis. Table 3 provides assessment of measurement model fit, standardized loadings, and the uniqueness or R^2 for each indicator. All variables were scaled so that higher scores indicated higher levels of the resource. In the appendix, we provide a nontechnical summary of our results, listing the recommended questions for each indicator of the five OARS resources.

We used full-information maximum likelihood (FIML) to estimate our models [28, 29]. For our latent variable analyses we used *M*plus 6.11 [30] and employed FIML with the estimator MLR (maximum likelihood parameter estimates with standard errors and a mean-adjusted chi-square test statistic that are robust to nonnormality).

Exploratory factor analyses were conducted using SPSS 18.0, whereas confirmatory factor analyses and structural equation modeling were conducted with *M*plus [30]. Overall model fit was assessed by employing the Satorra-Bentler chi-square test statistic. This type of chi-square test statistic provided maximum likelihood parameter estimates with standard errors and a mean-adjusted chisquare test statistic that is robust to nonnormality of measures. Because the chisquare goodness of fit test and its corresponding probability value are sensitive to sample size, often making it difficult to accurately assess model fit when limited to this single statistic [31, 32], other measures of model fit were reported including the Comparative Fit Index (CFI) [33], the Tucker-Lewis coefficient (also called the NNFI) (TLI) [34], Browne and Cudeck's [35] root mean squared error of approximation (RMSEA), and the standardized root mean squared residual (SRMR). It has been suggested that values close to .95 for TLI and CFI, .08 for SRMR, and .06 for RMSEA are necessary before concluding that a relatively good fit between the observed data and the hypothesized model exists [36, 37].

Table 3: OARS resources latent variable measurement model results.

Construct/indicators	Loadings (λ)[a]	Uniqueness (R^2)	Loadings (λ)[a]	Uniqueness (R^2)
	T1*		T2**	
Economic Resources				
Sufficient Income	.81[b]	.66	.96[b]	.93
Overall Income	.70	.49	.61	.37
Meet Payments	.63	.40	.30	.09
Mental Health				
Exciting	.60[b]	.36	.53[b]	.28
Overall Mental Health	.53	.29	.49	.24
Life Satisfaction	.50	.25	.69	.47
IADLS				
Getting Out	.89[b]	.80	.94[b]	.88
Housework	.88	.78	.94	.88
Medicine	.65	.42	.77	.59
Physical Health				
Low Troubles	.70[b]	.49	.86[b]	.73
Overall Physical Health	.66	.44	.49	.24
Comparative Health	.46	.21	.48	.23
Social Resources				
Phone Talk	.64[b]	.41	.94[b]	.89
Visit Network Number	.47	.22	.08	.01
Visits With Others	.42	.17	.29	.08

[a] Parameter estimates are from the standardized solution. [b] These indicator loadings were fixed to 1.0 (unstandardized) for model identification; all estimated loadings $P < .01$; except Time 2 Social Resources.
*T1 Fit Indices: MLR χ^2 ($N = 321$; df = 80) = 144; CFI = .94; TLI = .92; RMSEA = .05; SRMR = .05.
**T2 Fit Indices: MLR χ^2 ($N = 201$; df = 80) = 136; CFI = .93; TLI = .90; RMSEA = .06; SRMR = .07.

3. Results

Economic Resources included six items. We conducted an exploratory factor analysis (principal axis factoring) with an oblique rotation and extracted three factors, accounting for 76 percent of the variance. Based upon these results, we constructed three indicators. First, we summed the three dichotomous items tapping the sufficiency of the respondent's economic resources to meet emergencies and provide extras currently and in the future (Cronbach's alpha = .81). This indicator, *Sufficient Income*, was recorded so that the scores ranged from 0 to 2. (Because we summed these indicators to create a manifest variable in other analyses, we recorded the indicators for equal weighting.) Second, two items loaded on a second factor, both asking the respondents how well they were doing financially. These two items were then averaged to create a second indicator, *Overall Income*, and assessed how well the respondents felt they were doing relative to their overall financial well-being (Cronbach's alpha = .59). Finally, the last item, *Meet Payments*, assessed the participant's expenses, was recorded to 0–2, and used as a third indicator. This item tapped the respondents, ability to meet payments. The three indicators loaded significantly and substantively on the latent variable, Economic Resources, at Time 1 and Time 2 (Table 3).

Inspection of the *Mental Health* assessment revealed that five items had 90% or more respondents scoring alike, five had 80% or more of respondents scoring alike, and three had 70% or more of respondents scoring alike. Thus, we did not use these items and specified a latent variable with three single-item indicators: (a) "In general, do you find life exciting, pretty routine, or dull?" (b) "How would you rate your mental or emotional health at the present time?" and (c) "Taking everything into consideration how would you describe your satisfaction with life in general at the present time?" These three indicators, *Exciting*, *Overall Mental Health*, and *Life Satisfaction*, loaded significantly and substantively on the latent variable Mental Health at Time 1 and Time 2 (Table 3).

Activities of Daily Living (IADL) consisted of instrumental activities of daily living (seven items) and physical activities of daily living (six items). Because descriptive statistics demonstrated that for those in their 60s and 80s few difficulties with physical activities of daily living were encountered, we did not include this subscale but created three indicators for IADL based upon an exploratory factor analysis of the seven items of IADL. The first indicator, labeled *Getting Out*, included items assessing (a) "Can you use the phone?" (b) "Can you get to places out of walking distance?" and (c) "Can you go shopping for groceries or clothes?" Cronbach's alpha for these three items was .76. The second indicator, *Housework*, was comprised of three items (Cronbach's alpha = .88) assessing: (a) "Can you prepare your own meals?" (b) "Can you do your own housework?" and (c) "Can you handle your own money?" The third indicator, *Medicine*, was a single item, "Can you take your own medicine?" The three indicators loaded significantly and substantively on the latent variable IADL at Time 1 and Time 2 (Table 3).

Physical Health consisted of three single-item indicators assessing subjective health perceptions. First, for the indicator *Low Troubles*, respondents were asked, "How much do your health troubles stand in the way of your doing the things you want to do?" Second, the question for the indicator *Overall Health* asked "How would you rate your overall health at the present time?" A third question for the indicator *Comparative Health* asked, "Is your health now better, about the same, or worse than it was five years ago?" These three indicators loaded significantly and substantively on the latent variable Physical Health at Time 1 and Time 2 (Table 3).

Social Resources included seven items. Because three dichotomous items did not provide much variance (over 90% of respondents scored "yes"), we did not use them. We then conducted an exploratory factor analysis on the remaining questions. Four items were used in our initial latent variable: (a) "How many times did you talk to friends, relatives, or others on the phone in the past week?" (b) "How many people do you know well enough to visit in their homes?" (c) "How many times in the past week did you spend some time with someone who does not live with you?" and (d) "Do you find yourself feeling lonely?" (recorded so that high scores reflected low loneliness). Thus, a latent variable was specified with *Phone Talk* as the first indicator, with *Visit Network Number* as a second indicator, *Visits With Others* as a third indicator, and *Loneliness* as a fourth.

Based on the previous exploratory factor analyses, we specified and tested a measurement model using confirmatory factor analysis and comprised of the five factors and their respective indicators as previously discussed. However, in the first test of the measurement model, loneliness did not significantly load on the latent variable for Social Resources at Time 1 ($t = 1.62$); this item was dropped and not used as an indicator in further analyses. Next, we conducted a similar analysis and these indicators loaded on the latent factor, Social Resources, significantly and substantively at Time 1 (see Table 3 for the results). However, at Time 2 the second and third indicators did not load significantly or substantively, although the overall measurement model fit to the data was adequate. This indicates that the construct might have changed over time, and the results for Time 2 Social Resources need to be stated with caution (Table 3).

The five latent variables were significantly correlated with one another at each measurement occasion with a few exceptions at Time 2 (Table 4). For example, at Time 2 Social Resources was only significantly associated with IADL; also, Physical Health was not significantly associated with either Mental Health or Social Resources at Time 2. Also, power issues may have influenced the results as the sample size was $N = 321$ at time 1 and $N = 201$ at Time 2, resulting in a lack of findings that may have existed. For example, consider the correlation between Social Resources and Mental Health at Time 2: $r = .25$, $P > .05$. However, at Time 1, with the larger sample size, two correlations close to the same magnitude as that between Social Resources and Mental Health at Time 2—the correlation between Economic Resources and IADL ($r = .25$, $P \leq .01$) and the correlations between Economic

Table 4: Correlation Matrix of OARS Resources Latent Variables (Time1 below the diagonal; Time 2 above the diagonal).

	1	2	3	4	5
1. Economic Resources	—	.26**	.43**	.27**	.08
2. Physical Health	.46**	—	.15	.58**	.14
3. Mental Health	.60**	.83**	—	.38**	.25
4. IADLS	.21**	.56**	.42**	—	.45**
5. Social Resources	.27**	.34**	.35**	.50**	—

** $P < .01$.

Resources and Social Resources ($r = .27$, $P \leq .01$)—are significant, indicating a likely reduction in power at Time 2. Table 5 presents the final correlations and descriptive statistics for all indicators of the OARS measurement model.

Finally, we attempted a nested model test for factorial invariance over time by constraining the loadings of each indicator at Time 1 equal to the same indicator at Time 2. Also, the residual for each indicator at Time 1 was correlated with its counterpart at Time 2. This constrained or nested model did not fit the data well: MLR χ^2 (354, $N = 201$) = 527.03, $P = .001$, CFI = .91, TLI = .89, RMSEA = .05, and SRMR = .07. However, despite increasing the number of iterations and specifying starting values, we were not able to get the unconstrained or base model to converge. This measurement model included the Social Resources latent construct at Time 2 that did not have significant loadings for its estimated indicators. Thus, the overall poor model fit may be due to a poor measurement model for Social Resources.

As a follow-up, we decided to fit a measurement model without the Social Resources latent variable. The unconstrained or base model, including the four latent variable resource constructs (without Social Resources at Time 1 and Time 2), specified with correlated residuals across time, fit the data well: MLR χ^2 (211, $N = 201$) = 289.09, $P = .001$, CFI = .95, TLI = .94, RMSEA = .04, and SRMR = .06. Next, we added across time constraints to the factor loadings for each corresponding indicator and ran the model. This constrained or nested model with eight more degrees of freedom fit the data well also: MLR χ^2 (219, $N = 201$) = 300.18, $P = .001$, CFI = .95, TLI = .94, RMSEA = .04, and SRMR = .07. Finally, we performed a nested model chi-square difference test following the specifications provided by B. Muthén and L. Muthén [30] for the MLR chi-square. In this case, the chi-square difference was 11.06 with eight degrees of freedom, $P = .20$. Thus, no significant difference was found between these two models and it is reasonable to assume factorial invariance over time.

4. Discussion

The focus of this study was a widely used integral part of the *Multidimensional Functional Assessment of Older Adults: The Duke Older Americans Resources and Services Procedures* [7]. To date, few studies have specified one or more of the five OARS resources as latent variables [20–22] and we found no studies with older adults, especially centenarians, specifying

TABLE 5: Correlation matrix of indicators for OARS measurement model (Time 1 below the diagonal; Time 2 above the diagonal).

Variables	1	2	3	4	5	6	7	8	9	10	11	12	13	14	15	16		
(1) Age Group	—	−.18**	.02	−.08	−.22**	−.23**	−.13	−.72**	−.71**	−.47**	−.27**	−.10	−.09	−.40**	−.18**	−.03		
(2) Sufficient Income	−.05	—	.58**	.28**	.17**	.18**	.32**	.27**	.25**	.12	.19**	.30**	.04	.14	−.02	.16		
(3) Overall Income	.07	.56**	—	.22**	.07	.14	.21*	.02	.04	−.01	.02	.16*	.04	.08	.10	.09		
(4) Meet Payments	−.04	.55**	.41**	—	.09	.06	.14	.12	.10	.06	.21**	.10	.13	−.02	−.06	−.01		
(5) Exciting	−.24**	.22**	.27**	.20**	—	.29**	.35**	.23**	.17	.22**	.05	.13	−.09	.14*	.06	.20**		
(6) Overall Mental Health	−.08	.28**	.31**	.16**	.27**	—	.33**	.16**	.21**	.07	.00	.33**	.01	.07	.13*	.03		
(7) Life Satisfaction	−.10	.22**	.24**	.24**	.38**	.23**	—	.19*	.26**	.20*	.09	.18**	−.02	.16**	.04	.17**		
(8) Getting Out	−.69**	.17**	.11	.18**	.33**	.13**	.20**	—	.88**	.73**	.46**	.32**	.17*	.40**	.13	.02		
(9) House Work	−.63**	.04	.07	.16**	.29**	.11	.14**	.79**	—	.72**	.48**	.27**	.16*	.40**	.07	.07		
(10) Medicine	−.38**	.19**	.00	.02	.21**	.03	.07	.55**	.61**	—	.38**	.27**	.14	.31**	.07	.05		
(11) Low Troubles	−.26**	.19**	.25**	.21**	.32**	.26**	.28**	.41**	.35**	.30**	—	.40**	.41**	.09	−.14*	.00		
(12) Overall Physical Health	−.16**	.30**	.29**	.22**	.33**	.48**	.20**	.28**	.24**	.17**	.45**	—	.33**	.16*	.03	.08		
(13) Comparative Health	−.28**	.08	.12	.11	.25**	.17**	.13**	.29**	.27**	.19**	.35**	.28**	—	.10	−.13	−.03		
(14) Phone Talk	.23**	.04	.18**	.03	.16**	.08	.11	.35**	.30**	.20**	.15*	.20**	.01	—	.07	.27**		
(15) Visit Network Number	−.21**	.03	.07	.09	.11**	.05	.04	.32**	.21**	.19	.10	.13	.09	.24**	—	.19		
(16) Visits With Others	−.03	.14**	.05	−.01	.10	.09	.11	.10	.00	.08	.11	.09	−.01	.31**	.25**	—		
Means	Time 1	$N = 321$	1.14	1.52	1.44	1.78	1.41	2.06	1.75	1.63	1.58	1.83	1.29	1.89	.86	2.41	2.86	2.16
	Time 2	$N = 201$	.99	1.52	1.42	1.72	1.42	1.97	1.77	1.55	1.47	1.77	1.17	1.83	.78	2.41	2.87	2.08
SD	Time 1	$N = 321$	.78	.78	.52	.50	.57	.70	.47	.46	.59	.40	.76	.77	.62	.85	.49	.77
	Time 2	$N = 201$	.83	.78	.77	.58	.57	.72	.49	.55	.67	.51	.78	.80	.61	.89	.48	.88

$^*P \le .05$. $^{**}P \le .01$.

all five OARS resources as latent variables. Thus, empirical and clinical attention to multidimensional assessments of older adults and their successful aging, especially those in their 80s and 100s, and the continued popularity of the OARS instrument as a standardized scale motivated this study development of a measurement model of psychosocial resources essential to successful aging for very old adults.

Five latent variables with three indicators each, corresponding to the five OARS resources, were specified; the combined measurement model fit the data adequately using a sample of older adults in their 60s, 80s, and 100s. Three results from the measurement analyses are noteworthy. First, because of advances in SEM programs and techniques allowing specification of measurement error and latent factor modeling, a comprehensive measurement model of the five OARS resources would prove useful to researchers and those assessing and caring for older adults. With the exception of Social Resources at Time 2, researchers employing the OARS may confidently specify the measurement model tested in this study. The measurement model tested in this study fit the data well at Time 1 and Time 2. Factor loadings (except those of Social Resources at Time 2) were significant and substantive, providing adequate evidence of an acceptable latent variable measurement model for the five OARS resources.

Second, supplementary analyses of factorial invariance over time, conducted without Social Resources at Time 2, revealed that in this sample, the four latent variables (i.e., Economic Resources, IADL, Physical Health, and Mental Health) fit the data well and did not change significantly over time. It is noted that for the younger participants (i.e., those in their 60s and 80s), five years elapsed between measurement occasions, whereas, for the centenarians, 20 months. Researchers interested in developmental questions of change over time are encouraged to employ the measurement model verified by this study and to extend this work by carefully considering the time intervals necessary for proximal and distal influences to unfold among older adults.

Third, Social Resources tended to have the lowest loadings per indicator. In this sample, relative to the other indicators, talking on the phone is the main indicator tapping the respondent's Social Resources. Burholt and colleagues [38] investigated OARS Social Resources in a population-based study of older adults living independently in six Western European countries and argued that the items demonstrated a breadth of conceptual assessment. It is our contention that such is the case with the three single-item indicators for the latent variable Social Resources. These indicators may assess a breadth of structure and at times the items may not be related. These three items may better serve as a checklist of social resources structure. Expecting relatively high factor loadings for such a construct may be unfounded (see [39], for a discussion regarding why checklist assessments often exhibit low internal consistency). Thus, other valid and reliable assessments of social support might be examined to augment or supplant the items included in the OARS assessment. Finally, empirical work investigating the relationship between measures of social support and loneliness has demonstrated discriminant validity; despite the strong association these measures tap different constructs [40, 41]. This is consistent with the finding of this study; the loneliness item did not load significantly on the Social Resources latent variable and was not included in the final measurement model.

4.1. Limitations and Direction for Future Research. Several limitations, however, exist that affect the generalization of this study's results. First, the participants were Southeastern older adults in reasonably good health, mentally competent, and community-dwelling. Second, the younger age groups (those in their 60s and those in their 80s) were randomly selected by race and gender to approximate older adults in Georgia. However, in contrast, centenarians were selected using convenience sampling through state and local agencies. Also, the sexagenarians and octogenarians were assessed in testing locations; centenarians completed their assessments at home. In addition, for the two younger age groups, measurement occasions were five years apart, but for the centenarians the measurement occasions were approximately 20 months apart. With only two waves of data, longitudinal results are to be interpreted with caution. Future research will want to employ other valid assessments of similar assessments of the five resources for comparison, particularly with larger, more homogeneous samples. This would provide opportunity to compare the relationships between the revised OARS latent resources based on our results and other known measures. Also, using a more homogenous sample of older adults might mitigate some of the methodological difficulties inherent in our heterogeneous sample that includes three age groups of old (60s and 80s) and very old adults (100s).

Finally, the items used for Social Resources in this study could be improved in future research. All the latent variables except Social Resources were fairly consistent across measurement occasions. In fact, for the models tested without the Social Resources latent variable, the overall measurement model fit the data well and factorial invariance of the latent variables over time was substantiated. Future research is encouraged to consider other measures of Social Resources (see [42], for 12 different measures assessing social support).

This study employed data from the Georgia Centenarian Study and used the popular Duke OARS [7] to develop a measurement model consisting of latent variables for Economic Resources, Instrumental Activities of Daily Living, Physical Health, Mental Health, and Social Resources. The model was specified and affirmed using longitudinal (two waves) data from a sample of sexagenarians, octogenarians, and centenarians, further substantiating the robustness of these latent variables in research with older adults. The results of this study allow reduction of the numerous items used in assessing the five OARS resources. This has valuable and practical implications because increased difficulties with hearing, vision, and fatigue in older adults may require extended time or multiple interviewer sessions to complete the extensive battery of questions in the OARS. Thus, researchers conducting etiological investigations, health professionals conducting intake and out-patient assessments, and other practitioners wishing to employ the OARS with older populations and the resources essential to successful aging will benefit from using this reduced version.

Acknowledgment

This research was supported in part by NIH grant RO1-43435 and PO1 AG17533-01A1.

References

[1] P. B. Baltes, "On the incomplete architecture of human ontogeny: selection, optimization, and compensation as foundation of developmental theory," *American Psychologist*, vol. 52, no. 4, pp. 366–380, 1997.

[2] P. B. Baltes and M. M. Baltes, *Successful Aging: Perspectives from the Behavioral Sciences*, Cambridge University Press, Cambridge, UK, 1990.

[3] M. Von Faber, A. Bootsma-Van Der Wiel, E. Van Exel et al., "Successful aging in the oldest old," *Archives of Internal Medicine*, vol. 161, no. 22, pp. 2694–2700, 2001.

[4] S. E. Hobfoll, "Social and psychological resources and adaptation," *Review of General Psychology*, vol. 6, no. 4, pp. 307–324, 2002.

[5] L. W. Poon, P. Martin, A. Bishop et al., "Understanding centenarians' psychosocial dynamics and their contributions to health and quality of life," *Current Gerontology and Geriatrics Research*, vol. 2010, Article ID 680657, 13 pages, 2010.

[6] P. Martin, "Individual and social resources predicting well-being and functioning in the later years: conceptual models, research, and practice," *Ageing International*, vol. 27, no. 2, pp. 3–29, 2002.

[7] G. G. Fillenbaum, *Multidimensional Functional Assessment of Older Adults: The Duke Older Americans Resources and Services Procedures*, Lawrence Erlbaum Associates, Hillsdale, NJ, USA, 1988.

[8] H. B. Bosworth and K. W. Schaie, "The relationship of social environment, social networks, and health outcomes in the Seattle longitudinal study: two analytical approaches," *Journals of Gerontology*, vol. 52, no. 5, pp. P197–P205, 1997.

[9] M. Martin, M. Grünendahl, and P. Martin, "Age differences in stress, social resources, and well-being in middle and older age," *Journals of Gerontology*, vol. 56, no. 4, pp. P214–P222, 2001.

[10] M. Pinquart and S. Sörensen, "Influences of socioeconomic status, social network, and competence on subjective well-being in later life: a meta-analysis," *Psychology and Aging*, vol. 15, no. 2, pp. 187–224, 2000.

[11] R. A. Pruchno, M. Wilson-Genderson, M. Rose, and F. Cartwright, "Successful aging: early influences and contemporary characteristics," *Gerontologist*, vol. 50, no. 6, pp. 821–833, 2010.

[12] D. G. Blazer, "Psychiatry and the oldest old," *American Journal of Psychiatry*, vol. 157, no. 12, pp. 1915–1924, 2000.

[13] C. McCamish-Svensson, G. Samuelsson, and B. Hagberg, "Correlated and prevalence of loneliness from young old to oldest old: results from a Swedish cohort," *Hallym International Journal of Aging*, vol. 3, pp. 1–24, 2001.

[14] R. M. Suzman, D. P. Willis, and K. G. Manton, *The Oldest Old*, Oxford University Press, New York, NY, USA, 1992.

[15] A. J. Selim, G. Fincke, D. R. Berlowitz et al., "Comprehensive health status assessment of centenarians: results from the 1999 large health survey of veteran enrollees," *Journals of Gerontology*, vol. 60, no. 4, pp. 515–519, 2005.

[16] M. L. Stek, J. Gussekloo, A. T. F. Beekman, W. Van Tilburg, and R. G. J. Westendorp, "Prevalence, correlates and recognition of depression in the oldest old: the Leiden 85-plus study," *Journal of Affective Disorders*, vol. 78, no. 3, pp. 193–200, 2004.

[17] C. Bailey, J. Corner, J. Addington-Hall, D. Kumar, M. Nelson, and J. Haviland, "Treatment decisions in older patients with colorectal cancer: the role of age and multidimensional function," *European Journal of Cancer Care*, vol. 12, no. 3, pp. 257–262, 2003.

[18] P. Krach, S. DeVaney, C. DeTurk, and M. H. Zink, "Functional status of the oldest-old in a home setting," *Journal of Advanced Nursing*, vol. 24, no. 3, pp. 456–464, 1996.

[19] M. C. Tierney, J. Charles, G. Naglie, S. Jaglal, A. Kiss, and R. H. Fisher, "Risk factors for harm in cognitively impaired seniors who live alone: a prospective study," *Journal of the American Geriatrics Society*, vol. 52, no. 9, pp. 1435–1441, 2004.

[20] A. J. Bishop, P. Martin, and L. Poon, "Happiness and congruence in older adulthood: a structural model of life satisfaction," *Aging and Mental Health*, vol. 10, no. 5, pp. 445–453, 2006.

[21] B. S. Fees, P. Martin, and L. W. Poon, "A model of loneliness in older adults," *Journals of Gerontology*, vol. 54, no. 4, pp. P231–P239, 1999.

[22] P. Martin, B. Hagberg, and L. W. Poon, "Predictors of loneliness in centenarians: a parallel study," *Journal of Cross-Cultural Gerontology*, vol. 12, no. 3, pp. 203–224, 1997.

[23] P. A. Holtsberg, L. W. Poon, C. A. Noble, and P. Martin, "Mini-Mental State Exam status of community-dwelling cognitively intact centenarians," *International Psychogeriatrics*, vol. 7, no. 3, pp. 417–427, 1995.

[24] P. Martin, M. V. Long, and L. W. Poon, "Age changes and differences in personality traits and states of the old and very old," *Journals of Gerontology*, vol. 57, no. 2, pp. P144–P152, 2002.

[25] L. W. Poon, G. M. Clayton, P. Martin et al., "The georgia centenarian study," in *in The Georgia Centenarian Study: A Special Issue of the International Journal of Aging and Human Development*, L. W. Poon, Ed., vol. 34, pp. 1–18, Baywood Publishing, Amityville, NY, USA, 1992.

[26] M. F. Folstein, S. E. Folstein, and P. R. McHugh, "'Mini mental state'. A practical method for grading the cognitive state of patients for the clinician," *Journal of Psychiatric Research*, vol. 12, no. 3, pp. 189–198, 1975.

[27] B. Reisberg, S. H. Ferris, M. J. De Leon, and T. Crook, "The global deterioration scale for assessment of primary degenerative dementia," *American Journal of Psychiatry*, vol. 139, no. 9, pp. 1136–1139, 1982.

[28] A. C. Acock, "Working with missing values," *Journal of Marriage and Family*, vol. 67, no. 4, pp. 1012–1028, 2005.

[29] P. D. Allison, "Missing data techniques for structural equation modeling," *Journal of Abnormal Psychology*, vol. 112, no. 4, pp. 545–557, 2003.

[30] B. Muthén and L. Muthén, *Mplus User's Guide*, Muthén & Muthén, Los Angeles, Calif, USA, 3rd edition, 2004.

[31] B. M. Byrne, *Structural Equation Modeling with LISREL, PRELIS, and SIMPLIS: Basic Concepts, Applications, and Programming*, Lawrence Erlbaum Associates, Hillsdale, NJ, USA, 1998.

[32] J. B. Ullman and P. M. Bentler, "Structural equation modeling," in *Handbook of Psychology: Research Methods in Psychology*, J. A. Schinka and W. F. Velicer, Eds., vol. 2, pp. 607–634, John Wiley & Sons, New York, NY, USA, 2003.

[33] P. M. Bentler, "Comparative fit indexes in structural models," *Psychological Bulletin*, vol. 107, no. 2, pp. 238–246, 1990.

[34] P. M. Bentler and D. G. Bonett, "Significance tests and goodness of fit in the analysis of covariance structures," *Psychological Bulletin*, vol. 88, no. 3, pp. 588–606, 1980.

[35] M. W. Browne and R. Cudeck, "Single sample cross-validation indices for covariance structures," *Multivariate Behavioral Research*, vol. 24, pp. 445–455, 1989.

[36] L. T. Hu and P. M. Bentler, "Cutoff criteria for fit indexes in covariance structure analysis: conventional criteria versus new alternatives," *Structural Equation Modeling*, vol. 6, no. 1, pp. 1–55, 1999.

[37] R. C. MacCallum and J. T. Austin, "Applications of structural equation modeling in psychological research," *Annual Review of Psychology*, vol. 51, pp. 201–226, 2000.

[38] V. Burholt, G. Windle, D. Ferring et al., "Reliability and validity of the Older Americans Resources and Services (OARS) social resources scale in six European countries," *Journals of Gerontology*, vol. 62, pp. S371–S379, 2007.

[39] T. B. Herbert and S. Cohen, "Measurement issues in research on psychosocial stress," in *Psychosocial Stress: Perspectives on Structure, Theory, Life-Course, and Methods*, H. B. Kaplan, Ed., pp. 295–332, Academic Press, San Diego, Calif, USA, 1996.

[40] D. W. Russell, "UCLA Loneliness Scale (Version 3): reliability, validity, and factor structure," *Journal of Personality Assessment*, vol. 66, no. 1, pp. 20–40, 1996.

[41] D. W. Russell, C. Kao, and C. E. Cutrona, "Loneliness and social support: same or different constructs?" in *Proceedings of the Iowa Conference on Personal Relationships*, Iowa City, Iowa, USA, June 1987.

[42] N. Krause, "Assessing change in social support during late life," *Research on Aging*, vol. 21, no. 4, pp. 539–569, 1999.

Permissions

All chapters in this book were first published in JAR, by Hindawi Publishing Corporation; hereby published with permission under the Creative Commons Attribution License or equivalent. Every chapter published in this book has been scrutinized by our experts. Their significance has been extensively debated. The topics covered herein carry significant findings which will fuel the growth of the discipline. They may even be implemented as practical applications or may be referred to as a beginning point for another development.

The contributors of this book come from diverse backgrounds, making this book a truly international effort. This book will bring forth new frontiers with its revolutionizing research information and detailed analysis of the nascent developments around the world.

We would like to thank all the contributing authors for lending their expertise to make the book truly unique. They have played a crucial role in the development of this book. Without their invaluable contributions this book wouldn't have been possible. They have made vital efforts to compile up to date information on the varied aspects of this subject to make this book a valuable addition to the collection of many professionals and students.

This book was conceptualized with the vision of imparting up-to-date information and advanced data in this field. To ensure the same, a matchless editorial board was set up. Every individual on the board went through rigorous rounds of assessment to prove their worth. After which they invested a large part of their time researching and compiling the most relevant data for our readers.

The editorial board has been involved in producing this book since its inception. They have spent rigorous hours researching and exploring the diverse topics which have resulted in the successful publishing of this book. They have passed on their knowledge of decades through this book. To expedite this challenging task, the publisher supported the team at every step. A small team of assistant editors was also appointed to further simplify the editing procedure and attain best results for the readers.

Apart from the editorial board, the designing team has also invested a significant amount of their time in understanding the subject and creating the most relevant covers. They scrutinized every image to scout for the most suitable representation of the subject and create an appropriate cover for the book.

The publishing team has been an ardent support to the editorial, designing and production team. Their endless efforts to recruit the best for this project, has resulted in the accomplishment of this book. They are a veteran in the field of academics and their pool of knowledge is as vast as their experience in printing. Their expertise and guidance has proved useful at every step. Their uncompromising quality standards have made this book an exceptional effort. Their encouragement from time to time has been an inspiration for everyone.

The publisher and the editorial board hope that this book will prove to be a valuable piece of knowledge for researchers, students, practitioners and scholars across the globe.

List of Contributors

Emam M. M. Esmayel, Mohsen M. Eldarawy, Mohamed M. M. Hassan and Hassan Mahmoud Hassanin
Department of Internal Medicine, Faculty of Medicine, Zagazig University, Zagazig 44519, Egypt

Walid M. Reda Ashour and Wael Mahmoud
Department of Neurology, Faculty of Medicine, Zagazig University, Zagazig 44519, Egypt

Rachael C. Stone, Brad A. Meisner and Joseph Baker
School of Kinesiology & Health Science, York University, Toronto, ON, Canada M3J 1P3
Department of Psychology, Ryerson University, Toronto, ON, Canada M5B 2K3

Bryan D. James
Rush Alzheimer's Disease Center, Department of Internal Medicine, Rush University Medical Center, Chicago, IL 60612, USA

Thomas A. Glass
Department of Epidemiology, Johns Hopkins Bloomberg School of Public Health, Baltimore, MD 21205, USA

Brian Caffo and Jennifer F. Bobb
Department of Biostatistics, Johns Hopkins Bloomberg School of Public Health, Baltimore, MD 21205, USA

Christos Davatzikos
Department of Radiology, University of Pennsylvania School of Medicine, Philadelphia, PA 19104, USA

David Yousem
Department of Radiology, Johns Hopkins School of Medicine, Baltimore, MD 21205, USA

Hongjie Liu, Xin He, Judith A. Levy, Yongfang Xu and Chunpeng Zang
Department of Epidemiology and Biostatistics, School of Public Health, University of Maryland, College Park, MD 20742, USA
Health Policy and Administration, School of Public Health, University of Illinois, Chicago, IL 60612, USA

Xinqin Lin
Nanning Center for Disease Control and Prevention, Nanning 530023, China

Shilpa Dogra and Liza Stathokostas
School of Recreation Management and Kinesiology, Acadia University, Wolfville, NS, Canada B4P 2R6
Centre for Activity and Aging, University of Western Ontario, London, ON, Canada N6G 2M3

Sandro S. Ferreira, Ragami C. Alves, Mariana L. Benites, Paulo E. Redkva, Tácito P. Souza-Junior and Sergio G. da Silva
Department of Physical Education, Federal University of Parana, Caixa Postal 92, mJD Botänico, 80215-370 Curitiba, PR, Brazil

Kleverton Krinski
Federal University of Sao Francisco Valley, 56304205 Petrolina, PE, Brazil

Hassan M. Elsangedy
North York General Hospital, 4001 Leslie Street, Toronto, ON, Canada M2K 1E1
Center for Health Sciences, Federal University of Rio Grande do Norte, Caixa Postal 3000, Lagoa Nova, 59078970 Natal, RN, Brazil

Cosme F. Buzzachera
University Norte of Parana, Caixa Postal 675, JD Piza, 86041-100 Londrina, PR, Brazil

Kam-Tong Yeung
North York General Hospital, 4001 Leslie Street, Toronto, ON, Canada M2K 1E1

Silvia Duong
North York General Hospital, 4001 Leslie Street, Toronto, ON, Canada M2K 1E1
Herzl CRIUWalk-In Centre, Jewish General Hospital, 5858 Côte-des-Neiges, Suite 500, Montreal, QC, Canada H3S 1Z1

Feng Chang
School of Pharmacy, University of Waterloo, 200 University Avenue West, Waterloo, ON, Canada N2L 3G1

Catherine W. Yeckel
The John B. Pierce Laboratory, Yale School of Medicine, New Haven, CT 06519, USA
Department of Epidemiology and Public Health, Yale School of Medicine, New Haven, CT 06519, USA

Loretta Di Pietro
The John B. Pierce Laboratory, Yale School of Medicine, New Haven, CT 06519, USA
Department of Epidemiology and Public Health, Yale School of Medicine, New Haven, CT 06519, USA
The George Washington University, 817 23rd Street, NW, Washington, DC 20052, USA

Andrei Gribok
Beltsville Human Nutrition Research Center, The United States Department of Agriculture, Beltsville, MD 20705, USA

D. Kuh and M. Richards
MRC Unit for Lifelong Health and Ageing, London WC1B 5JU, UK

D. Cadar and H. Pikhart
Faculty of Population Health Sciences, University College London, London WC1E 6BT, UK

G. Mishra
School of Population Health, University of Queensland, Herston, QLD 4006, Australia

A. Stephen
MRC Human Nutrition Research, Elsie Widdowson Laboratory, 120 Fulbourn Road, Cambridge CB1 9NL, UK

Xin Qi Dong and E-Shien Chang
Chinese Health, Aging, and Policy Program, Rush Institute for Healthy Aging, Rush University Medical Center, 1645West Jackson Blvd, Suite 675, Chicago, IL 60612, USA

Esther Wong
Chinese American Service League, Chicago, IL, USA

Melissa Simon
Northwestern University, Feinberg School of Medicine, Chicago, IL, USA

Roberta Semprini, Adele Lubrano and Giulia Misaggi
Clinica Neurologica, Dipartimento di Neuroscienze, Universitàdi Roma "Tor Vergata", Via Montpellier, 00133 Rome, Italy

Alessandro Martorana
Clinica Neurologica, Dipartimento di Neuroscienze, Universitàdi Roma "Tor Vergata", Via Montpellier, 00133 Rome, Italy
IRCCS Santa Lucia, Via Ardeatina, 00179 Rome, Italy

Treena Wu and Angelique Chan
Health Services & Systems Research, Duke-NUS Graduate Medical School, Level 4, 8 College Road, Singapore 169857

Lena Dahlberg
School of Education, Health and Social Studies, Dalarna University, Dalarna, Sweden
Aging Research Center, Karolinska Institutet & Stockholm University, Stockholm, Sweden

Ming-Ming Lai and Shi-Ying Lein
Faculty of Management, Multimedia University, Persiaran Multimedia, 63100 Cyberjaya, Selangor, Malaysia

Siok-Hwa Lau
Faculty of Business, Multimedia University, Jalan Ayer Keroh Lama, 75450 Bukit Beruang, Melaka, Malaysia

Ming-Ling Lai
Faculty of Accountancy, Universiti Teknologi MARA, Level 14, Menara SAAS, 40450 Shah Alam, Selangor, Malaysia

Evangelia Chrysikou
Faculty of the Built Environment, UCL Bartlett School of Architecture, 140 Hampstead Rd., London NW1 2BX, UK

Richard Rabnett
AM-GAR, Hashdera Hamerkazit 15, Ligad 1, 7173003 Modi'in, Israel

Chariklia Tziraki
MELABEV-Community Elders Club, Research and Evaluation Department and Hebrew University of Jerusalem, Israel Gerontological Data Center, 9190501 Mount Scopus, Israel

Erik Lykke Mortensen
Department of Public Health, Section of Environmental Health, Medical Psychology Unit, University of Copenhagen, Øster Farimagsgade 5 A, 1353 Copenhagen K, Denmark
Center for Healthy Aging, Faculty of Health Science, University of Copenhagen, 2200 Copenhagen N, Denmark
Institute of Preventive Medicine, Copenhagen University Hospital, Copenhagen, 1353 Copenhagen K, Denmark

John Calvin Barefoot
Institute of Preventive Medicine, Copenhagen University Hospital, Copenhagen, 1353 Copenhagen K, Denmark
Department of Psychiatry and Behavioral Sciences, Duke University, Medical Center, Durham, NC 27710, USA

Kirsten Avlund
Department of Public Health, Section of Social Medicine, University of Copenhagen, 1353 Copenhagen K, Denmark
Danish Aging Research Center, Universities of Aarhus, Copenhagen and Southern Denmark, Denmark

Mohammed K. Shakeel
Department of Psychology, University of Calgary, 2500 University Drive NW, Calgary, AB, Canada T2N 1N4

Vina M. Goghari
Department of Psychology, University of Toronto, 1265 Military Trail, Toronto, ON, Canada M1C 1A4

Mei-Lan Chen
Byrdine F. Lewis College of Nursing and Health Professions, Georgia State University, Atlanta, GA 30303, USA
Gerontology Institute, Georgia State University, Atlanta, GA 30303, USA

Jie Hu
College of Nursing, the Ohio State University, Columbus, OH 43210, USA

Thomas P. McCoy and Susan Letvak
School of Nursing, University of North Carolina at Greensboro, Greensboro, NC 27402, USA

Luba Ivanov
College of Nursing, Chamberlain University, Downers Grove, IL 60515, USA

Ulla Svantesson and Carin Willén
Department of Health and Rehabilitation, Institute of Neuroscience and Physiology, University of Gothenburg, Gothenburg, Sweden

Hadeel Halaweh
Department of Health and Rehabilitation, Institute of Neuroscience and Physiology, University of Gothenburg, Gothenburg, Sweden
Department of Physiotherapy & Rehabilitation, Faculty of Health Professions, Al Quds University, Jerusalem, State of Palestine

Synneve Dahlin-Ivanoff
Department of Health and Rehabilitation, Institute of Neuroscience and Physiology, University of Gothenburg, Gothenburg, Sweden
Centre for Ageing and Health, AGECAP, University of Gothenburg, Gothenburg, Sweden

Pornpun Manasatchakun
Boromarajonani College of Nursing, Udonani, Thailand

Åsa Roxberg
School of Health and Welfare, Halmstad University, Halmstad, Sweden VID Specialized University, Bergen, Norway
Centre for Ageing and Health, AGECAP, University of Gothenburg, Gothenburg, Sweden

Margareta Asp
School of Health, Care and Social Welfare, Mälardalen University, Eskilstuna, Västeras, Sweden

G. Kevin Randall
CC Wheeler Institute, Bradley University, 05 Bradley Hall, 1501 W. Bradley Avenue, Peoria, IL 61625, USA

Peter Martin
Gerontology Program, Iowa State University, 1096 Le Baron Hall, Ames, IA 50011 1120, USA

Mary Ann Johnson
Department of Foods & Nutrition, The University of Georgia, 143 Barrow Hall, 115 DW Brooks Dr, Athens, GA 30602, USA

Leonard W. Poon
Institute of Gerontology, College of Public Health, The University of Georgia, 255 E. Hancock Avenue, Athens, GA 30602-5775, USA

Index